ADAPTED PHYSICAL ACTIVITY

From Theory to Application

This volume contains selected papers from the Third International Symposium on Adapted Physical Activities, held in New Orleans, Louisiana, November 1981, and is a publication of the International Federation of Adapted Physical Activity.

ADAPTED PHYSICAL ACTIVITY

From Theory to Application

EDITORS

Robert L. Eason, EdD
University of New Orleans
New Orleans, Louisiana

Theresa L. Smith, PhD
University of New Orleans
New Orleans, Louisiana

Fernand Caron, PhD
Université du Québec
Trois-Rivières, Québec

HUMAN KINETICS PUBLISHERS
Box 5076
Champaign, Illinois 61820

Publications Director
Richard D. Howell

Production Director
Margery Brandfon

Editorial Staff
Dana Finney
John Sauget

Typesetters
Sandra Meier
Carol McCarty

Text Layout
Lezli Harris

Cover Design
Margery Brandfon

ISSN: 0736-2943
ISBN: 0-931250-40-4

Copyright © 1983 by Human Kinetics Publishers. All rights reserved. Except for use in a review, the reproduction or utilization of this work in any form or by any electronic, mechanical, or other means, now known or hereafter invented, including xerography, photocopying, and recording, and in any information storage and retrieval system is forbidden without the written permission of the publisher. Printed in the United States of America.

9 8 7 6 5 4 3 2 1

Human Kinetics Publishers, Inc.
Box 5076
Champaign, Illinois 61820

Contents

Third International Symposium on Adapted Physical Activities	ix
History of the International Federation on Adapted Physical Activities	xi
Officers and Board of Directors	xi
Preface	xiii
KEYNOTE ADDRESS	1
Third International Symposium on Adapted Physical Activities *by Eunice Kennedy Shriver*	3
SECTION 1: **ADAPTED PHYSICAL EDUCATION IN EUROPE**	11
In-Service Training in Physical Education for Teachers in Inner London Schools for the Educationally Subnormal (Severe) *by Eileen McLeish*	13
Physical Education Programs for Mentally Retarded Children in Germany *by Gudrun M. Doll-Tepper*	19
Adapted Physical Education in Germany *by Ernst Kiphard*	25

SECTION 2:   33
DEVELOPING CURRICULA FOR SPECIAL POPULATIONS

Quality Programming in Physical Education and   35
    Recreation for All Handicapped Persons
    by Janet A. Wessel

Individualized Instruction for Special Students: 53
    A Challenge for Change in Physical Education
    by Claudia Jane Knowles

Physical Activity for the Severely Handicapped: 63
    Theoretical and Practical Considerations *by John M. Dunn*

Pedagogy in the Psychomotor Domain for the Severely   74
    Handicapped *by Claudine Sherrill*

How to Include Blind Children in Vigorous Public School   89
    Physical Education *by Charles Buell*

SECTION 3:   93
RECREATION AND ADAPTED PHYSICAL ACTIVITY

Recreation for Handicapped in the United States: 95
    A Historical Perspective *by John A. Nesbitt*

Recreation Unlimited: Responding to Persons with   111
    Severe Disabilities *by Janet Pomeroy*

Development and Validation of a Leisure Diagnostic   124
    Battery for Handicapped Children and Youth *by*
    David M. Compton, Peter A. Witt, and Gary D. Ellis

The Effects of Increased Recreation Opportunities on   139
    Life Satisfaction and Physical/Mental Health of the
    Elderly—A Reconnaissance Evaluation *by Jean Tague*

SECTION 4:   151
THEORY AND RESEARCH IN MOTOR DEVELOPMENT

Factors Affecting Motor Development Delays   153
    by Jean Pyfer

An Ecological Approach to Perceptual-Motor Learning   162
    by Walter E. Davis

Evaluation of Motor Skills of the Handicapped: 172
    Theory and Practice *by Hollis Fait*

Generalization of Motor Skills from Training to   180
    Natural Environments *by David Auxter*

Bridge over Troubled Waters — Research Review and 189
Recommendations for Relevance *by Julian U. Stein*

SECTION 5: 199
RESEARCH TOPICS IN ADAPTED PHYSICAL ACTIVITY

The Motor Performance of Autistic Individuals 201
by Greg Reid, Doug Collier, and Brian Morin

A Comparison of the Qualitative Motor Performance 219
of Normal, Educable, and Trainable Mentally
Retarded Students *by Dale A. Ulrich*

Discriminatory Response Time and Heart Rate Differences 226
Between Gifted and Learning Disabled Children *by
Leighton E. Stamps, Bobby L. Eason, and Theresa L. Smith*

Effects of Uncertainty of Time and Occurrence on 230
Reaction Time *by Paul R. Surburg*

A Comparison of Two Sensory Motor Intervention 236
Programs for Elementary Children Diagnosed as Specific
Learning-Disabled *by Joey Cowden, Robert Eason, and
Jennifer Wright*

Discriminant Analysis in Adapted Physical Education 244
by Gabie E. Church and Geoffrey D. Broadhead

SECTION 6: 251
CONSIDÉRATIONS SUR L'ACTIVITÉ PHYSIQUE
POUR LES HANDICAPÉS

La Plasticité du Muscle Vieillissant *by Clermont P. Simard* 253

Réaction à la Conférence du Dr. Clermont Simard Portant 267
sur la "Plasticité du Muscle Vieillissant" *by André Quirion*

Modèle de Programme d'Education Plein Air Adapté 270
aux Personnes Agées *by Georges A. Nadeau et
Clermont P. Simard*

Evaluation des Compétences Motrices de Déficients 281
Mentaux *by Jean-Claude De Potter*

Considérations sur l'Enseignement de l'Activité Physique 287
aux Élèves en Difficulté d'Adaptation et d'Apprentissage *by
Michel Lirette, Claude Paré, Fernand Caron, et Pierre Black*

Attitude des Educateurs à l'Egard de la Personne 300
Handicapée *by Pierre Potvin*

Stress Cardiaque Produit par Deux Activités Physiques 311
  Chez des Personnes Agées *by Clermont P. Simard,
  Jean Jobin, Julien Vallières, Henri Bessette, Renée Caron,
  et Martine Dupuis*

SECTION 7: 323
SUMMARY PAPERS

Summary of Pedagogy Sessions *by G. Lawrence Rarick* 325

Research Directions in Adapted Physical Activity 329
  by Geoffrey D. Broadhead

Third International Symposium on Adapted Physical Activities

Officials and Committees

Sponsors

Honorable Kelly Nix, Superintendent of Education, State of Louisiana
Dr. Henry Smith, Assistant Superintendent of Special Education Services
Dr. Leon Richelle, Chancellor, University of New Orleans
Dr. Clermont Simard, President of the International Federation on Adapted Physical Activity

Executive Committee

Robert L. Eason, Executive Chairman
Jo E. Cowden, Executive Coordinator
Fernand Caron
Janice Fruge
Billy Ray Stokes

Scientific Committee

Theresa Smith, Chair
Geoffrey Broadhead
Charles Buell
Fernand Caron
Gail Clark
Carol Ann Peterson

Organization Committee

Julian Stein, Administration
Earl Harrison, Exhibits
Vane Wilson, Hospitality
Jennifer Wright, Media Consultant
Anthony Esposito, Administrative Assistant

Special Commendation

Of the many individuals whose contributions led to the acknowledged success of the Symposium, one is worthy of special commendation—Dr. Billy Ray Stokes of the Louisiana Department of Health and Human Resources. Dr. Stoke's power of thought and process was very instrumental in both the conceptual and financial success of the Third International Symposium on Adapted Physical Activities.

Robert L. Eason
Jo E. Cowden

History of the International Federation of Adapted Physical Activities

The International Federation on Adapted Physical Activities originated in the Canadian Province of Quebec in 1973. Since then it has rapidly expanded into a worldwide organization with an international charter. It has sponsored three international meetings in Quebec, Brussels, and New Orleans; in 1983, the Federation will convene in the British Isles. Its objective as an organization is to give global focus to professionals who use adapted physical activities for instruction, recreation, remediation, and research. It solicits membership from adapted physical educators, therapeutic recreators, and therapists from the disciplines of allied health. Please write for membership details to Robert L. Eason, Department of Physical Education, University of New Orleans, New Orleans, LA 70148, USA.

Officers and Board of Directors

Clermont Simard, President
Laval University
Quebec, Canada G1K7P4

Gudrun M. Doll-Tepper
Institüt für Sportwissenschaft
Freie Universität Berlin
1000 Berlin 33, West Germany

Robert L. Eason, Vice-President
University of New Orleans
New Orleans, Louisiana 70148,
USA

David Ernest Jones
Brisbane College of Advanced
 Education
Kelvin Grove, Queensland,
Australia

Jean Claude Pageot, Secretary
1034 Avignon Court
Orleans, Ontario, Canada K1C2R2

Eileen McLeish
46 Warwick Road
Bishops Stortford
Herts CM235WW England

Fernand Caron
Université du Quebec
Trois-Rivieres, Quebec G8Y-3M7

John A. Nesbitt
University of Iowa
W612A Seashore
Iowa City, Iowa 52242, USA

Jean-Claude De Potter
Université Libre De Bruxelles
B-1050 Bruxelles, Belgium

Julian U. Stein
1832 Dalmation Drive
McLean, Virginia 22101, USA

Preface

> But when the sun came up it burned the young plants; and because the roots had not grown deep enough, the plants soon dried up. . . . But some seeds fell in good soil, and the plants bore grain. *From the Parable of the Sower.*

Within human history, the concept of adapted physical activity is a freshly planted seed. It is an international idea with adapted physical education and recreation programs "springing up" in many countries. The basis of the idea is the awareness that handicapped individuals have the right to experience meaning from purposeful movement, and also the right to participate in movement for remediation and normalization.

But, as in the parable, not all of the seeds are falling on good soil. Once sympathetic legislatures are now yielding to other forces with anti-spending themes. School authorities in some local education and recreation agencies are ignoring requirements to provide adapted physical activity. State agencies are not developing regulations that insure compliance with newly passed legislation, and many universities are not preparing professionals with the skills to adequately teach or lead recreation for the handicapped. And often, teachers and recreators are not sensitive to the unique developmental differences of the atypical.

But there is good soil as well as bad. Professional educators and practitioners from physical education and recreation are joining those in the fields of medicine and allied health to provide quality programs and services. Around the globe bold new legislation is providing legal mandates and financial assistance for adapted physical activity programs and many states in the US have passed model legislation for adapted physical education and recreation. Physical education is interwoven into school law so that handicapped children are guaranteed the right to full participation in physical education, school recreation, and athletics.

The logo for the IIIrd International Symposium on Adapted Physical Activity was a heavily foliaged plant with the initials APA imposed in the leaves to resemble fruit or grain. Indeed, the Symposium provided good soil for growth. The theme was "Adapted Physical Activity: From Theory to Implementation," providing a forum for information dissemination concerning the physical, psychological, and sociological needs of the handicapped. It focused attention of leaders from countries in all parts of the world on the role of physical activity in meeting the needs of the handicapped. Innovative and creative ideas from pedagogy and research were presented. Of significance to this world which is rapidly growing smaller, the Symposium enabled individuals from all countries who specialize in adapted physical activity the opportunity to interact. What will surely transpire are better services and understanding for handicapped individuals.

The Symposium's scope included adapted physical activity research, model programs, and legislation as they relate to atypical populations. Professionals in the field presented specific information for those working with the severe and profoundly retarded, the mentally retarded, the learning disabled, the emotionally disturbed, and other educationally handicapping conditions. Attention also was directed toward physically handicapped children and adults, the sensory-impaired, the aged, and other classifications of impaired and disabled individuals.

As you read these proceedings, assume the leader's role—a curriculum coordinator of adapted physical education, a recreation program director, or a director of occupational therapy. In all cases we will have the challenging responsibility of conceptualizing and implementing movement programs for children and adults with handicapping conditions. With such a mind set, we will find these proceedings to be rich soil indeed. To assist the conceptualization, the proceedings have been organized into seven sections: (1) International Adapted Physical Activity, (2) Adapted Physical Education Curriculum, (3) Recreation and Adapted Physical Activity, (4) Theoretical and Research Considerations, (5) Research Papers, (6) Papers in French, and (7) Summary.

Until recently, educators were little concerned with the moral or legal rights of the handicapped to receive instruction in either the purpose or process of movement. Administrators, teachers, and parents alike ignored the fact that physically, emotionally, and mentally disabled children require physical activity for health related fitness. A related fact, that handicapped individuals profit psychologically when they experience meaning from purposeful movement, was also discounted. Therefore, very little support from precedent or from the professional literature is available to guide us, the specialists, in the conceptualization process.

Careful readers will determine that they must go beyond traditional understanding of the role of movement to accomplish the conceptualization process. Many of the articles imply that forces other than recreation or education operate within the community or nation, and it is those political, financial, and socioeconomic forces that determine school and recreation policy. Adapted physical activity cannot exist without the force of public demand or, similarly, public awareness. Thus, understanding public attitude coupled with awareness of the law and the legislative process is the point of departure for the adapted specialists. Federal and state dollars are available in unprecedented amounts, but only the politically energetic coordinators are receiving the grants. Funding is the key to successful programs.

Continuing in our role as coordinators for the atypical, we must be knowledgeable of sound pedagogical principles. The formulation of valid, reliable assessment plans is one of the great challenges of the adapted physical activity director. Atypical individuals must be located, screened and placed. We must develop, monitor, evaluate, and reconceptualize our programs if necessary.

As leaders we must predetermine what activities, facilities, equipment and safety measures are required. We must develop curriculum and program guides which include specific knowledge about the atypical. With pedagogical considerations in mind, the reader will find helpful advice in the pages that follow.

The adapted physical activity theorists will be especially interested in the research and theory section of these proceedings. In recent years several new, well conceived books and articles have attempted to draw into focus a body of knowledge for adapted physical activity. This literature, along with the manuscripts presented in these proceedings, should arouse the creative energy in each of us to test the ideas, principles, and methods presented. Undoubtedly, we will find many of them to be excellent, but others to be untenable. Most important, we can discover new ideas and approaches to be tried. In such a process new projects will be crystallized, research conducted, legislation inspected, and the net result will be a dynamic burst of growth for the seedlings of adapted physical activity. With proper nourishment the fruit yielded will be excellent programs for the handicapped populations of the world.

Robert L. Eason
Theresa L. Smith
Fernand Caron

KEYNOTE ADDRESS

Third International Symposium on Adapted Physical Activities

Eunice Kennedy Shriver
Joseph P. Kennedy, Jr., Foundation

Amost 20 years ago, I was talking to Mary Switzer who was the head of the Office of Vocational Rehabilitation. I was telling her about ways of helping the mentally retarded develop and strengthen their bodies. I had become very aware of the fact that most mentally retarded people were fat, awkward, and uncoordinated. For the most part, they sat around in the back wards of institutions doing nothing. You remember, I am sure, that in those days most mentally retarded people were in institutions.

Frankly, I was looking for money to begin a camping program which would show what the mentally retarded could do if they were given a chance to exercise and become physically fit.

Mary Switzer listened to me and then she said, "I am no doctor, Eunice, but I can't believe that this is a natural condition of the mentally retarded. I can see that if these young people become fit, they can get out of institutions. They can become more independent. They can do better in school. They can get a job, and they can become a part of their communities."

So Mary Switzer gave me the money. We started very small, training teachers to work with mentally retarded children in the summer camp program. And the more we saw mentally retarded people in the swimming pools, throwing a ball, running, and jumping, we were convinced that they could become strong and well-coordinated. They could become more independent. They could get out of the institutions and live and work in their communities.

With the help of Larry Rarick, Bryant Cratty, Frank Hayden, and many others in the field of adapted physical education, we worked to develop fitness activities and proficiency tests for the mentally retarded.

Then, we came to the conclusion that if we would adapt regular sports and games to the mentally retarded, we could adapt the mentally retarded to society. And that is how, with the help of so many of you, a theory, an idea, a goal, was transformed into Special Olympics.

And that single idea which began so small has spread and has changed the lives and thoughts of millions.

What is this idea? It's more than games and exercises.

It is the simple, obvious idea that when we speak of human rights we mean rights for all. When we speak of opportunity we mean opportunity for all, not just some. Not just the best. Not only the brightest, the fittest, the most promising, but all.

Yet for generations, even while civil rights were being won by racial and religious minorities, very few had thought to apply this idea, this central moral value of our American democracy, to 6 million of our fellow citizens, the mentally retarded.

Then, 11 years ago, in Chicago, not far from the scene of the first controlled nuclear chain reaction, we gave that idea a practical test. There on Soldier Field a track meet for 1,000 mentally retarded boys and girls took place.

This was an act of some daring because never before had retarded persons taken part in a public event like this, in a public arena.

And many experts, the best and the brightest in their fields, said it couldn't, and shouldn't, be done.

They said that retarded people couldn't understand the meaning of competition. . . .

The retarded couldn't run 300 yards or swim the length of a pool. . . .

The retarded couldn't take part in team sports. . . .

The retarded would get sick, get hurt, get lost.

On every count, they were wrong. Because almost no one except a few of you in this room today had ever thought of retarded people as athletes! They had been regarded only as case histories. They had been tested over and over again for intelligence, the one quality in which they could not measure up to norms. But they had never been tested for courage. For determination. For skill. For the capacity of joy and for growth—qualities that make us truly human.

Since then, this idea has spread to every continent. It is called "Special Olympics" and millions of people who once did not consider the mentally retarded as even human have been witness to the marvelous gifts of courage, of fidelity, of love they bring to us.

For in "Special Olympics" it is not the fastest time or the longest distance that matters, but the unconquerable spirit of the athletes; the joy of taking part; the courage to overcome; the generosity to share.

The overwhelming significance of this great idea, which is so much a symbol of your life's work, was brought home to me forcefully this summer in an extraordinary trip I made to the country of my ancestors — the wounded, suffering, terrible beauty of northern Ireland. In northern Ireland, set against the amazing beauty of the country, I watched men dying for what they felt was right, their right to be Irish and not British. But, at the same time, I saw British men and women working hard, loving passionately, and sacrificing much to change the lives of the mentally retarded in Ireland.

But the most incredible experience in Ireland came not through patriots or politicians, leaders of government or the church, but through Special Olympics. Yes, I saw Catholics and Protestants in northern Ireland and in southern Ireland working together in Special Olympics, many speaking to one another for the first time.

I saw people of the north and south coaching athletes together; doctors examining Special Olympians together; parents and teachers comparing experiences and sharing their pride and dedication.

I saw businessmen working together, not for profit but to organize bus trips from northern Ireland to Dublin in the south for 700 athletes taking part in the All-Ireland Special Olympics Games. I saw a coaching clinic open to northern and southern Protestants and Catholics alike. All this was for a common cause under the yellow and blue banner of Special Olympics.

What I saw in Ireland has been repeated over and over in many other parts of the world: the skill of professionalism joining forces with the spirit of volunteerism and the pride and love of families to bring health and strength to thousands, once abandoned and given up for lost.

In El Salvador, another country torn by war, Special Olympics continues to develop and more than 1,000 athletes took part in their national games this last August.

In Ecuador, which is in political and social turmoil with students rioting against the government, these same students have forgotten their political differences and volunteered in record numbers to coach Special Olympians.

In Honduras, a country that is one of the poorest in the Western Hemisphere, more than 8,000 parents and friends of the mentally retarded came out as spectators for their national games last July.

In France, a nation with no tradition of volunteerism, a volunteer organization for Special Olympics has flourished since 1968.

I relate these examples not because they tell us something flattering about Special Olympics, but because they illustrate something significant about the work we all share, that idea which has swept the world.

Every day, in our schools and universities, our playgrounds and our gymnasiums, we both teach and learn the lesson that a healthy, skilled, and joyous child in a loving family and a welcoming society is a vibrant desire and a common goal.

To create that child, to sustain that family, to strengthen that society is the work we do, under the dull and colorless title of "Adapted Physical Activity."

Is this an overstatement? I think not. For the facts are that what we do really works. The living, human proof is there for everyone to see.

For example, every piece of research done on Special Olympics—by the most distinguished people in the field, like Bowers, Cratty, and Rarick; by Simpson and Meany; and in a 3-year study by the Research and Training Center at Texas Tech University—has proven this: Training and participation in sports produces not only social and emotional gains for the participants, but important growth in pride, self-esteem and acceptance among their families, friends, and communities.

In other words, the influence of teachers and coaches extends far beyond the improvement of motor skills into the very fabric of society and the quality of life.

Yet everywhere in the world there is more to be done. More teaching, more training, more coaching, by the people best qualified to bring to the mentally retarded the gifts of skill, strength, and coordination. In other words, by you.

Thousands of members of your profession at every level have become a part of Special Olympics' rapidly growing training program. In the past year alone, with the help of many of you, we have created coaching manuals in almost every sport. Using these, we have conducted 98 training schools in track and field, winter sports, softball, basketball, soccer, gymnastics, volleyball and general fitness activities. They are all based on the idea that mentally retarded people can grow in ability and improve in performance when they are well-trained.

Eleven thousand coaches have taken part in this program and have guaranteed that they in turn will train Special Olympians in their communities. But this is only a beginning.

We need thousands more of you to work with the volunteer coaches, teachers, and families of the mentally retarded. It is a fact that of the 11,000 coaches we have trained, over half are from professions other than adapted physical education. And throughout Special Olympics this same ratio holds true.

Why is your participation so important? Because professionals in adapted physical activity are the most essential single ingredient in

Special Olympics. Because, increasingly, we are finding that the level of skill, strength, endurance, and speed of the handicapped can be extended beyond all our expectations, if there is a high quality of professional coaching and training.

Let me tell you about a few athletes who are proof of the ability of mentally retarded people to change and grow, if we believe in them and work with them.

Toni Marie Chillemi lives in Florida. She is a Downs' Syndrome child with an I.Q. of about 35. If not for Special Olympics, she would be shut up in an institution. But she had loving parents and coaches who taught her gymnastics. She has won gold and silver medals, performed on national TV and now teaches gymnastics to others, even normal children.

Or take Brian Loeb. He could not speak and had trouble even learning to walk. Then a coach of the high school swimming team began to teach Brian to swim. His unused body grew strong. Now he teaches others to swim and last year on national television, Brian Loeb received a medal from Bob Hope as the most courageous athlete of the year.

Think of Loretta Claibourne. They said she couldn't compete in any race longer than the 100-meter dash. But she was determined to run further, much further. And this year, through Special Olympics coaching and her own efforts, she finished the Boston marathon in 3 hours and 9 minutes, far ahead of 500 other competitors, male and female.

The examples are legion, so much so that they have become commonplace. Now, we focus our efforts on raising the level of performance of all those who are still outside our programs because there have not been enough professionals, enough skilled coaches and teachers to construct the strong foundations on which parents, friends, and volunteers can then build.

You may think this will be difficult to do in a time of shrinking budgets, fewer grants, and diminished government support. But I believe that the work we do will become ever stronger; ever larger; because the need is so evident and the cause is so just.

For example, in July 1983, the Sixth International Special Olympics Games will be held here in Louisiana with 4,000 athletes and 1,000 coaches from every state and 40 countries. Why Louisiana? Because the governor and the legislature recognized the power of an idea. They came up with the best facilities. The best housing. The best game directors. They have already appropriated a large sum of money, with more to come.

Civic organizations such as the American Legion and Civitan have inspired their members to volunteer to help Special Olympics in their own communities.

And business has been moved by this idea to contribute money, volunteers, and equipment needed to make the games a success.

Right now, in more than 19,000 communities in America, coaching and training are taking place, so that one million Special Olympians will be able to do their very best in the local and state competitions leading up to the 1983 Games.

And the media are getting behind this idea.

On the night of January 4, 1982, on the NBC television network, millions of Americans—I hope all of you among them—will see at first hand the everyday miracles that can come about through the devotion of a parent, the skill of a physical educator, and the capacity of a child who has been called handicapped, to learn and grow.

This beautiful, 2-hour motion picture was inspired by Special Olympics. In addition to recognized stars such as Beau Bridges, Susan St. James, and Loretta Swit, it features Ricky Wittman, a Special Olympian. The title of the film is "The Kid from Nowhere," and that title speaks volumes about what you do, and the people you work with. For without your professional contribution to the lives of the handicapped, they are indeed people from nowhere; fitting in nowhere; and going nowhere. But with you and because of you, millions of people all over the world have found a place, and the strength and ability to claim it as their own.

In closing, I would like to give all of you, and especially those of you from other nations, an invitation and a challenge to help us strengthen Special Olympics in your own communities or, if a program does not now exist, to help us get one started there.

More than 52 nations of the world, on every continent, are now involved in developing an international Special Olympics program. About one-third of these are well along the way; one-third have limited development and the remainder have done little more than express interest. Huge areas of the world have been left untapped. No program exists today behind the Iron Curtain. And yet we know that interest does exist there, that programs could succeed.

If any of you will agree to carry the message of Special Olympics to your own nation, we will help identify both the promise and the problems in your country and assist you in every way possible by providing materials, technical assistance, and possibly even a small grant. But even without knowing what state or nation you come from, I can tell you this: Special Olympics needs you. It needs your professionalism, your knowledge, and your skill. And if you are willing to give us just a portion of these, the rest will follow, because this is an idea which knows no limits and cannot be stopped.

At the 1983 games we would like to get every one of these 52 nations represented with a professionally trained delegation. Not just a token group, but well-coached, skilled athletes who have won the right to come to the games through year-round training by professionals and participation in local and national events.

We share a huge undertaking but it is one we must approach with great joy. It is not too much to say that we are all engaged in the true pursuit of happiness which is the striving for excellence. Together we can bring to the world a new concept of justice, of unity and of love, which in time will bring peace to all our families and nations.

In our giving to others or failing to give—in our caring or failing to care—we inch mankind forward or let it fall back. The love we give to our friends, our parents, our children, to the sick, the aged, the poor, the powerless, becomes a part of each of us and multiplies.

SECTION 1:
Adapted Physical Education in Europe

Adapted physical activity specialists will have had their sensitivity for the needs of the handicapped renewed after reading the keynote address by Mrs. Shriver. In this section specialists from Europe describe the progress of adapted physical activity in each of their countries.

In England, as the reader will discover, professional preparation can be effectively conducted even with a limited amount of funds or university support. Eileen McLeish explains an in-service process for Inner London schools for the severely handicapped. She demonstrates again that the British can "muddle through" even the most perplexing problems and achieve excellent results. The final entries of the section deal with physical activity in Germany. Doll-Tepper relates the status and philosophy of adapted physical activity and ideas related to programming. Kiphard, in splendid theoretical style, explains the importance of a multi-disciplined approach for using movement to educate the handicapped. As you read his paper, take a test: Compare your ability and training to his criteria for a "motologist." Do you qualify?

In-Service Training in Physical Education for Teachers in Inner London Schools for the Educationally Subnormal (Severe)

Eileen McLeish
Inner London Education Authority

Background

Exactly 10 years ago, mentally handicapped children came, by law, from the social services, with their emphasis on training skills, into the care of education authorities and teachers with different attitudes and expectations. The switch did not occur overnight, as teachers had to be recruited and new courses devised. Many educationalists had studied the care of mentally handicapped children theoretically and explored the literature available but it took time before that theory could be satisfactorily married with the practice and strategies could be established. It is only 4 years since we could say that all our schools in Inner London were staffed by teachers and during the last 3 years that the surplus social service personnel were phased out.

The largest of our schools has about 150 pupils, the smallest about 40 pupils. Obviously, such numbers do not allow the luxury of a fully qualified specialist physical educator to cover just those specific aspects of the curriculum. Table 1 presents a comparison of the number of schools and populations for normal, subnormal, and subnormal severe.

Table 1
Inner London Education Authority School Population as of September 1980 with Special Students Instructed

Type of school	No. of schools	Number of full-time pupils	
Nursery	45	1,724	
Primary	816	152,429	
Secondary	178	157,013	
Special[a]	80	6,957	(2.186%)
	Total	318,123	

[a]Educationally Subnormal (Severe) Schools

No. of day schools	No. of boarding schools	Number of full-time pupils
15	1	1,425[b]

[b]E.S.N. (Severe) pupils compose 20.48% of the special schools population and 0.45% of the total school population.

The teachers appointed to the severe subnormal schools usually have 3 years of training in basic subjects, including a special course of about 6 months. These courses vary among training institutes. At one college, for example, the students have 1 day per week in the first year and 2 days per week in the second year on work specifically related to the mentally handicapped. The students are able to opt for other related units such as movement training or physical education. For the first teaching practice, the students visit a nonhandicapped school, then visit weekly a "severe" school for 13 weeks, and finally have a teaching practice of 4 continual weeks in that school.

During the training period, a student may have no practical experience in movement training. Where it is available, the number of aspects studied and the depth in which these are treated vary widely. In general, theoretical perceptual-motor concepts and motor assessment seem to be emphasized, so that the majority of teachers come into the schools with little idea of what kind of material to take in physical education terms. Fortunately, many teachers do have a personal interest in a particular sport or recreative activity, and participate at their own level.

The inspectorate of the Inner London Education Authority mounts a very wide program of in-service courses for all teachers, from the gymnastics, game skills, and expressive movement activities in the infant school to the most advanced coaching awards in all activities. All teachers in special schools have been encouraged to attend these courses and to adapt the activities for their own needs. It is also important for these teachers to see the nonhandicapped child in action so that they can remain in touch with what is "normal."

In-Service for Teaching Adapted Physical Activity

In October 1979 I took over as inspector/adviser in physical education for 75% of all special schools in the Authority. As I visited various areas of handicap, I became very aware of how isolated the teachers felt in their schools and their need to have a forum to share achievements, concerns, and strategies. The teachers in the severe subnormal schools had had enough of being talked to in theoretical concepts and having disability emphasized. They wanted to know how to educate, what material to give, how to "tap" the potentiality of their pupils. We decided to run an 8-week course for these 16 schools by "homing-in" to those teachers already employing good practice in a particular aspect and using, for tuition, the professional expertise of the advisory teachers attached to the physical education inspectorate. In the morning of each session, the children participated in lessons and the teacher explained how the activity was introduced, how this particular stage had been reached, and the expectations of the next stage. After lunch at a typical English "pub" of a pint and a pie, where perhaps some of the most valuable exchange of ideas took place, the teachers returned to the school and had a practical session taken by the professional physical educator. In this session the teachers analyzed material, shared their own strategies, and, we hope, departed at the end of the day with a lot of valuable material tucked up their sleeves. Each school was asked to send one staff member to each session. Some sent a different teacher each week and others sent three or four teachers to cover all the aspects.

Illustrative Examples

One very successful course was the "basic games skill course." The organizers were teacher adviser and the teacher in the school responsible for that area of the curriculum. They produced a booklet which would be a handbook for the teachers in that particular school as well as for the in-service course. By preparing the booklet, both teachers learned much from each other. The adviser became more aware of the needs of these special children and the teacher found a rich source of material to add to his program. Much of the literature they used came from America.

Materials included in the booklet are:
1. Introduction
2. Framework

3. Vocabulary
4. Sample lesson plan
5. Safety aspects
6. Material for lessons
7. Equipment list
8. Evaluation and assessment
9. Bibliography

A statement of the aims and how these should be carried out is given after the contents page. Then the framework is described—the stages, classic now, and the application of these for each of the groups in this particular school. The vocabulary section is an analysis of words that can and should be used in relation to the activities. These are discussed with the class teacher so that at a certain period of time a particular vocabulary is used by all teachers with certain children in all their learning experiences. A sample lesson plan is included in the booklet so that teachers implementing the course can clearly understand the actual process. During the in-service, two sample lessons from the "basic games skill course" were taught to the participating teachers. Afterward, the lessons were discussed in terms of planning and content.

The booklet also contains safety aspects and "material for lessons" to show the variety of activities to be taught. Another section is a list of useful equipment, where it can be obtained in England, and how much it costs. The penultimate section is not a scientific assessment but a descriptive list of problems which could be encountered in the teaching of children, some guidelines for the mild-to-moderate children, and some for the more severely handicapped. The assessment was put out in a list of questions which the teacher should consider. These were taken freely from the literature which the teacher-authors had studied at an earlier in-service course and were included in the booklet as important reminders to all teachers in such schools. Table 2 is a list of general suggestions for teaching students with subaverage intellectual functioning at a severe degree.

A second highly successful in-service course during the 8-session series was in the area of gymnastics. All schools in the Inner London Education Authority have this booklet of lower primary guidelines in gymnastics. The teachers preparing the gymnastic section used this booklet as the reference point for the discussion of tasks and themes. They decided to take one theme, jumping, plan six lessons, and one of the teachers would teach the stage he had reached with the children after 6 weeks. That was lesson number 3. He was then able to describe to the other teachers where the problems had been, the sticking points, where progress was very slow, where it flowed a little more easily, and where adaptations had to be made. He then discussed how he would approach the next lesson.

Table 2
General Suggestions for Teaching Students with Subaverage Intellectual Functioning at a Severe Degree

1. Apply suggestions common for the mild-to-moderately involved.
2. Have a full understanding of students' medical records. Any limitations to activity should be noted. Additional information may be obtained from other personnel such as physical or occupational therapists.
3. Make no assumptions of students' knowledge or performance levels. A complete appraisal should be given to determine individual needs.
4. Work with the physical and occupational therapists in designing the program for individuals. The therapists can indicate specific movement or positioning needs of each student and may request repetition of particular exercises.
5. Provide activities that acquaint students with environmental concepts.
6. Provide a high level of stimulation. This motivation must be geared to the needs and interests of each participant. All students have one thing that will interest or prod them into action.
7. Expose individuals to events that will help them understand cause and effect — particularly the effects of their own actions upon various events and objects.
8. Maintain an understanding of strict discipline though the situation itself may be free and unstructured.
9. Give rewards freely and promptly for good performance.
10. Alternate short periods of work, play, and rest. The interest span of these pupils is very short. The fitness levels are often very low.
11. Start with the simple task to encourage and assure a degree of success.
12. Provide enough stress to stimulate continuous improvement.
13. Keep directions brief. Emphasis should be on demonstration. Manipulation and guiding of students though the movement may be necessary.
14. Repeat directions so that students know exactly what is expected of them.
15. Elicit any possible purposeful movement from the individuals. Make them aware that they are moving. Explore every possible way of moving. Even though someone has been confined to bed for years, he/she still has a developmental need to move.
16. Remember that successful experiences, even the smallest achievement, are more helpful to learning than failure.

Conclusion

This paper has briefly explained the results of many hours of preparation by the session leaders for in-service training in physical education for teachers in Inner London schools for the educationally severely subnormal. It demonstrated first that through cooperation of the physical educator and the curriculum teacher, excellent physical activity instruction can result, even when ideal professional training is missing. Strategies were presented which enabled this cooperation to be shared with and used by other schools through in-service. Finally, it briefly explained how existing curriculum materials designed for normal children could be modified for use with the severely subnormal.

Physical Education Programs for Mentally Retarded Children in Germany

Gudrun M. Doll-Tepper
Freie Universität Berlin

During the past few years research has increased in the domain of mental retardation. Schools and public and voluntary organizations also have intensified and improved their efforts with opportunities for mentally retarded children. A large number of problems remain to be solved, however.

Present Situation of the Retarded in the School System

The school system in the Federal Republic of Germany (FRG) is quite different from that in the US, especially for the education of handicapped and retarded children. The German school system provides 10 different types of schools for these children to serve their specific needs. Schools exist for the blind, the partially seeing, the deaf, the auditory defective, the physically disabled, the mentally retarded, and the socially deviant, as well as for children with speech disorders or learning disabilities. In addition, special classes are provided for the ill and private lessons are given at home by special teachers.

On November 12, 1981, a complete program for physical education and sports for handicapped children and young adults was published in the FRG. It contains common recommendations developed by the Permanent Conference of the German State Ministers of Education and the German Sport Federation. It deals with sports and physical education for handicapped children at special schools and describes the goals and new programs in this field.

Recently, a controversy arose about whether the German special school system should be changed to avoid increasing isolation of the handicapped. Although a complete change of the school system cannot be expected within the near future, strong reformatory efforts are underway.

Teachers, psychologists, physicians, and the politicians in charge of education are interested in experiments done with "mainstreaming," "individual education programs," and "least restrictive environment" in the US and with new school concepts in the Scandinavian countries aimed at better integration of the handicapped. They are also following reports that deal with the situation of handicapped children in Italy after the abolition of all special schools and other special institutions.

Despite the difference in attitudes of institutions and organizations responsible for physical education and sports for the mentally retarded in different countries, most people agree on the necessity of an exact knowledge of the individual's capacities, and on the need for development of programs which include a wide variety of physical, creative, and social activities.

Program Planning and Evaluation

Physical education programs should be carefully planned with regard to the specific problems of the mentally retarded. Each child has to undergo a detailed examination for assessment of intellectual dysfunctioning, motor disturbances, and impaired adaptive behavior. It has been shown that mentally retarded children show striking impairment of gross and fine motor coordination, balance and body control, movement accuracy, and controlled use of physical strength (Brandenstein, Brandenstein, & Fleck, 1977; Irmischer, 1980; Kraus, 1973; Schilling, 1980; Theile, 1974; Vannier, 1977).

Schilling (1979) has described mentally retarded children as being far behind "normal" children in speed, reaction time, body experiences such as body structure, sensation of movement and position, as well as spatial and temporal orientation. The examination should therefore include sensory-motor factors. A multidimensional and interdisciplinary diagnosis is necessary. Procedures necessary for planning and evaluation include anamnesis; observation; medical, neurological, and psychological examinations; motor skill and physical fitness tests; checklists; and parent-teacher conferences (Irmischer, 1980; Rarick, 1981).

Only on the basis of the results of the individual program can planning be efficient. It must include the goals and the contents of the program: teaching suggestions should be based on practicality regarding the frequency and length of the physical education lessons, the group structure and size, the equipment available, the sports ground and gymnasium, and the number of specialized teachers and instructors.

In the course of the program, different methods of evaluation must be used periodically to help check the progress of the applied program in relation to the child's development, the teacher's ability, and the program's advantages and disadvantages.

Goals and Content

The main intent of education, in general, and of physical education, in particular, is to help individuals develop their personalities efficiently. Children need help and guidance to develop individual behavior. They must be enabled to adapt to the environment and they must be given the opportunity to alter environmental conditions if necessary. This is a goal for the mentally retarded, as well.

Within present physical education programs for mentally retarded children, it must be emphasized that they need stimulation in three main types of learning. These are perceptual learning, motor learning, and social learning. In Germany, several programs have been developed which put these into practice. Such programs use the term "movement education" or better, "motopedagogy" (Irmischer, 1980; Kiphard, 1979) and are based on the so-called psychomotor education which "emphasizes the identity of psychological processes and movement expression" (Kiphard & Leger, 1975).

All of these programs are developed on the basis of the results of diagnostic procedures. When remedial and therapeutic aspects are of great importance, the program is entitled "mototherapy." This type of exercise program can be found in special schools for the handicapped and retarded as well as in the remedial and medical fields.

The most important goal is to improve the individual's motor, cognitive, and social processes and their resulting behavior, which can be acquired on three closely connected levels: self-awareness, awareness of material environment, and social competence (Irmischer, 1980). Children must receive a variety of stimuli to improve their capacities. It has been found that in many cases, neither the traditional sport discipline nor its particular equipment has been sufficient.

This finding initiated a change in curricula and the development of new, imaginative types of equipment for the handicapped. As Kiphard

(1981) has pointed out, this new equipment has to meet the following requirements: It should be attractive in shape and color, warm and cozy on the skin, light and handy, easy to take apart, and not dangerous. Even more, it should be possible for the children to combine all parts in many different ways and it should function efficiently. In general, this concept is characterized by a certain departure from traditional physical education and sports programs (De Potter, 1978; Kiphard & Huppertz, 1977).

Today, many persons propose an opposite approach; they have been influenced by the idea of normalizing and adapting the handicapped to a so-called "normal" standard and therefore plead for programs offering traditional forms of sport with fixed rules and competition. A combination of these two positions extended by some additional aspects seems to be the most beneficial approach. Within the early part of physical or movement education the following subordinate goals can be reached by particular exercises and games: improvement and control of the movement of the body; improvement of the perceptive faculty (e.g., spatial orientation); improved knowledge and use of different kinds of equipment; and improved adaptability and capacity to cooperate in exercises and games with other children (Adolph, 1981; Der Kultusminister, 1980; Deutscher Sportbund, 1977; Rieder, Buttendorf, & Höss, 1981). In addition to these goals, it is important to help mentally retarded children to enlarge their knowledge and competence by becoming acquainted with particular learning conditions (Kapustin, 1981): gymnasium, sports ground, playground, swimming area, and experiences in open air, such as games, hikes, bicycle trips, canoeing, coasting, skiing, and ice-skating.

At an advanced level of physical education, it is possible to introduce traditional sports and perhaps competition. Authors such as Kraus (1973) and Schilling (1981), however, indicate the danger of overemphasizing competitive sports for the mentally retarded.

Teaching Suggestions

Educators generally agree that certain modifications of physical education programs are necessary such as a change in rules, a shortening of time periods, and an increase in the size of targets and projectiles. If modified teaching procedures are used, the following suggestions may be helpful:

1. Offer motivating activities in various forms.
2. Use praise as often as possible, even for the slightest success.
3. Progress slowly and use repetition.
4. Postpone competition during the early part of the program.
5. Allow the children to have their own choice of activities and games.
6. Offer rhythmical and creative activities.

7. Aim at a better control of psychic and motor behavior.
8. Get the children accustomed to occasional failures to make them more resistant to conflicts.
9. Strive for a better social integration and cooperation by offering partner and group activities.
10. Be kind, patient, and clear in your instructions.

For additional information, see Daughtrey & Woods (1971), Kiphard (1979), and Irmischer (1980).

Conclusions

A large amount of research has examined the causes and prevention of mental retardation. In addition, research with the mentally retarded has been aimed at studying motor behavior and motor learning as well as the effects of special physical education and recreational programs. However, transferring the results of research into practical work has serious disadvantages. There are still many complaints about the marked gulf between researchers and practitioners (Jochheim & Van der Schoot, 1981; Kraus, 1973). A better understanding and collaboration among scientists, researchers, lecturers, teachers, and therapeutic and recreational staff should be achieved.

Proceeding from today's level of research and considering the different physical education programs for mentally retarded children, it is necessary to work for a better knowledge of the motor and learning behavior of mental retardates, the connection between motor and psychosocial development, the effects of special physical education, therapeutic and/or recreational programs in relation to specific characteristics of personality and behavior, and the relationships and interactions of different kinds of programs. In addition, greater efforts are needed to improve program planning and evaluation and to develop adequate curricula in adapted physical activity.

The schools, as well as public and private organizations and institutions, should provide greater opportunities for the mentally retarded and should try to intensify relationships between these people and their environment. Improved and further training and education for people working in the field of adapted physical education is needed.

References

ADOLPH, H. *Sport mit geistig behinderter.* Bad Homburg: Limpert Verlag, 1981.

BRANDENSTEIN, Ge., Brandenstein, Gu., & Fleck, D. Vergleichende Untersuchungen zur Entwicklungsdiagnostik bei geistig Behinderten. *Psychomotorik,* 1977, **2**, 57-60, 65-66.

DAUGHTREY, G., & Woods, J.B. *Physical education programs: Organization and administration.* Philadelphia: W.B. Saunders, 1971.

DE POTTER, J.-C. (Ed.). *Psychomotricité—Psychomotor learning.* Bruxelles: Editions de l'Université de Bruxelles, 1978.

DER KULTUSMINISTER des Landes Nordrhein-Westfalen (Ed.). *Sport mit geistig Behinderten.* Köln: Greven Verlag, 1980.

DEUTSCHER Sportbund (Ed.) *Sport für geistig behinderte Kinder,* Frankfurt/M., 1977.

IRMISCHER, T. *Motopädagogik bei geistig behinderten.* Schorndorf: Hofmann Verlag, 1980.

JOCHHEIM, K.-A., & van der Schoot, P. (Eds.). *Behindertensport und Rehabilitation.* Schorndorf: Hofmann Verlag, 1981.

KAPUSTIN, P. In Deutsche Sportjugend (Ed.), *Symposium Behindertensport—Heidelberg 1981.* Frankfurt/M., 1981.

KIPHARD, E.J. *Motopädagogik.* Dortmund: Verlag Modernes Lernen, 1979.

KIPHARD, E.J. Sind unsere Turn- und Sportgeräte kindgemäß? In *Praxis der Psychomotorik,* 1981, **2**.

KIPHARD, E.J., & Huppertz, H. *Erziehung durch Bewegung* (4th ed.). Bonn-Bad Godesberg: Verlag Dürrsche Buchhandlung, 1977.

KIPHARD, E.J., & Leger, A. *Psychomotorische Elementarerziehung.* Ein Bildband, Gütersloh: Flöttmann-Verlag, 1975.

KRAUS, R. *Therapeutic recreation service, principles and practices.* Philadelphia: W.B. Saunders, 1973.

RARICK, G.L. In H. Rieder, T. Buttendorf, & H. Höss (Eds.), *Förderung der Motorik geistig Behinderter.* Berlin: Carl Marhold Verlagsbuchhandlung, 1981.

RIEDER, H., Buttendorf, T., & Höss, H. (Eds.). *Förderung der Motorik geistig Behinderter.* Berlin: Carl Marhold Verlagsbuchhandlung, 1981.

SCHILLING, F. In H.D. Bach (Ed.), *Pädagogik der Geistigbehinderten.* Berlin: Carl Marhold Verlagsbuchhandlung, 1979.

SCHILLING, F. In Der Kultusminister des Landes Nordrhein-Westfalen (Ed.), *Sport mit geistig Behinderten.* Köln: Greven-Verlag, 1980.

SCHILLING, F. In Deutsche Sportjugend (Ed.), *Symposium Behindertensport Heidelberg 1981.* Frankfurt/M., 1981.

THEILE, R. *Frühförderung geistigbehinderter Kinder.* Berlin: Carl Marhold Verlagsbuchhandlung, 1974.

VANNIER, M. *Physical activities for the handicapped.* Englewood Cliffs, NJ: Prentice-Hall, 1977.

Adapted Physical Education in Germany

Ernst Kiphard
Frankfurt University

Adapted or remedial physical education as we understand it in West Germany covers a wide range of approaches. Within our special education we have special physical education programs in the schools for exceptional children, that is, those who are mentally retarded, slow learning, or emotionally disturbed. Besides the school programs in physical education, we have sport clubs especially for the handicapped. Public sport clubs currently are open to these children either by establishing special departments or groups for them or by trying to integrate them into the sessions with the normal children and young adults.

A number of alternate programs such as perceptual and psychomotor training methods for children with motor impairments have been developed recently. These additional rehabilitation measures are offered in different institutions, for example, child guidance clinics or child psychiatric institutions. In our regular primary and secondary schools, selected children have the opportunity to participate in a physical corrective program. Details about this subject are presented in this chapter.

Corrective Physical Education for School Children

This approach has a rather long tradition. It started before the Second World War as an "Orthopedic Turnen" to help school children with slight orthopedic deficiencies. Later it became institutionalized in the schools with the intention of letting the children overcome their muscular, organic, and coordinative inefficacies by means of special corrective exercises. At first, the physical educator could specialize in corrective training as an option. But since the end of the 1960s these courses have been required for everyone studying physical education. Generally, it was not at all easy to motivate the students to go into "prescribed" training routines, and the effectiveness of such programs was rather doubtful. Thus, we have developed more innovative ways to interest children in physical activities.

On the Way to a New Approach

Orthopedic research opened the door for a new development. Scientific investigations over several years revealed that the so-called postural weaknesses and defects cannot be improved by compensatory measures. Various efficiency controls have shown that muscular weakness is a temporary phenomenon which normally disappears during puberty. On the other hand, some children have abnormal posture patterns of the back which have been considered bad habits that should be altered. According to the results of recent research, however, the lordotic or kyphotic curves of the spine seem to be biologically satisfactory individual adaptations, Obviously, it is needless to compensate posture patterns which are normal (Clauss, 1981; Rompe & Sommer, 1981).

Today we are experiencing basic changes in principles, in selective criteria, and in goals and compensatory techniques. In each classroom we find an increasing number of clumsy children who are deeply frustrated and show various disturbances in behavior. Recently, an expert commission of physical educators, psychologists, orthopedic physicians, and child psychiatrists have concluded that the former selective criteria should be altered. Rather than concentrating on the postural weakness, the focus now is on the motor and behavioral problems of the children who suffer from their inability to compete motorically with their classmates (Clauss, 1981).

Psychomotor Education and Therapy

In the search for adequate remedial physical education content, experiments with emotionally disturbed, hyperactive, and uncoordinated children were valuable in designing appropriate methods. The concept behind this new approach is "education through movement." It is not a training *of* movement, *of* motor skills, or *of* sport techniques. Extensive movement exploration (and not rigid sportive movement patterns) is the basic element of psychomotor education. Especially at the beginning, the adapted physical education teacher focuses on the children's strong points rather than on their weaknesses. He or she considers the students' needs, meets their personal problems, and encourages and strengthens their personalities as much as possible. This method has improved their physical education performance and very frequently their academic standard as well (Kiphard, 1979).

The Remedial Movement Specialist

Well-trained motor experts are needed to do this kind of psychomotor work. Five years ago, we began to offer a 1-year training program for physical education teachers which leads to a final diploma. We call these specialists "licensed motopedes." They have gained knowledge about early motor development. They are able to observe, assess and judge deviations, slight disturbances, and also the pathological impairment of sensory-motor performance. According to that particular diagnostic evaluation, the "motopede" develops individual programs and applies them to the children. At present, several hundred of these specialists are working with thousands of motor-impaired children in West Germany. But we still need many more for the future (see Figure 1). According to statistical evidence, 17.5% of the uncoordinated children in regular schools need special physical education. Among emotionally disturbed children, 47% need a special program. Children with speech disturbances need to be treated in 52% of the cases. With slow learners, the percentage increases to 70%, and with the mentally retarded, up to 98% (Schilling, 1981).

Motor Assessment as "Furthering Diagnosis"

During the psychomotor exercise treatment, the motor diagnosic process continues. The training program has to be adapted to the respective progress or stagnation of the students. That means the assessment procedures should be considered as "furthering diagnosis" which shows how this particular child should be treated for optimal training results. The child's potential could not be reached by rigid planning. The motopede must always be aware of the child's reactions to the training stimuli. In this sense, psychomotor education not only stresses the dimension of sensory-motor functioning, but also the emotional, social, and cognitive aspects of the child's personality (see Figure 2).

Knowledge and Experiences

→ Motor Development—normal and abnormal (motopathology)
→ Perceptual Development (psychology of perception)
→ Cognitive Development (also: learning theory)
→ Emotional and Social Development (vital needs, neurosis, etc.)
→ Movement and Behavior Observation Techniques
→ Motor Assessment Tools (motoscopic/motometric tests)
→ Motor Program Planning, Execution, and Efficiency Control
→ Information about other treatment methods (as a supposition for team work)

Figure 1—The movement specialist (Motologists, Motopede).

Motor Activity = Functional Unity of Perception
➡ Affection
Cognition
Action within social context.

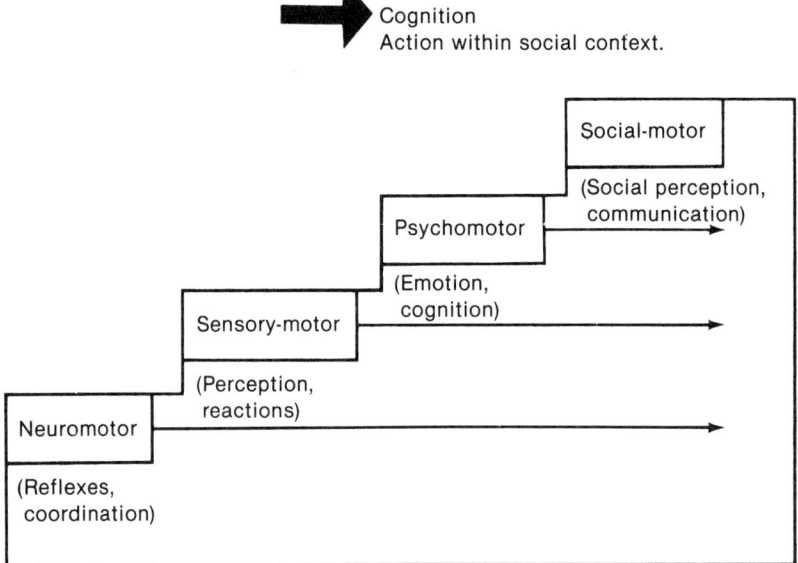

Figure 2—The main aspect of human movement.

Training Results with Handicapped Children

This psychomotor or remedial movement approach has also shown unexpectedly high results with various groups of handicapped and retarded children. For instance, trainable mentally retarded youth displayed a remarkable increase in their motor development quotients at the end of a remedial physical education training program even at the ages of 14 to 16 years. The results show that perceptual-motor development programs with the mentally retarded should start early and should be applied as long as possible.

Slow learners who received regular remedial physical education lessons every day showed a negative reaction at first. They were tired and displayed even greater difficulties in academic learning. But after 6 weeks of subsequent training, they became more attentive and their concentration endurance increased. Similar results have been reported with a class of emotionally disturbed children. In total it took nearly a whole year, with two lessons of adapted physical education training per week, for these children to change their misbehavior and to cooperate during the lessons in the classroom.

The German Model of Motology

In 1976, after extensive work of many experts in motor development and motor behavior, an official working group was established in West Germany. This "Association for Psychomotor Activity" is an interdisciplinary union of physical educators, special educators, pediatricians, child neurologists, psychologists, and physiotherapists, all interested and engaged in the field of motor activity. Within the association, a special board was formed to develop the foundation for a fundamental doctrine of motology or kinesiology (Kiphard, 1979) (see Figure 3).

The philosophy behind the model is the theory of motor adaptation. As the children live and develop in relation to their surroundings, they must first develop the means to adapt to their world. But as the children grow older they must also learn to adapt the environment to their own needs. This applies to things as well as people. It means that children should learn by means of various movement situations how to get along with themselves and with their surrounding material and social world.

The interaction between the human organism and the environment occurs in the form of a "homeostatic" process—the permanent maintenance of a biological equilibrium. Each environmental object sends off "acting directions" or "movement questions" to the child. And the child, after perceiving the situation, responds via movement. The environment, therefore, actually determines perceptual and motor patterns.

Motor-impaired children are unable to integrate their personalities into the environment. Here, they need special help to enable them to develop their motor abilities as far as possible, in spite of their handicaps. This can be done by multiple variations of motor situations and

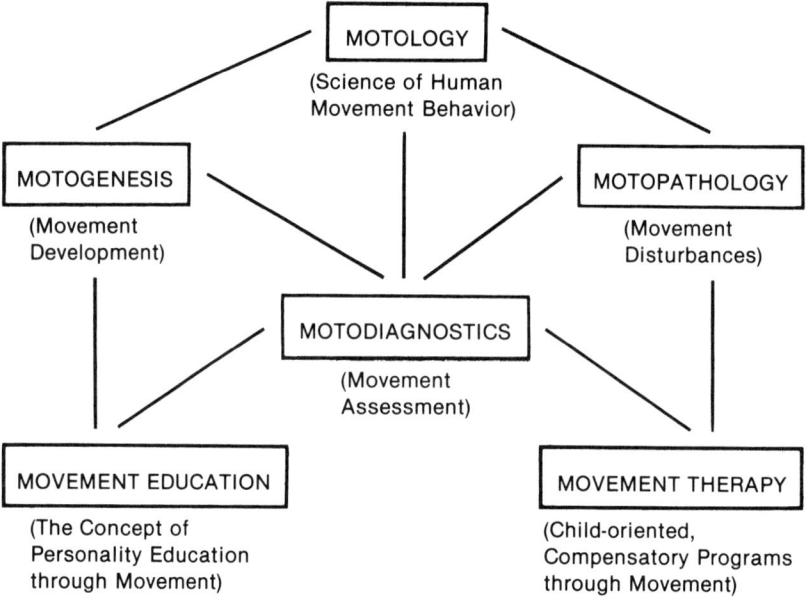

Figure 3 — The model of motology.

conditions. Each time these children are forced to adapt their perceptual and motor patterns and alter their strategies of motor behavior, they will increase their ability to generalize their own perceptual-motor patterns. This means they will be able to find a way to cope with each new situation.

Traditional physical education aims at the improvement of motor achievement. Psychomotor education goes further. It uses movement to educate the general personality. Overpowering joy, encouragement, confirmation, and success form the pillars of an inner ability to bear difficulties and to tolerate conflict. Thus, the children are assisted in finding their individual modes of expression in a basic joy of movement. In this way, they form a link between ego and environment (see Figure 4).

Children in the program enjoy answering the repeated but varied movement problems with their own way of finding a solution. The movement problem can come from a piece of equipment if it attracts the child to try it out. Or the children themselves may hit on the idea of combining various pieces of equipment. By this we mean the whole range of aids which the teacher offers: ribbons, ropes, bobbins, small boards, sticks, laths, foam rubber bags of sand, beanbags, balloons, and also balancing equipment, equipment for rolling, riding, climbing, overcoming obstacles, and jumping.

The movement task can also be set by the children themselves as they try out and "explore" the various possibilities of the respective situation.

ADAPTED PHYSICAL EDUCATION IN GERMANY / 31

Adaptation to environment ⟵⟶ Altering and changing environment

Thus the child achieves *3 stages of competence*:

→ 1. Ego Competence: body ego experiences and movement exploration as well as movement expression (miming, dance)
→ 2. Object Competence: material experiences, creative problem-solving
→ 3. Social Competence: adaptation to other individuals and groups, but also stressing own needs = communication

Figure 4 — Adaptation is a reciprocal process.

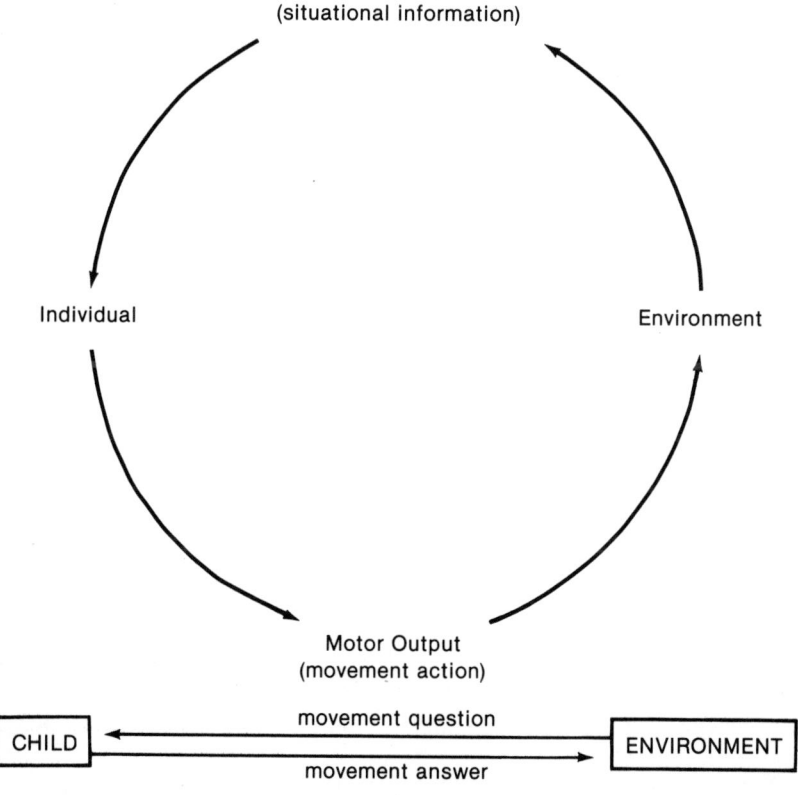

Figure 5 — Adaptation theory.

There is no norm, no force, and no obligation. The children will correct themselves if an attempt to solve the problem does not succeed immediately, and with time, they will be able to predict the results of their motor action by experience (see Figure 5). It will be necessary, in the near future, to revise the usual rigid equipment of the gym and to add new, fascinating, child-oriented equipment. We have just held a project seminar to find new posssibilities for combining old equipment pieces into an attractive "movement landscape."

References

CLAUSS, A. (Ed.). *Förderung entwicklungsgefährdeter und behinderter Heranwachsender*. Erlangen: Perimed, 1981.

KIPHARD, E.J. *Motopädagogik. Band 1 der Schriftenreihe, psychomotorische entwichlungsförderung*. Dortmund: Modernes Lernen, 1979.

ROMPE, G., & Sommer, H.M. Schulsonderturnen (kompensatorischer Sport) aus medizinischer Sicht. In A. Clauss (Ed.), *Förderung entwicklungsgefährdeter und behinderter Heranwachsender*. Erlangen: Perimed, 1981.

SCHILLING, F. Grundlagen der Motopädagogik. In A. Clauss (Ed.), *Förderung entwicklungsgefährdeter und behinderter Heranwachsender*. Erlangen: Perimed, 1981.

SECTION 2:
Developing Curricula for Special Populations

Adapted physical activity has made a significant impact on most of society's institutions, but none as dramatic and perplexing as the impact on education. Schools, either by special programs or by "mainstreaming," are providing physical education to special students. As very little precedent exists for program models, curriculum problems have multiplied. School systems and universities have combined efforts to conceptualize and test solutions to issues centered around the who, what, when, and where of teaching physical education to the handicapped.

One paper that is sure to become a classic for the curriculum specialists is provided by Janet Wessel. When she makes the claim that her I CAN is "a program that works," she's stating a fact. Somewhere out there is a person who has written down every "thorny" issue that faces adapted physical education teachers and specialists. We challenge that person to match the list against Wessell's article of solutions.

Inservice training is a continual problem in some parts of the world, but not in the Austin, Texas area. Claudia Knowles' paper is an explanation of how the teachers in Austin are providing individualized instruction for special students after receiving inservice. Dunn and Sherrill explain with specificity and power the solutions to the problem of programming for the severely mentally retarded. For specificity, Dunn teaches us how to use behavior modification and a data-based curriculum for providing developmental physical education. For power, Sherrill grips us with statements such as, "The aim in teaching dance [to severely mentally retarded] is physical education, *not therapy!*" Buell finishes the section with excellent advice for providing physical education for the blind and partially sighted. "Make them exert effort!" Perhaps his advice is good for all handicapped populations and for us, their teachers!

Quality Programming in Physical Education and Recreation for All Handicapped Persons

Janet A. Wessel
Michigan State University

Interest in the importance of and demands for instructional programs and services in physical education and recreation for handicapped persons at all ages increased dramatically after the middle 1970s. Today, however, simple expansion of existing programs is not an answer. Teaching performance and program accountability in meeting program objectives set for students, individual and/or groups of students, must be risks we are willing to take in this time of tax revolt, inflation, and economic constraints.

Three major changes and challenges will affect our programming services for the handicapped during the remainder of this decade. These include:

- Doing more with less
- Fluctuating national and local values and economic changes in education
- Rapid, complex changes bringing new techniques, new knowledge, and information overload that affect program, personnel, and services

Overriding these changes are at least two major challenges if we are to improve the quality of programming and services to the handicapped: documenting results and replication or adaptation of program models or key elements of proven value that "*work*." With these challenges has come efforts to link research to practice (universities and local educational program models). Through these efforts, pervasive components or elements of physical education and recreation programs that work must be identified and disseminated to consumers (students, parents, administrators, and others) concerned with equity and quality programming for all handicapped individuals. Instructional programs that work must demonstrate the parameters listed in Table 1.

In the past 10 years we have been involved in designing, developing, and validating model instructional programs (objective-based) for handicapped student populations, preschool through secondary levels. I CAN system and resource materials resulted from this work. I CAN was made feasible by grants from the United States Department of Education, Office of Special Education, and by the State of Michigan, 1971-81. It was validated and approved by the Joint Dissemination Review Panel for the National Diffusion Network (State Adoption) on June 11, 1981. I CAN is a program that works (Wessel & Vogel, 1981).

The major focus of this paper is to share with you program elements of proven value resulting from our studies. To accomplish this, the paper is designed to: (1) identify key requirements and design criteria to improve the quality of programming for handicapped individuals; (2) describe characteristics of an objective-based instructional system to improve the quality of programming for handicapped individuals; and (3) provide a base for international comparative studies and leadership development opportunities.

Table 1
Criteria Used to Judge Effectiveness of Instructional Programs

Program effects	Valid and reliable student performance gain scores
Educationally meaningful	Size of effect (group and individual)
Individual gain scores	Meaningfulness of gain to quality of life Cost of effect
Transportability	Reproducible program components (implementation model, competencies defined, resource materials) to other settings, with other implementers, and adaptable to available resources

Instructional Programs: Design Criteria to Improve Quality

Over the course of the identification of instructional design criteria, several different ways of clustering them have been used (Gagne, 1974). Initially the criteria statements were grouped by the three main categories of project activities: planning, implementation, and evaluation. Each of these major categories has similar criteria. In our final listing of the quality design criteria statements, we have used a different approach to clustering. Threaded throughout the criteria statements themselves is a focus on students and other participants who are immediate beneficiaries (e.g., teachers, parents, administrators, school board members, aides, support personnel, and others). Five design criteria of quality programming identified have impact on organizations as well as on individuals. The five design criteria are explained next.

1: Flexible

The program which is developed or selected, or selected and adapted, is supported by the organization within which it will function. The program represents a wide range of content derived from a set of educational goals for students which are based on findings of research, assumptions with rationale explicitly stated, and values of the participants within the organization. The program model defines a long-range program plan with content organized by levels tied to program goals common to all students (handicappers and nonhandicappers). This model is modifiable to meet the needs and capabilities of learners from near zero-competence to functional competence on a wide variety of content to be taught: cognitive, social, and motor. The model provides a dynamic and continuous systematic process which is responsive to changing needs of students, personnel, resources, new requirements, technology, or change in values. It also defines a systematic process for planning, implementation, and evaluation, not a methodology for teaching.

2: Communicable

The program is designed to result in instruction which is communicable and collaborative. Programs are most effective when they include participants (students, parents, teachers, administrators, and others in the community) in planning, delivery, and evelution. Program planning must provide opportunities for all school personnel to act as participants, as well as students and parents. Participants and others involved in the program provide the data for program planning and evaluation. Specific and long-range intentions (goals) and results of the program must be readily and regularly communicated and reported to students, parents, and other participants involved or affected by the program or from whom support is needed. Maximal communication and collaboration among teachers and related support personnel require all participants to know what is taught, when, to whom, what worked and did not work, and results of instruction in terms of student performance data on content taught.

Results of instruction communicated in terms of student performances and teaching-learning needs provide decision-making criteria for optimal learning and instructional placement for each student based on unique needs, not a categorical label. Momentary learning problems are communicated not as failures but as occasions for decision-making: extension of time to achieve, modification of content to be taught (task analysis), selection of different instructional procedures, or need for more in-depth evaluations to support the student's effort to achieve target objectives of instruction.

3: Efficient

The program is designed to result in instruction which is needs-based and responsive to changing needs. Programs are most efficient when they are organized to provide nonredundant, progressive instructional programs which are based on a set of program goals and student objectives. Continuous student assessment, entry status and evaluation of progress are embedded in content to be taught. The instructional activities are designed to meet the assessed needs of the student on content to be taught. Students' assessed needs identify needed instructional resources including personnel needed to implement the program. These assessed needs facilitate placement, implementation, and evaluation of quality instructional practices throughout the organization within which it functions, including students who are nonhandicappers.

Teacher competencies required to plan, implement, and evaluate the program are derived primarily from the program goals and instructional objectives set for students. Teachers can assess their strengths and needs, monitor their performances and design their inservice program to maintain quality and keep the program updated and responsive to new development.

4: Accountable

Program evaluation is designed and conducted in ways compatible to the underlying philosophy of the program approach. Program evaluation can help determine the degree of effectiveness of the program, provide instructional accountability at all levels of decision-making in the delivery of the program, and strengthen planning and implementation activities when data are systematically collected about context and operation of the program.

The evaluation design addresses both processes (planning, implementing, evaluation, and dissemination) and products of the program (student and teacher performances). This design includes plans to regularly report data on all program aspects to major participants: students, parents, administrators, boards of education, taxpayers, legislators, and others.

Information drawn from the evaluation yields data to develop cost-benefit analyses to properly document and/or define programmatic needs; to determine needs; to revise and redevelop the program or its components; as well as to judge its effects. Overall effectiveness of the program is judged in terms of significant numbers of students making meaningful performance gains on the content taught. The meaningfulness of the gain must be judged in terms of importance to the students' quality of life: health-fitness, lifetime leisure activities, personal and social competency, and other relevant program goals. Data from the evaluation are used for ongoing planning and implementation of inservice, competency-based programs for continuous staff development.

5: Compliant

The program is designed to result in instruction which is in full compliance with state and federal mandates and professional guidelines. Procedures exist to ensure inclusion of all students with handicapping conditions in equitable and quality programming based on students' assessed needs (learning characteristics, performances on content to be learned, health-safety considerations) and the instructional context.

Inservice education programs are readily accessible in time and location and are planned to provide the competencies defined based on assessed strengths and needs of teachers. Inservice education programs and support services are offered on an ongoing need basis.

Using these general design criteria to develop, select, or select and adapt quality program models, the program which invariably emerges is an objective-based instructional approach.

Quality Programs: An Objective-Based Instructional System

Characteristics

An important determinant of quality programming is the extent to which individualized instruction is proven to meet individual student needs. Individualized instruction places emphasis on matching the content to be taught (skills, knowledge, and values) and on designing instructional procedures to meet students' assessed needs (Dunn, Morehouse, Anderson, Fredericks, Baldwin, Blair, & Moore, 1980; Vodola, 1973; Wessel,

1977). At the core of this philosophy is the answer to seven key questions. Answers to these questions provide the distinguishing characteristics of an objective-based instructional system. To the right of each question in Table 2 are the characteristics of the system which relate to the seven key questions for individualizing instruction.

Typically, the system has two components. The first component is a set of program goals and objectives with related instructional resource materials from which appropriate selections can be made. The second component is an implementation model which identifies competencies required to improve the program and provides specific information about how to use the resource materials to plan, implement, and evaluate the program.

The system contributes to quality programming in three important ways by providing: (1) a model for implementation; (2) objectives for designing effective instruction; and (3) a systematic approach to inservice staff development. Each of these contributions will be briefly presented in the following discussion.

Contributions to Quality Programming

Implementation Model. The implementation model contributes to quality programming in three important ways. First, it provides a systematic model for planning, implementing, and evaluating instructional programs for handicapped students. Second, it provides a systematic approach to design and implement effective instruction for students with handicapping conditions. Third, it provides the basis for inservice program design directly linked to students' assessed needs on a set of educational goals and to teachers' strengths and needs in planning and implementing the program.

The implementation model presented in Figure 1 illustrates the series of sequential steps that teachers take to plan, implement, and evaluate the program. Each step required to implement the objective-based instructional system can be considered independently from all others. However, the steps are closely related and at the same time are mutually dependent on each other. This is the reason for the term "system" in the title of objective-based instructional program approaches.

Objectives for Designing Effective Instruction. The major premise underlying the objective-based instructional system is that the goal of teaching is to maximize effectiveness/efficiency and minimize the anxiety with which students achieve target objectives set for the unit (Kibler, Cegala, Watson, Barker, & Miles, 1981). The specific function of the system is to (1) guide the teacher in designing or selecting instructional procedures based on preassessment of student on content to be taught

Table 2
Characteristics of an Objective-Based Instructional System Related to Seven Basic Questions to Individualize Instruction

Question	Objective-based instructional system characteristics
1. What content should be taught and why?	1. Documented goals and program objectives specify the content to be learned during the school career.
2. When is the student to learn the content?	2. The objectives which operationally define each goal are sequentially arranged into appropriate levels of the program.
3. What is the student's present level of skill and what does the student need?	3. Criterion-referenced assessment of student's level of performance is derived from the program objectives subdivided into sequential instructional objectives. These objectives are stated in performance terms which range in skill level from near zero to functional competence.
4. What are the most appropriate instructional experiences to influence student learning?	4. Instructional activities are prescribed based on assessed needs of students on the instructional objectives to be taught.
5. How does the teacher know what each student has learned?	5. Assessment is a continuous, ongoing reassessment process documenting entry level and student achievement during and at the end of a lesson, unit, or other time period.
6. Is instruction effective or should it be modified?	6. Continuous monitoring and ongoing evaluation of student's progress on target objectives with modification during instruction and/or at the end of instruction is facilitated.
7. How can the results of the instruction be communicated to parents, students, and administrators?	7. Student performance data documenting both entry and progress on target objectives provide basis for lesson unit, yearly comprehensive reporting, and communication of program results in terms of student performances.

(instructional objectives of unit); (2) develop a sequential plan that takes students from where they are in the beginning of a unit to mastery of the unit objectives; and (3) provide teachers with structure for evaluating in-

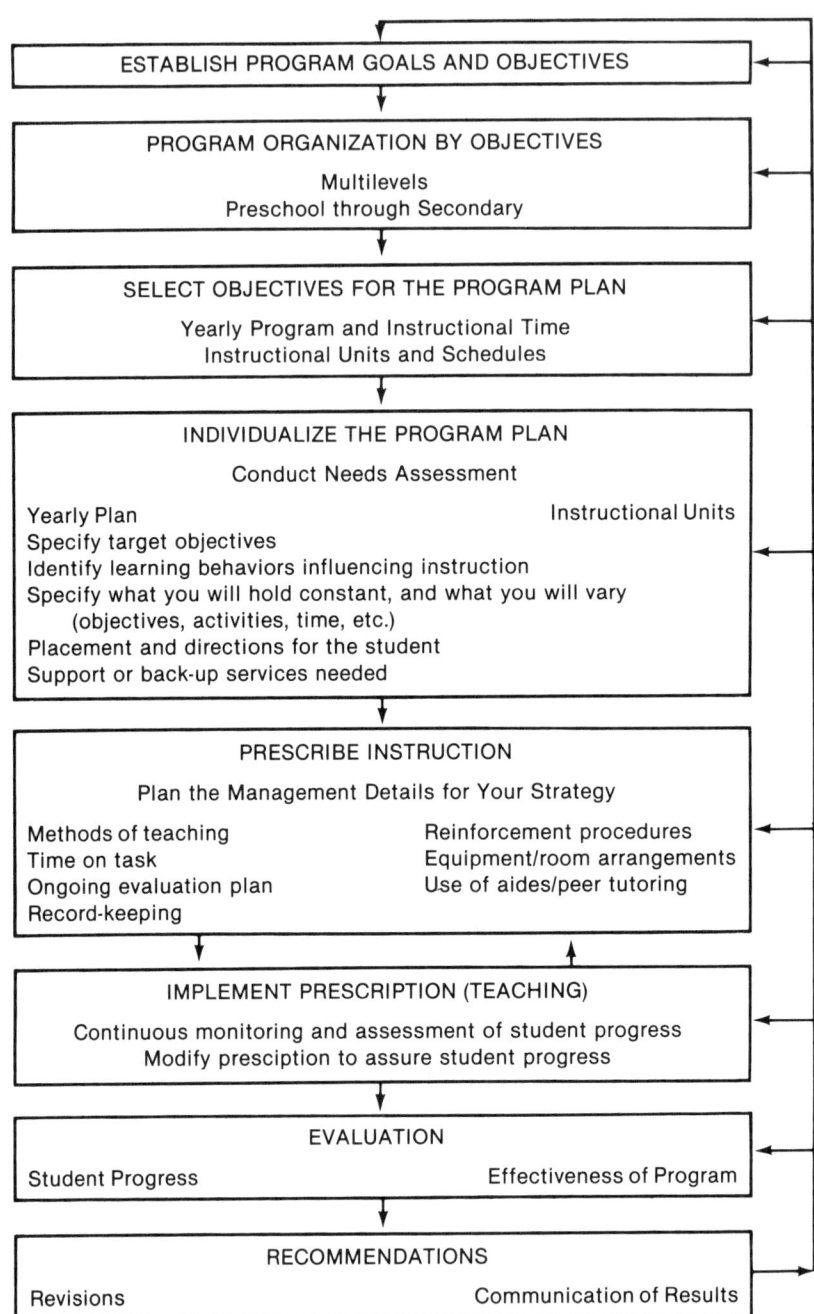

Figure 1 — Model for implementation of the objective-based instructional program approach.

struction (e.g., modify instruction, consider possible reasons for failure, such as objectives, cues, activities, motivation, feedback and corrective procedures, prerequisites, expectancy level, and time).

Data gathered from preassessment should provide teachers with information for planning and implementing instruction geared toward high student achievement on specified objectives. It is the teachers' judgments and skills that provide the criterion for what is meant by "appropriate" or quality instruction. Objective-based instruction based on student needs and instructional procedures based on such research evidence geared to these needs provide teachers with guidelines for effective instruction.

Clearly defined instructional objectives help teachers in prescribing and evaluating instruction according to whether the objectives are achieved. It appears logical that students will learn more easily if they know what they are expected to learn and how they will be expected to demonstrate that learning has occurred. Table 3 provides examples in the use of instructional objectives to plan, implement, and modify instruction. The statements highlight instructional procedures that have been shown to be highly related to student achievement.

Inservice Staff Development. The implementation model provides that the program is developed and implemented in a manner consistent with current knowledge about learning and effective instruction. The evaluation component, accountability-based instructional system, provides for improving the program at the unit level or across school years. Students must be able to demonstrate what they have learned as a result of their instruction. Accordingly, instructional accountability can be implemented successfully only if program goals and objectives are identified and stated before instruction begins. The objectives provide reliable measure of the effectiveness of instruction implementing these goals. The resultant program should represent the best of what is known about delivering quality services to students with handicapping conditions, regardless of type, severity, or placement setting.

Inservice programs as well as college courses can be based on the discrepancies between "what is" and "what should be" with respect to defined competencies required to implement the system. The teaching competencies defined become the content of a needs assessment instrument. In this way, inservice instructional activities can be tailored to participants' strengths and needs, now or on an ongoing self-monitoring basis.

The system facilitates the use of computer-teacher support systems. It is an instructional management system providing a combination of procedures, guidelines, and tools for the teacher who is teaching, plus objectives that are instructionally appropriate for each student. The system will vary in content and instruments, and it should, as no one particular system will meet the needs of all teachers in the variety of instructional settings. It is important that the system selected, or selected and adapted,

Table 3
Quality Programs: Using the System to Maximize Teaching Effectiveness/Efficiency

Plan instruction	Implement instruction	Modify instruction to meet students' needs
More able to . . .	Provided for more . . .	More often . . .
1. Assess students or instructional objectives and set appropriate learning tasks.	1. On-task time for students to engage in assigned learning tasks.	1. Use a variety of instructional cues to direct student's attention on learning tasks.
2. Prescribe instruction based on preassessment.	2. Positive feedback and corrective procedures specific to learning tasks (class and individual student).	2. Adjust instructional time needed to accomplish different objectives for individual students.
3. Focus lesson on students' target learning tasks and develop a sequential learning plan.	3. Active student participation rather than absorption of knowledge.	3. Anticipate learning problems and make instructional changes during lesson to meet students' learning needs.
4. Continually reassess, monitor, report and communicate results of instruction for students on instructional objectives.	4. Motivation, high-interest activities, and orderly class routine to manage disruptive behaviors.	4. Modify instructional and game activities to different skill levels of students in class.
5. Evaluate instruction, modify for student to achieve, consider possible causes for failure, represcribe based on students' needs.	5. Positive commitment of teachers' expectations that students can and will learn.	5. Modify instructional objectives (task analyze) breaking down learning tasks into smaller, teachable objectives for students to achieve success as they progress toward goal.

or developed by a school or district, contain the following six basic, common elements:

Goals: Defensible, representative of subject matter, provide intent and direction of the program.

Objectives: Sequenced/clustered/leveled as this relates to program level, unit of study, lesson or objective.

Assessment: Objective/criterion-referenced assessment instruments for: instructional needs assessment (locater, placement, inventory) pre-/post-tests. Procedures for using the instruments and procedures for teacher observation assessment strategies.

Resources: Instructional materials/activities matched to objectives and organized for ease of application by the teacher (resource index/file system, etc.).

Records: Forms and procedures for recording student information matched to objectives (individual profiles, group matrix).

Reports: Forms and procedures for reporting student achievement matched to objectives (parents, students, teachers, and administrators).

The school or district sets guidelines for the use of each component for the system to work in a well-orchestrated manner. Without common guidelines, the system's output would not be useful to everyone concerned: for the next teacher, for common record-keeping and reporting practices, for data needed in analysis for improvement, and for accountability—demonstrating what students learned as a result of instruction.

The instructional management system helps teachers prescribe appropriate instruction. The system should not confine, but rather support/facilitate the teachers' styles of instruction and their ability to implement a variety of learning experiences to meet a range of students' learning styles, abilities, achievements, and interest levels.

Comparative International Studies and Leadership Development Opportunities

Objective-based instructional system provides a structure for conducting international comparative studies and designing leadership development opportunities. The system was developed using the previously described design criteria for quality requirements. It is a data-based instructional management system which teachers can use to adapt the system to alternative populations. It is an accountability-based system for teachers or school/community systems to demonstrate what participants have learned as a result of their instruction.

I CAN provides such a system. It is an instructional physical education system that works. Although the initial validation studies focused on trainable mentally retarded students 3 to 25 years of age, other studies have demonstrated the effectiveness of the program with other student populations (e.g., severely/profoundly mentally retarded, autistic, deaf-blind, educable mentally retarded). At present, we are involved in implementing, adapting, and evaluating the I CAN system and resource materials with other population groups in middle city school districts in Michigan. These populations include learning-disabled, physically or otherwise health-impaired, as well as the previously mentioned student population. I CAN system was approved by the Joint Dissemination Review Panel (National Institute of Education-USDE) for the National Diffusion Network (approved for adoption as an educational program that works) in June 1981.

Overview of the I CAN System Components

The three major components of the I CAN system consist of a teacher's implementation guide, instructional resource materials, and inservice procedures and materials. The teacher's implementation guide provides the information necessary to use the instructional materials and implement the system appropriately. The instructional resource materials for preschool (2-5 years), primary (5-14 years), and secondary (15-25 years) levels guide the systematic teaching of a large variety of independent physical education content (performance objectives) in the program. Inservice procedures and materials also have been developed to guide the education of teachers and teacher consultants in implementing the system.

Implementation

The implementation guide provides the information necessary to conduct (1) program planning, (2) long-term planning, (3) assessment of student status, (4) prescription of instruction based on assessed needs, (5) implementation of teaching-learning activities associated with prescriptions, and (6) student and program evaluation of the results of instruction. Program planning and long-term planning are concerned with the derivation and appropriate placement of relevant program goals and objectives. Assessment, prescription, and teaching chapters describe the mechanics of systematic teaching. The evaluation section describes the procedures necessary for reassessing and reporting student achievements and for deciding on instructional and program plan modifications.

Instructional Resource Materials

Instructional resource materials are divided into preschool, primary, and secondary skills (I CAN, 1976, 1979, 1980a, 1980b). The preschool content includes 29 performance objectives (POs) for ages 2 through 5 years. Primary content includes 71 POs for ages 5 through 14, and 79 secondary level POs for ages 15 through 25. The PO is the basic element of the materials used in program planning. The preprimary, sport-leisure, and recreation POs with content categories are given in Table 4.

Performance objectives with criterion-referenced test items are included for all skill objectives. Each skill objective is divided into sequential instructional levels which range in performance competence from near zero to functional. The levels can be generically stated as: (1) assisted performance, (2) rudimentary performance, (3) qualitative pattern (biomechanically efficient), (4) qualitative pattern plus a distance and/or control criterion, and (5) functional performance (a qualitative pattern plus distance and/or control and accuracy at a criterion level enabling participation in sports of the culture). The instructional levels of all POs are stated in behavioral terms and have both qualitative and quantitative standards. The standards are operationally defined by focal points (discrete, measurable elements of skill) within each instructional level. Focal points are thus the units on which assessment, teaching, and performance improvements are based. Figure 2 illustrates an objective.

Implementation of the instructional system requires selection of POs from the primary and/or secondary resource bank in accordance with either existing or program goals derived using the implementation guide. Selected objectives are then systematically placed at appropriate program levels and ordered into a teaching sequence based on identified criteria. Student assessment regarding their performance status (zero to functional) is followed by prescription and teaching (i.e., students at level 1, 2, 3, or 4 on a PO are taught the focal points necessary to achieve level 2, 3, 4, or 5, respectively). Reassessment documents the degree to which the intended achievements in fact occurred and provide the data necessary to plan subsequent instruction and report student progress. Daily lessons can focus on one, two, three, or more POs depending on the content and/or circumstances present in a local setting.

Inservice Training

Inservice training system includes: the *Leadership Training Manual,* 16-mm films and overheads portraying key aspects of the materials and implementation process, workshop and follow-up schedules, and assorted evaluation forms for assessing knowledge and application of knowledge in planning, implementing, and evaluating the I CAN system.

Table 4
Preprimary, Primary, and Sport-Leisure Performance Objectives (POs) and Resource Materials of the I CAN System

Preprimary POs		Primary POs		Sport-leisure POs	
Body management		Body management		Backyard/neighborhood activities	
Body control	(5)	Body control	(10)	Badminton	(7)
		Body awareness	(7)	Croquet	(2)
Fundamental skills		Fundamental skills		Horseshoes	(2)
Locomotor	(7)	Locomotor and rhythm	(12)	Roller skating	(4)
Object control	(6)	Object control	(11)	Tetherball	(2)
Health/fitness		Health/fitness		Outdoor activities	
Physical fitness	(2)	Physical fitness	(11)	Backpacking	(2)
		Postural	(9)	Camping	(4)
Play participation	(2)	Aquatics		Hiking	(2)
		Basic skills	(6)	Cross-country skiing	(6)
Play equipment	(6)	Swimming	(7)	Dance and individual sports	
				Bowling	(3)
				Folk dance	(7)
				Gymnastics	(11)
				Track and field	(6)
				Team sports	
				Basketball	(8)
				Kickball	(3)
				Softball	(4)
				Volleyball	(6)
PO totals	(28)		(73)		(79)

SKILL LEVELS	CRITERION-REFERENCED TEST ITEM
1. To run with assistance.	Given a verbal request, a demonstration of mature running pattern, and physical assistance, the student with ability to walk can exhibit consistent periods of nonsupport (both feet temporarily off the ground) for at least half the strides taken over a distance of 50 feet, without resistance.
2. To run without assistance.	Given a verbal request and a demonstration of mature running pattern, the student with ability to run with assistance can exhibit consistent periods of nonsupport for at least half of the strides taken over a distance of 50 feet, unassisted.
3. To demonstrate a mature run. 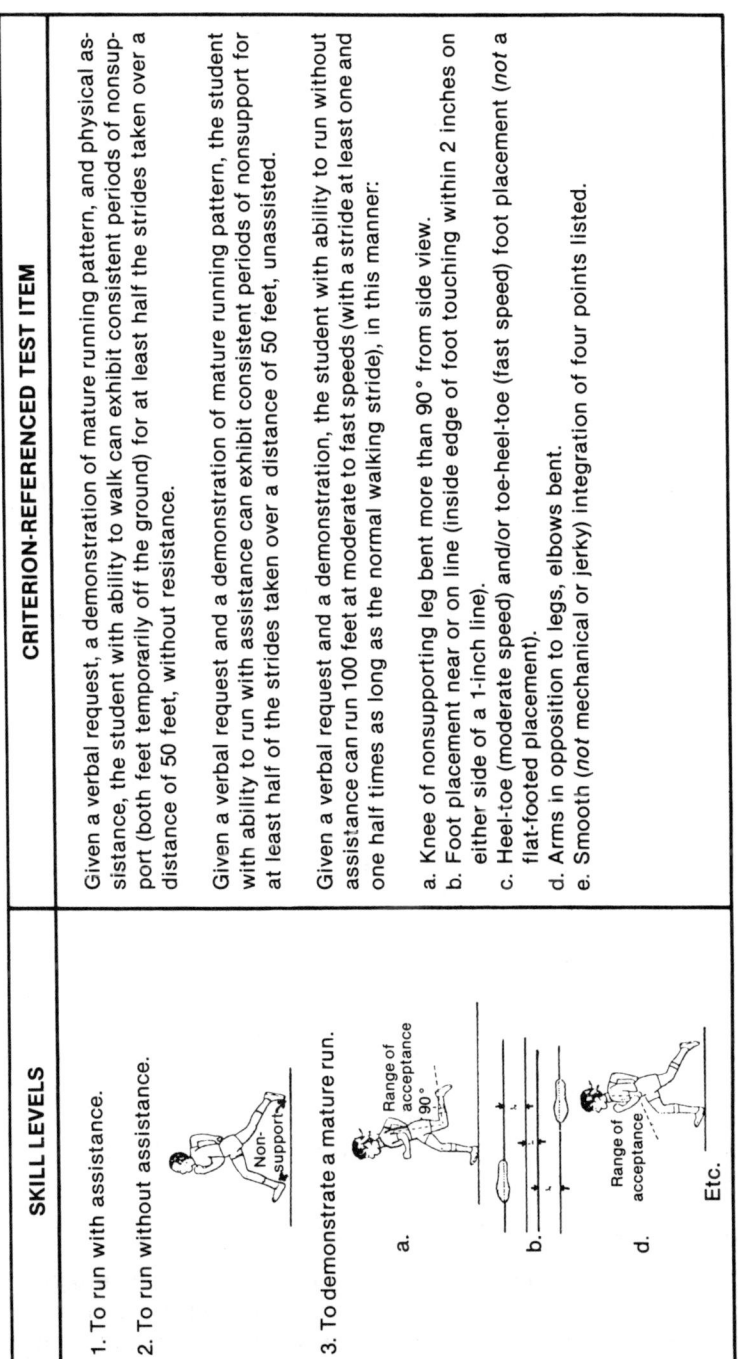	Given a verbal request and a demonstration, the student with ability to run without assistance can run 100 feet at moderate to fast speeds (with a stride at least one and one half times as long as the normal walking stride), in this manner: a. Knee of nonsupporting leg bent more than 90° from side view. b. Foot placement near or on line (inside edge of foot touching within 2 inches on either side of a 1-inch line). c. Heel-toe (moderate speed) and/or toe-heel-toe (fast speed) foot placement (*not* a flat-footed placement). d. Arms in opposition to legs, elbows bent. e. Smooth (*not* mechanical or jerky) integration of four points listed.

Figure 2 – Example program objective, instructional objective skill levels and criterion-referenced assessment: run.

The *Leadership Training Manual* is appropriate for training teachers, teacher consultants, and/or instructors of teacher consultants. All the major processes involved in implementing I CAN are explained with reference to when and how to use films, overheads, worksheets, examples, etc. Time allotment to workshop activities and implementation follow-up visits on-site are specified to achieve an efficient and replicable training system. The inservice training program is competency-based and result-focused.

Field Service Unit in Physical Education and Recreation for the Handicapped

The Field Service Unit (FSU) at Michigan State University is organized to improve the delivery of physical and leisure education program services for special populations, preschool through secondary. The major objectives include: (1) the conversion of the body of knowledge into instructional materials and/or processes which can positively influence educational practice; (2) the testing of the effects of such conversions; and (3) the dissemination of promising practices to potential users. Projects are selected in accordance with the needs identified in the field. The unit seeks to facilitate university, public school, and community agencies' collaboration in solving problems of mutual concern in the delivery of services to their respective clientele. An overview of information linkage between public school and university is presented in Figure 3.

Master Data Base Plan

One of the primary activities of the FSU staff is the establishment of a master data base plan along with technical assistance for systematic collection and analyses of valid, reliable data from people who have used the system. Those people have selected or selected and adapted the I CAN system and resource materials with alternate populations of persons with handicapping conditions in diverse settings. Technical assistance is available from personnel in the I CAN consultant network, as well as from staff at the FSU unit. We have just initiated these efforts in two other countries through the support and development of the University Center for International Rehabilitation-Michigan State University.

Leadership Development Opportunities

The preparation of personnel to effectively implement quality programs in physical education and recreation demands continuous and meaningful contact with the field by university faculty. This is one of the underpinnings of the Field Service Unit.

```
    ┌─────────────┐                    ┌─────────────┐
    │    FIELD    │                    │ UNIVERSITY  │
    │Program planning,│  Information   │  Research,  │
    │implementation,  │                │ development,│
    │evaluation and   │     flow       │ evaluation, │
    │ modification    │                │inservice and│
    │                 │                │  preservice │
    └─────────────┘                    └─────────────┘
```

Figure 3 — Master data base system.

The Field Service Unit has liaison with the University Center for International Rehabilitation (UCIR) at MSU. We work together to make international information available and useful to domestic service providers. Special emphasis is placed on physical education and recreation programs (formal and informal) designed to meet the unique needs of international students. Those interested in UCIR-FSU goals and activities are invited to contact the author. Such preparation programs include MA, PhD, and a specially designed Leadership Development Program.

The Leadership Development Program is for physical educators and recreation personnel who wish to develop competencies required to improve the effectiveness/efficiency of their school or community programs. A critical need is for leadership skilled in instructional design and program evaluation for handicapped persons which links together the field and university faculty.

Summary

To improve the quality of programming in physical education and recreation for all handicapped persons requires us to meet two major challenges: documenting results and replication/dissemination of programs of proven value that work. Pervasive programs that work must demonstrate program effects, meaningfulness, and transportability to all locales.

Through our review of literature and promising practices in the field, five major design criteria for developing, selecting, or adapting quality programs have been identified: flexible, communicable, efficient, accountable, and compliant. Using these design criteria, the program which invariably emerges is an objective-based instructional system. Characteristics of the system relevant to individualizing instruction were presented. The components of an objective-based instructional system and ways that it contributes to quality programming were identified: implementation model, objectives for designing effective instruction, and competency-based inservice staff development.

The role of an objective-based instructional system in providing a structure for data-based comparative studies was discussed with the I CAN system described as an example. The functions of a Field Service Unit in Physical Education and Recreation, linking together research and practice (university and field) as a potential for such collaborative studies, were identified. Opportunities for leadership development (postgraduate or institutes) to promote international studies and to institute data-based programs (students and teachers) were briefly outlined.

References

DUNN, J.M., Morehouse, J.W., Anderson, R.B., Fredericks, H.D., Baldwin, V.L., Blair, F.L., & Moore, W.G. *A data based gymnasium: A systematic approach to physical education for the handicapped.* Monmouth, OR: Instructional Development, 1980.

GAYNE, R.M. *Principles of instructional design.* New York: Holt, Rinehart, & Winston, 1974.

I CAN Instructional Resource Materials. *Primary Skills.* Northbrook, IL: Hubbard, 1976: *Sport, leisure & recreation skills.* Northbrook, IL: Hubbard, 1979; *Adaptation manual for teaching physical education to severely handicapped individuals preprimary through adulthood.* East Lansing: Michigan State University Instructional Media Center Marketing Division, 1980(a): *Preprimary motor and play skills.* East Lansing: Michigan State University Instructional Media Center Marketing Division, 1980(b).

KIBLER, R.J., Cegala, D.J., Watson, K.W., Barker, L.L., & Miles, D.T. *Objectives for instruction and evaluation* (2nd ed.). Boston: Allyn & Bacon, 1981.

VODOLA, T.M. *Individualized physical education program for the handicapped child.* Englewood Cliffs, NJ: Prentice-Hall, 1973.

WESSEL, J.A. (Ed.). *Planning individualized education programs in special education with examples from I CAN physical education.* Northbrook, IL: Hubbard, 1977.

WESSEL, J.A., & Vogel, P. *National Institute of Education—Joint Dissemination Review Panel, Project I CAN proposal report.* Field service Unit in Physical Education and Recreation for Special Populations, Michigan State University, June 1981. (Available from Hubbard, PO Box 104, Northbrook, IL 60062.)

Individualized Instruction for Special Students: A Challenge for Change in Physical Education

Claudia Jane Knowles
The University of Texas at Austin

National and state commitments for preparing educational personnel to work with handicapped students have, in the past decade, led to the creation of numerous staff development programs. The Division of Personnel Preparation (USOSE) has targeted 12 different areas of personnel need. One of these priority areas is physical education. Therefore, many of these new staff development programs have focused on the physical education content area. Not only are the processes contained in these programs innovative, but the procedures for personnel development itself involve new techniques. The challenge and concern of staff developers now is to personalize development of educational staff in a way similar to how instruction is individualized for school-age children.

The extensive educational changes required by law are difficult to make, particularly if we accept present practices in teacher education and in the public schools (Meyen, 1978). Meyen states that inservice training has had a history of inadequacies with regard to teacher needs in today's schools and argues that practicing teachers should be involved in determining inservice needs and in providing retraining. In any case, the teacher trainer, whether a faculty member from an institution of higher education, a practicing teacher, an administrator, or a school district consultant, must be aware of the inservice trainees' needs to facilitate change.

This paper includes a presentation of techniques for systematically planning training, diagnosing needs, and documenting the impact of a change effort, along with examples of the practical application of these techniques. The problems in attempting to measure student change as a result of teacher training programs will be addressed.

Overview of the Inservice Training Program

The purpose of the inservice training program was to prepare teachers to individualize instruction in physical education as specified by Public Law (PL) 94-142. Content of the program included:

- overview of PL 94-142;
- psychomotor assessment;
- individual educational programming in physical education; and
- managing individualized instruction in the least restrictive environment in physical education.

The training program consisted of two to three formal group sessions and four individual consultant visits during a 4-month block. The program materials were replicable and were adapted from the "I CAN" training modules developed at the Field Research Unit in Physical Education for the Handicapped at Michigan State University (Wessel, 1979).

The training activities during the 4 months focused on the first two phases of the following three-phase model: *Phase 1*—developing the physical educator's awareness of the implications of PL 94-142 in the physical education setting, interest in establishing a quality program, and the awareness of needs assessment at the local education agency level; *Phase 2*—developing the physical educator's skills in using the individualized process in the least restrictive alternative environment; and *Phase 3*—developing the physical educator's skill as a demonstrator and/or trainer of other teachers.

Training Plan

The specific interventions that were used to implement the teacher training program are outlined in Table 1. This game plan is the overall plan of actions that is taken to implement the new program (Hall et al., Note 1). It contains all aspects of the change effort, covers the full time-period of the change process, and affects all persons directly or indirectly involved.

A game plan has six components, which are:

(1) *Developing supportive organizational arrangements*—actions taken to develop policies; plan, manage staff, fund, and restructure

roles; and provide space, materials, and resources to establish and maintain use of the innovation. Examples would be to hire new staff, seek or receive funding, and provide equipment.

(2) *Training*—actions taken to develop positive attitudes, knowledge, and skills in role performance in relation to use of the innovation through formal, structural, and/or preplanned activities. Examples are workshops and modeling or demonstrating use of a new program.

(3) *Providing consultation and reinforcement*—actions taken to encourage use and to assist individuals within the user system in solving problems related to the implementation of the innovation. Examples of such actions are consultant sessions with one or several users, arranging small problem-solving groups, and organizing peer-support groups.

(4) *Monitoring and evaluation*—actions taken to gather, analyze, or report data about the implementation and outcomes of the change effort. Examples might be end-of-workshop questionnaires, periodic assessment of concerns, use of the innovation, or configuration of the innovation.

(5) *External communication*—actions taken to inform and/or gain the support of individuals or groups of individuals external to the users. Ex-

Table 1
Game Plan for Training with an Example of Each Component[a]

Game plan components	Interventions	
	Strategy	Tactics
Developing supportive organizational arrangements	Each on-site coordinator schedules consultant follow-up visits with all teachers during 4-month period.	For the first follow-up visit, coordinator schedules meeting for consultant with each teacher in a physical education setting that includes handicapped children.
Training	Consultant provides training for all teachers on implementing P.L. 94-142 in a physical education setting.	(1) Consultant provides awareness session at field site for each cluster of teachers. (2) A 2-3-day group training session is provided at each field site for each cluster of teachers by consultants.
Providing consultation	(1) Consultant takes calls, responds to teachers' problems by phone during 4-month period. (2) Four times during 4-month period consultant visits each teacher trainee individually to provide support.	For the first follow-up visit, consultant observes each teacher in physical education setting with handicapped children.

continued

Table 1, continued

Monitoring and evaluation	Consultant assesses teachers' skills and needs periodically.	(1) Stage of Concern questionnaire and Levels of Use interview are administered to teachers after awareness workshop. (2) Knowledge test is administered by consultant to all teachers at the end of 4-month period. (3) Anecdotal records are kept by consultant on informal observations of teachers.
External communication	Consultant maintains periodic communication with Office of Education project officer.	
Dissemination	Consultant mails brochures monthly to potential adopters.	(1) Special education and physical education directors receive brochure during the summer. (2) Overviews of program are presented by consultants at state and national meetings.

[a]Policy: PL 94-142 and its mandate of individualized programming in physical education; Special Education for Regular Teacher Competencies from Texas Register (July 15, 1977).

amples are reports to the board of education, presentations at conferences, and public relations campaigns.

(6) *Dissemination*—actions taken to broadcast innovation information and materials to encourage others to adopt the innovation. Examples are regular mailing of descriptive brochures to potential adopters, making charge-free demonstration kits available, training and providing regional innovation representatives, and presenting the innovation at administrator conferences.

Diagnosing Teacher Needs

Teacher needs were measured across a variety of areas: knowledge, concerns, skills, and behaviors. The instrumentation used to assess teacher skills in each of these areas is discussed below, along with examples of how the data from these assessment instruments were used to design intervention strategies for teachers.

Knowledge

A written test was used to assess the teachers' knowledge of the program content. Teachers completed the test independently, and were then presented the answer key in order to self-check their responses. Any incorrect responses were discussed with the trainer. For example, if the teacher felt unsure of the test questions focusing on a particular handicapping condition, the trainer provided clarification of correct answers and additional resources relative to the handicap. Teachers repeated the test until 90% of the items were answered correctly.

Concerns

Concerns of teachers about individualized physical education were measured prior to and immediately following the training program using the Stage of Concern questionnaire. Concerns are the feelings, attitudes, thoughts, ideas, or reactions an individual has related to an innovation. The work of Frances Fuller (1969) is the basis for the Stages of Concern. An early result of research was the realization that all teachers faced with a new program or innovation have concerns that are identifiable and developmental, similar to those documented by Fuller. From this research on change, seven Stages of Concern about the Innovation have been identified (see Figure 1).

Stages of Concern about the Innovation (SoC) (Hall & Rutherford, 1976) describes the kinds of concerns which the individual may experience, across time, related to the innovation. They range from initial *self-*concerns (Stages 1 and 2) — "In what ways will I be affected by this innovation?" — to concerns related to *task* (Stage 3) — "How can I make this innovation work?" — and then to concerns for *impact* (Stages 4, 5, and 6) — "How will using this innovation affect my students?" Individuals experience a variety of concerns at any one point in time. However, the degree of intensity of different concerns about an innovation will vary, depending on the individual's knowledge or experience. Whether teachers are using or not using, whether they are preparing for use, have just begun use, or are highly skilled with the innovation will contribute to the relative intensity of different concerns.

Thus, teachers seldom have concerns at only one stage. Teachers who are nonusers of an innovation generally have concerns high on Stages 0, 1, and 2. They are more concerned with gaining information (Stage 1) or with how using the innovation will affect them personally (Stage 2). As they begin to use an innovation, Stage 3 (management) concerns become higher and more intense. And, when teachers become experienced and skilled with an innovation, the tendency is for concerns at Stages 4, 5, and 6 to become more intense, with a decrease in Stages 0, 1, 2, and 3 (Hall, George, & Rutherford, 1977).

Although several ways to assess concerns have been developed, the Stage of Concern about the Innovation Questionnaire (SoCQ) (Hall,

Impact

┌ 6 REFOCUSING: The focus is on exploration of more universal benefits from the innovation, including the possibility of major changes or replacement with a more powerful alternative. Individual has definite ideas about alternatives to the proposed or existing form of the innovation.

5 COLLABORATION: The focus is on coordination and cooperation with others regarding use of the innovation.

└ 4 CONSEQUENCE: Attention focuses on impact of the innovation on students in his/her immediate sphere of influence. The focus is on relevance of the innovation for students, evaluation of student outcomes, including performance and competencies, and changes needed to increase student outcomes.

Task

3 MANAGEMENT: Attention is focused on the processes and tasks of using the innovation and the best use of information and resources. Issues related to efficiency, organizing, managing, scheduling, and time demands are utmost.

Self

┌ 2 PERSONAL: Individual is uncertain about the demands of the innovation, his/her inadequacy to meet those demands, and his/her role with the innovation. This includes analysis of his/her role in relation to the reward structure of the organization, decision-making and consideration of potential conflicts with existing structures or personal commitment. Financial or status implications of the program for self and colleagues may also be reflected.

└ 1 INFORMATIONAL: A general awareness of the innovation and interest in learning more detail about it is indicated. The person seems to be unworried about himself/herself in relation to the innovation in a selfless manner such as general characteristics, effects, and requirements for use.

Unrelated

0 AWARENESS: Little concern about or involvement with the innovation is indicated.

CBAM Project
Research and Development Center for Teacher Education
The University of Texas at Austin

Figure 1 — Stages of concern about the innovation.

George, & Rutherford, 1977) was the technique used in this program. Teachers respond by indicating their degree of concern on a Likert scale for each of the items. Scoring these data by computer program, or manually, results in percentile scores and a profile of concerns for the individuals or for the group.

Skills and Behaviors

Observer monitor forms provided anecdotal information about observed teacher skills with regard to the inservice program. These forms also were used as an assessing device for individual teacher needs. In other words, the trainer planned follow-up activities based on observed skills of teacher trainees in a variety of areas: planning, assessing, managing instruction, and evaluation. For example, if the trainer were monitoring the teacher's use of a selected student evaluation device, the techniques used to implement the instrument would be noted. Procedures which enhanced and/or inhibited successful use were discussed. At the teacher's request, the trainer would demonstrate ways to enhance the use of the observed technique.

In addition to the monitor forms, the Level of Use Interview technique was used for a more systematic measure of actual teacher behaviors with regard to the training goals. Levels of Use describes how performance changes as the individual becomes more familiar with an innovation and more skillful in using it. Eight distinct Levels of Use have been identified (Hall, Loucks, Rutherford, & Newlove, 1975). In general, individuals first "orient" themselves to the innovation. Usually, they begin to use an innovation at a "mechanical" level, that is, planning is short-term and organization and coordination of the innovation are disjointed. As experience increases, innovation use becomes routine, and eventually it may be refined. At the three refinement levels—LoU IVB Refinement, LoU V Integration, LoU VI Renewal—changes are made in the individual's use based on formal or informal assessments of students' needs.

Documenting Program Impact on Students

Two basic methods have been devised to document the impact of an inservice training program. One deals with the educational process (What did teachers do?) and the other deals with the educational product (What was the result of what teachers did?). Inservice education must be designed so that it incorporates educational processes which will ultimately effect student change (the product). However, it is questionable whether student change data should be used to evaluate the effectiveness of such a program.

Since 1970, the number of investigations conducted in the area of teacher effectiveness in the classroom has increased. Almost all of these studies used a process-product analysis, that is, teacher behaviors and classroom characteristics were observed and then correlated to measures of student achievement. One outcome of these studies was that a large number of variables seemed to be consistently related to achievement. These variables included, for example, goal-setting by the teacher, time spent engaged in academically focused material, teacher monitoring, use of academic specific feedback, and classroom environments. Berliner (1979) concluded that teachers who could find ways to keep their students in contact with the academic curriculum and who still maintained a warm and caring atmosphere were successful in promoting scholastic achievement.

Although the majority of investigators of teacher effectiveness since 1970 have used the process-product strategy, Siedentop, Birdwell, & Metzler (Note 2) suggested that, because it is difficult to find reliable and valid measures of student achievement in physical education, this strategy may not be appropriate in physical education research. Physical education students rarely produce permanent products from which a teacher can assess retention of a concept. Students do not turn in written work or "completed" assignments as they do in math or reading. For this reason, Siedentop, Birdwell, & Metzler suggested that researchers and evaluators in physical education needed to examine available process variables that seemed to be related directly to learning (Note 2).

Academic learning time (ALT) is one of these process variables. It is defined as the amount of time a student spends engaged in an appropriate task that can be performed with high success. The basic components of ALT are allocated time, student-engaged time, and student success rate or task difficulty level. An underlying assumption is that ALT may be related to improved performance. Time-on-task, which has been seriously neglected in teacher effectiveness research in the past, is a major component of ALT. Teachers influence student time-on-task, which in turn may affect student performance (Berliner, 1976). A number of investigators (Berliner, 1976; Hall, Delquadri, & Harris, Note 3) found a positive relationship between academic learning time and achievement in elementary school reading and math classes.

The observational system used in this project to determine the effect of the training on children is the ALT-PE (Academic Learning Time-Physical Education) system developed by Daryl Siedentop at Ohio State University. ALT-PE data were obtained for 60 regular and 60 mildly handicapped elementary school students. The students were selected from seven teachers classified as users of individualized instruction and from seven teachers classified as nonusers of individualized instruction. Although the ALT-PE of the regular students of both users and nonusers was slightly higher than that of the handicapped students, the difference was not statistically significant. Because these data indicated that both handicapped and regular students had similar opportunities to learn, the concept of mainstreaming was supported. The data also indicated that students in the classes of teachers who used individualized instruction engaged in a significantly greater amount of ALT than students in classes of teachers who were nonusers. Because higher ALT-PE students had greater opportunities to respond and were likely to be learning more, support was thus generated for the use of individualized instruction in mainstreamed physical education classes.

Conclusion

The specification for individualized programming for special students has presented a challenge for change in physical education. This presentation focused on the way that one change facilitator systematically planned and implemented training interventions to address the need for individualized physical education programming. The techniques used in planning, implementing, and evaluating the staff development effort to personalize activities to the needs of teachers were overviewed.

Reference Notes

1. Hall, G.E., Zigarmi, P., & Hord, S.M. *A taxonomy of interventions: The prototype and initial testing.* Paper presented at the American Educational Research Assn., San Francisco, 1979.
2. Siedentop, D., Birdwell, D., & Metzler, M. *A process approach to measuring teacher effectiveness in physical education.* Paper presented at AAHPER National Convention, New Orleans, March 1979.
3. Hall, R.V., Delquadri, J.C., & Harris, J.W. *Opportunity to respond.* Paper presented at the Midwest Association of Applied Behavior Analysis, Chicago, May 1977.

References

BERLINER, D.C. Impediments to the study of teacher effectiveness. *Journal of Teacher Education,* 1976, **1**, 5-13.

BERLINER, D.C. Tempus educare. In P.L. Peterson & H.G. Walber (Eds.), *Research on teaching: Concepts, findings, and implications.* Berkeley, California: McCutchan, 1979.

FULLER, F.F. Concerns of teachers: A developmental conceptualization. *American Educational Research Journal,* 1969, **6**(2), 207-226.

HALL, G.E., George, A.A., & Rutherford, W.L. *Measuring stages of concern about the innovation: A manual for use of the SoC questionnaire.* Austin, TX: Research and Development Center for Teacher Education, the University of Texas, 1977.

HALL, G.E., Loucks, S.F., Rutherford, W.L., & Newlove, B.W. Levels of use of the innovation: A framework for analyzing innovation adoption. *Journal of Teacher Education,* 1975, **26**(1), 52-56.

HALL, G.E., & Rutherford, W.L. Concerns of teachers about implementing team teaching. *Educational Leadership,* 1976, **34**(3), 227-233.

MEYEN, E.L. Inservice implications for implementing P.L. 94-142. *Journal of Special Education Technology,* 1978, **2**, 4-14.

WESSEL, J.A. *I CAN leadership training manual.* East Lansing, MI: The Field Service Unit in Physical Education and Recreation for the Handicapped, Michigan State University, 1979.

Physical Activity for the Severely Handicapped: Theoretical and Practical Considerations

John M. Dunn
Oregon State University

Educators have long recognized that the motor development needs of the severely handicapped require specially designed physical activity programs. Unfortunately, however, little information has been presented to assist teachers in responding to the unique behavior and motor patterns of students with severe mental, emotional, and sensory impairments. The lack of appropriate educational programs was clearly emphasized with the passage of the Education for All Handicapped Children Act of 1975, Public Law 94-142 (USDHEW, 1977). This law emphasizes that special education programs, including physical education experiences, must be available for all handicapped children, including the severely handicapped.

Oregon State University's Department of Physical Education, in cooperation with the Special Education Department of Teaching Research in Monmouth, OR has developed over the past 5 years a data-based physical education program for the severely handicapped (Dunn, Morehouse, Anderson, Fredericks, Baldwin, Blair, & Moore, 1980). Through federal funds supplied by the United States Office of Special Education, a special curriculum and an instructional process have been developed to teach physical education to the severely handicapped. A unique inservice training program also has been developed to assist teachers in implementing the data-based system within their own school system (Note 1).

The purpose of this paper is to provide a general overview of the instructional system used and the materials which have been developed. Within this paper, sections on the philosophical basis of the model, as well as elements found in the model, will be presented. A discussion of the inservice training system used also will be described.

Philosophy of the Model

The design of the Oregon State University Data-Based Model was developed through extensive field testing with severely handicapped students enrolled in the National Model Program for Severely Handicapped Children conducted by Teaching Research in Monmouth, OR. Concepts which form the foundation of the model include the following:

1. Every student, regardless of handicapping condition, can learn. If a student is not learning, the fault lies not with the student but with the educational setting. Students will learn at their maximal rate or potential if the teacher has identified and utilized the correct combination of environmental factors. If the student is not learning, the teacher must experiment by modifying either the cue or consequence or by reducing the behaviors desired to smaller steps (task analysis) so that the student is able to achieve. These modifications to the environment must be done systematically. The data which result from the student's attempt to perform the desired task should be recorded carefully so that an analysis of effects produced by the various changes in cue, behavior, and consequence can be made.
2. Handicapped students learn in accordance with the same learning principles as normal students, only usually slower. Because handicapped students learn more slowly than normal students, they require more extensive and intensive education to compensate. This implies a longer period spent on education activities, but because it is generally impossible to extend the time of the school day, the extended period of education must be implemented in after-school activity with the parents assuming the responsibility of conducting part of the instruction.
3. We have no way of determining the extent to which a student will progress. Therefore, no ceiling is placed on the curriculum; the teacher must be prepared to take the student as far and as fast as one can go. Thus, the curriculum extends from very basic skills such as executing various body actions in a standing position, to more advanced game skills such as catching and throwing.
4. Because the range of individual abilities among a handicapped pop-

ulation is usually greater than the range of abilities among a nonhandicapped population, the physical education teacher of the severely handicapped must conduct individualized programs. All materials must be sequenced to meet the wide range of individual needs.
5. Because of the wide range of individual differences in the severely handicapped population and oftentimes their unmanageability due to previous ineffective training, effective instruction usually can be achieved only in a one-to-one relationship. Therefore, having trained volunteers to provide individualized instruction in the gymnasium is considered mandatory.
6. Physical education is an integral component of the educational curriculum for severely handicapped students. As an important area, it is essential, therefore, that physical education curricular materials adhere to the same standards expected of other academic areas. Instructional programs should be sequenced, task-analyzed, and data-based so that performance changes in physical education skills can be determined.

Elements of the Data-Based Model

The Oregon State University (OSU) Data-Based System contains certain elements which are essential components of the instructional model. These address such critical areas as the methods used to present information, reinforcement procedures, curriculum material, management approaches, and personnel needed. In the following paragraphs, some of the ingredients which comprise the OSU Data-Based System for severely handicapped students will be discussed.

Learning Approach

The basic approach underlying many effective instructional programs for the moderately and severely handicapped is known as behavior modification. The essence of this approach is that the instructor systematically makes maximal and efficient use of the environment to assist a student in learning a behavior or in extinguishing an undesirable behavior.

The foundation of behavior modification has three essential elements: (a) the stimulus, also known as the cue which is the instruction or material presented to the student, (b) the behavior, or the task which the student is to learn or do, and (c) the consequence, or the feedback that the student receives after responding. These elements will be examined repeatedly in relation to their use in the OSU Data-Based System.

Cue. The cue is the sign, signal, request, or information that calls for the occurrence of a behavior. It is synonymous to the instructions or materials presented to the student. Cues are those things in the environment that "set the occasion" for the student to behave. For instance, "Come to me, Johnny" is a cue for the student to respond to verbal instructions and to move toward the teacher. The presentation of a ball which the student is to throw is a cue. Thus, a cue can take the form of any instructional materials—verbal, printed, or gestural—that are presented to a student. The concept of cue includes all the verbal instructions by the teacher. It includes the teacher's gestures as well as the way in which objects or materials are presented.

Behavior. The second major element of this approach is behavior. Behavior is anything which a person does such as lifting a little finger, blinking an eye, kicking a ball, or climbing a rope. In the teaching of students a behavior is a particular task which the student is to learn. Behavior can be something as simple as having students extend their arms or as complex as having them bat a pitched ball.

When you are teaching a behavior, however, you should constantly keep in mind that most behaviors can be divided into smaller behaviors or pieces of behavior, and it is these pieces of behavior which make up the teaching sequence. Take, for instance, batting a pitched ball. Batting a ball is called a terminal behavior, yet it is composed of a number of smaller behaviors—placing each foot in the proper position, grasping the bat with the left hand and the right hand, putting the bat back over the shoulder, fixing the eyes on the pitcher, then following with the eyes the pitched ball, and so on, step by step through the procedure until the ball is batted. The smaller or less difficult behaviors are called "enabling" behaviors, and learning them enables the student to learn the terminal behavior.

This process of breaking down a terminal behavior into the enabling behaviors is called analysis of behavior. The physical education teacher is taught to analyze behavior—to break down the behavior to minute sequences and to teach each part as though it were a separate and distinct behavior to be learned. With each new part that is learned, the student must be taught to chain the parts together so they form a smooth-flowing, larger terminal behavior.

Consequences. Consequences are the third major element of concern and can be likened to a feedback system. After the student performs a particular behavior, feedback or a consequence for that performance is provided. This consequence tells the student that what he or she did was correct or incorrect. In a school setting, one might think of the student taking a motor fitness test and having the test score interpreted as a consequence of the way the individual performed. The consequence can be either pleasing or displeasing to the person receiving it. A consequence that is pleasing to a person is called a reinforcer whereas a consequence that is displeasing is called a punisher. The basic concept underlying the delivery of consequences is that the reinforcers which are delivered following a behavior increase the probability of the behavior occurring again; punishers which follow a behavior decrease that probability.

A reinforcer must be pleasurable to the person experiencing it. Because it is pleasurable, and because the person desires that pleasure and associates a particular behavior with the receipt of the reinforcer, a reinforcer by definition increases the probability of a behavior recurring. Students who enjoy social praise may increase the quality or quantity of their performance after being told, "You're doing a nice job!" Consequently, reinforcers by definition must be individualized because what is pleasing and, therefore, reinforcing to one person may not be pleasing and reinforcing to another. The principle of individualization also applies to punishers. A verbal reprimand may be severely punishing (displeasing) to one student whereas another student may not perceive that same reprimand as punishing. Therefore, punishers, like reinforcers, must be individualized.

A basic rule in the use of consequences is to rely, if at all possible, on the natural consequences of the environment. Fortunately, in the physical education environment many activities and experiences are in themselves reinforcing: for example, watching the movement of a ball after it is pushed. For some, however, the natural consequences of the environment are not sufficient and it may be necessary to identify other types of reinforcers which are foreign or artificial to indicate to the students that their behavior is acceptable.

Game, Exercise, and Leisure Sport Curriculum

In response to the physical education needs of the severely handicapped, we developed and implemented a special *Game, Exercise, and Leisure Sport Curriculum* (Dunn, Morehouse, & Dalke, 1979). Recent efforts have focused on field-testing the curriculum to determine its appropriateness. The present revision has been found effective as a guide for teaching severely handicapped students basic physical education skills.

The curriculum is divided into four sections. The first section, Movement Concepts, deals with movement through space in one's immediate personal environment to movement skills in more complex environments. Section two includes skills found in many of our popular elementary games. Physical fitness skills essential for survival in modern society are included in section three. The last section focuses on some popular lifetime leisure skills. It is believed that this curriculum provides a bridge between therapeutically oriented motor programs and the more advanced physical education experiences which include highly organized game, sport, and physical fitness skills. The ultimate goal is to equip severely handicapped students with essential prerequisite skills to enable them to use these skills in more normal settings. The OSU/Teaching Research curriculum is systematic, data-based, and consistent with the definition of physical education in Public Law 94-142 (USDHEW, 1977). Unfortunately, in the area of physical education, very few curricula are specifically designed for the severely handicapped (Geddes, 1974), and those which have been reported are either geared too high or are entirely therapeutic in nature.

The *Game, Exercise, and Leisure Sport Curriculum* consists of a series of behavior analyses (task analyses) of basic physical education skills. The entire concept of task analysis is based on the observation that for a student to learn a complex skill, it may be necessary to break that complex skill into more simple skills and to teach each of those simple skills separately. This curriculum is designed to be used in a program in which individual objectives are designed for each student. It must be emphasized, however, that no curriculum can provide all the needed sequences and task analyses for any particular student. The responsibility for altering the sequences to fit the student's needs belongs to the teacher. We believe, however, that given this curriculum and the skills to make alterations as necessary, the teacher can provide appropriate physical activity experiences for handicapped students.

Personnel

As is true with any educational system, the skill of the personnel involved in the program frequently determines the quality of the program. This basic concept also is true as it applies to the OSU Data-Based System.

The person responsible for teaching physical education to the severely handicapped in the US varies among school districts and states. The options usually include one or two persons—the special educator or the physical educator. According to the Rules and Regulations for PL 94-142 (USDHEW, 1977) it could be argued that, technically, either person is qualified. However, if the local school district has physical educators available to instruct nonhandicapped students it would seem logical that these personnel should be available to instruct handicapped students. In the eventuality that a physical educator is available to teach physical education to the severely handicapped, it is essential that this person articulate closely with the special education teacher. In short, it is necessary for the physical educator to understand not only the student's movement needs, but also basic information such as the student's reinforcement schedule and language capabilities.

The teacher of physical education for the severely handicapped must assume a role as manager of the learning environment. Students with major disabilities require educational settings in which they are instructed individually or in small groups. Such an arrangement is possible only if the teacher has personnel who can assist with instruction. Implementation of the OSU Data-Based System requires the availability of trained volunteers, for it is these individuals who are frequently most responsible for conducting the individual skill acquisition program.

Parents also are an essential part of the instructional team, as they can carry out effective instruction in the home. Parents can serve not only to maintain the child's skills learned in physical education, but also can actually accelerate learning so that coordination with parents is an important element in enhancing the motor and physical fitness of severely handicapped students. The OSU Data-Based System offers a process by which parents and volunteers are trained to implement programs developed by teachers.

The Clipboard System

All of the elements presented above must be brought together so that they become a cohesive system, facilitating the instructional process of the student. The administrative device that accomplishes this coordination is the clipboard, established for each student. The clipboard describes in detail what to do with each student, where to record the information (data), and how to interact with the student. It is the communication channel through which all instruction to volunteers and parents is given and through which feedback comes to the teacher so that the student's individualized program can be modified.

Each student's clipboard contains the weekly cover sheet which specifies all programs, including the physical education programs, in which the student is currently engaged. A student may be a participant in as many as five to a dozen programs; examples are physical education (underhand throw); eating (finger foods); writing (reproducing a cross). The number of programs will be determined by the number of volunteers available to conduct each one.

Immediately following the weekly cover sheet on the clipboard is the consequence list of items that are reinforcing to the student. This list provides teachers and volunteers the information necessary in choosing reinforcers for the student. On the sheet with the consequence list is a section devoted to behavioral comments which also provides instructions on how to handle behavioral problems that may occur during an instructional period.

The third page on the clipboard is the language sheet, which is divided into three parts: (a) receptive language, (b) expressive language, and (c) new vocabulary. The receptive language section defines the degree of understanding the student has of spoken language. The expressive language section describes the degree of language complexity the student is able to emit.

The new vocabulary section includes new words or sounds the student has acquired that need to be reinforced. In all programs, including physical education, the consequence and language sheets must be used by all teachers, aides, and volunteers. Whether we are in the gymnasium or in the classroom, consistency in behavior treatment and communication procedures is essential for successful programming.

Following the language sheet are three sheets (a behavioral sequence sheet, a program cover sheet, and a data sheet) for each program listed on the weekly cover sheet. The behavioral sequence sheet (Figure 1) contains an example of a task analysis of one skill, and the program cover sheet (Figure 2) describes how a sample program is to be run.

In Figure 2, a trained volunteer can see what the verbal and nonverbal cue is, the correction procedure, materials to be used, the reinforcement ratio, and the criterion level of success. All this information helps a volunteer determine how a program is to be run.

The last form is the data sheet. Recording data assists the teacher in reviewing the student's performance so that an informed decision can be made to update the program appropriately for the following day.

Training Personnel in the OSU Data-Based System

Since fall 1979, through funds provided by the US Office of Special Education, Oregon State University in conjunction with Teaching Research has trained school personnel to implement the OSU Data-Based System. The format includes a 1-week intensive inservice training experience with both theoretical presentations and practical applications of the information provided. Follow-up visits are included in the inservice training model to ensure the successful transition of concepts learned to their application in the trainee's own school. Specific objectives of the inservice training experience include:

- Demonstrate knowledge of the OSU Data-Based System by answering questions over materials and activities presented.
- Administer a placement and baseline test to establish appropriate physical education experiences for severely handicapped students.
- Conduct prescriptive physical education programs.
- Modify and update prescriptive physical education programs based on data collected during the teaching session.
- Demonstrate the ability to conduct physical education programs with small groups of severely handicapped students.
- Demonstrate knowledge of behavior management and behavioral terminology.

Game Skills, Basic

A. Underhand Roll

Terminal Objective: Student, from a standing position, will perform an underhand roll by swinging the arm backward and then forward while stepping forward simultaneously with the opposite foot and releasing the ball at the end of the swing in the direction of the target.

Prerequisite Skills: Gross Motor, DD; Fine Motor Skills, A and G.

Phase I Sitting in a chair, swing arm backward and then forward releasing ball.

Phase II Standing with knees bent, swing arm backward and then forward releasing ball.

Phase III Standing with one foot forward and one foot back, and knees bent, swing arm backward and then forward releasing ball.

Phase IV Standing with knees bent, swing arm backward and then forward releasing ball while simultaneously stepping forward with the opposite foot.

Teaching Notes:
1. For those students in wheelchairs, the underhand roll can be performed with the student sitting in the wheelchair, thus eliminating the need for the above prerequisite body positions.
2. For nonambulatory students who are not in a wheelchair, ball rolling could be taught from a supported sitting position.
3. When students have problems with timing the step and throw, the teacher may choose to physically assist, and/or prompt the foot during the throw.

Suggested Materials: A tennis ball and a 3' × 3' target placed on the floor. Any type or size of ball may be used to facilitate learning.

Figure 1 — An example of one skill from the Oregon State University *Game, Exercise, and Leisure Sport Curriculum.*

- Demonstrate ability to use a volunteer observation form to provide feedback to other trainees.
- Implement the OSU Data-Based System at your own school using the information and skills gained during the 1-week training.

During the 1980-81 school year, 28 school personnel were trained. Ninety percent of those trained have maintained the criterion developed during training with the result that 167 severely and moderately handicapped students are now receiving appropriate physical education experiences.

PUPIL: John Q. DATE STARTED: October 3, 1981 DATE COMPLETED:	PROGRAM: Game Skills, Basic - A. Underhand Roll
SETTING (NONVERBAL CUE): Establish eye contact with John prior to delivering the cue.	MATERIALS: Clipboard Pencil Chair Ball 3' × 3' Target
INSTRUCTIONAL PROCESS: Verbal cue — John, roll the ball underhand. Model — Demonstrate if the response to the verbal cue is incorrect. Physical assistance — Provide assistance if the response to the verbal cue and demonstration is incorrect.	CRITERION: Three consecutive responses before moving to the next phase.

Figure 2 — Sample program cover sheet.

The Oregon State University Data-Based System is a continually evolving, dynamic approach for responding to the needs of severely handicapped students. In this paper, a brief overview of the model, some of its elements, and the efforts to train others, have been presented. Additional information related to the intricacies of the system are beyond the scope of this paper. It is hoped, however, that this paper will serve to inform others of the Oregon State University System so that effective dialog can be established with others interested in improving and enhancing the motor and physical fitness experiences for handicapped students.

Reference Note

1. Dunn, J.M. *Program assistance grant: Inservice training for physical educators and special educators in physical education for the severely handicapped*. Submitted by Oregon State University, Department of Physical Education, and funded by the United States Office of Special Education, 1980.

References

DUNN, J.M., Morehouse, J.W., Anderson, R.B., Fredericks, H.D., Baldwin, V.L., Blair, L., & Moore, W. *A data based gymnasium: A systematic approach to physical education for the severely handicapped.* Monmouth, OR: Instructional Development, 1980.

DUNN, J.M., Morehouse, J.W., & Dalke, B. *Game, exercise, and leisure sport for the severely handicapped.* Corvallis, OR: Oregon State University, Department of Physical Education, 1979.

GEDDES, D. *Physical and recreational programming for severely and profoundly mentally retarded individuals.* Washington, DC: American Alliance for Health, Physical Education, Recreation, and Dance, 1974.

UNITED States Department of Health, Education, and Welfare. Education of handicapped children: Implementation of Part B of the Education of the Handicapped Act. *Federal Register,* 1977, **42**, 163.

Pedagogy in the Psychomotor Domain for the Severely Handicapped

Claudine Sherrill
Texas Woman's University

Severely handicapped (SVH) children need physical education training as much as their higher functioning peers. In working with such children, however, we must develop pedagogy to meet their special needs. It is naive to say that SVH children develop fitness and learn motor skills in the same way as do the mildly and moderately impaired, that all we have to do is slow down instruction, increase the number of repetitions, and demonstrate patience and understanding. Yet little physical education research has been conducted on the SVH.

Public Law (PL) 94-142 defines physical education as "the development of physical and motor fitness, fundamental motor skills and patterns, and skills in aquatics, dance, and individual and group games and sports" (*Federal Register*, 1977). What do these terms mean in physical education programming for SVH students?

Long-Range Goals for SVH Students

The three parts of the PL 94-142 definition of physical education can be conceptualized as long-range goals which guide individualized educational programming (IEP) for the SVH. Each is therefore discussed in this section. Because psychomotor learning should not be isolated from associated cognitive and social learning, these will be presented as a fourth long-range goal.

Physical and motor fitness are those aspects of physiological, neuromotor, and psychological functioning necessary to carry out daily living tasks without pain and undue fatigue, with ample energy for play, socialization, and self-care. In severely handicapped persons, physical fitness encompasses the functioning of the postural reflex mechanism (i.e., muscle tonus); adequate strength to lift the head, roll over, sit, and ambulate in some manner; and sufficient range of motion (flexibility) to engage in play, self-care, and other activities requisite to learning, growing, and developing.

Fundamental motor skills and patterns include movements of isolated body parts and of the body as a whole; object manipulation; and stability (static and dynamic balance). Learning theorists do not define skill as an entity which occurs only after a certain level of central nervous system (CNS) maturation is present. Instead, a skill is something which must be learned through practice rather than something which evolves or appears naturally. A major characteristic of SVH children is delayed or abnormal motor development. They must be carefully taught the motor behaviors which evolve naturally in normal children, and they must practice these repeatedly before learning (a permanent change acquired through practice) can occur.

The adapted physical educator facilitates learning of whatever motor skill is needed—lifting the head, rolling over, crawling, creeping, sitting, or changing from one position to another. Ball handling activities for the SVH may be conceptualized as teaching object awareness, eliciting approach-and-avoidance reactions to objects, and developing reach, grasp, hold, and release mechanisms.

Learning skills in aquatics, dance, and individual or group games and sports through participation entails development of social and cognitive skills as well as those in the psychomotor domain. Most SVH children function in Piaget's sensorimotor and preoperational intelligence stages (i.e., ages 0-2 or 2-7 years). This characteristic limits games participation more than it affects motor skill. Delayed social development (i.e., the ability to interact with one or more others) also interferes with achievement of this long-range goal. It can be assessed by observing SVH children's play behaviors and classifying them according to play stages (unoccupied, onlooker, solitary, parallel, associative, cooperative). The adapted physical educator works to facilitate progression from one play stage to another.

Associative Cognitive and Social Learnings

A weakness in the PL 94-142 definition of physical education is its omission of associative cognitive and social learnings. These should be emphasized—especially in the education of SVH children. In the formation of body image, for instance (knowledge of self vs not-self and what the body and its parts can do), it is impossible to separate cognitive, psychomotor, and affective aspects of information processing. Likewise, learning self-care skills is intricately related to motor control and subsequent new understandings of the body. For persons in Piaget's sensorimotor intelligence stage (age 0-2), cognition is primarily through movement.

Essential to the adaptive behaviors needed for physical education is language functioning. SVH students often do not have sufficient language to respond to simple instructions and to understand movement, space, and time concepts. Adapted physical educators must therefore work on language development concurrent with psychomotor development. Progress from sensorimotor to preoperational intelligence is largely a matter of learning to link meaning to objects and to the symbols which represent these objects. With meaning comes language (inner, receptive, and expressive), the ability to communicate, and the beginning of interpersonal skills needed in games as well as in all facets of life.

For the SVH child, all teaching should be integrated and designed to bring meaning and organization to the body, the self, and ultimately the surrounding environment. Associative cognitive and social learnings, therefore, comprise a major long-range goal and should be carefully broken down into short-term behavioral objectives.

Adapted Physical Education Service Delivery

Adapted physical education, for the SVH child as for other students, is a "comprehensive service delivery system designed to identify and ameliorate problems within the psychomotor domain" (Sherrill, 1981, p. 10). Services within this delivery system are assessment, individualized educational programming, prescriptive and/or developmental teaching (intervention), counseling, and coordination of related services. These services may be delivered in the mainstream, in a separate setting, or in a combined placement—whatever is the least restrictive learning environment. The combined placement is perhaps best—a separate setting 5 days a week for intensive motor development with as small a pupil-teacher ratio as possible and a mainstream setting 1 or 2 days a week primarily for social development. The remainder of this paper will focus on two of the five areas of adapted physical education service delivery: assessment and developmental teaching. Information about the other services can be found in Buscaglia (1975) and Sherrill (1979, 1981).

Assessment

In order to comply with PL 94-142 requirements, every adapted physical education program must begin with assessment of the present level of functioning of each student. Assessment should be in relation to the four long-range goals discussed in the last section. Jansma's (1980) review of psychomotor tests for the SVH is excellent; this paper will therefore not duplicate his content. Instead, some additional SVH assessment tools that are taught at Texas Woman's University will be discussed.

To determine *physical and motor fitness,* particularly of persons with some degree of cerebral palsy, the Milani-Comparetti Developmental Scale (Milani-Comparetti & Gidoni, 1967) guides evaluation of four head postures, three body postures, rise to stand, locomotion, five primitive reflexes, four righting reactions, four parachute reactions, and five equilibrium reactions.

Physical educators should assess reflexes and reactions (Sherrill, 1981, pp. 107-121). It is naive to plan SVH physical education programs, especially for the nonambulatory, without an understanding of primitive reflexes and automatic postural reactions. Research indicates that 65-94% of nonambulatory subjects retain primitive reflexes, often throughout life (Bleck, 1975; Capute, Accardo, Vining, Rubenstein, Walcher, Harryman, & Ross, 1978). Teaching young cerebral palsied (CP) children as well as coaching the growing number of athletes in the National Association of Sport for Cerebral Palsied network entails helping CPs to cope with and/or use reflexes such as the asymmetrical tonic neck and the extensor thrust. In the delayed motor development of the mentally retarded (as opposed to the abnormal in CP) researchers are reporting that the problem is primarily in the evolution of postural adjustment reactions (Molnar, 1978). If physical educators are to start programming at the level of SVH children's needs, these findings have clear implications which cannot be ignored.

Lying, sitting, standing, and locomotor postures also are important in the assessment of fitness. The New York Posture Test has been found reliable with SVH persons, as have various checklists of static and dynamic postures (Sherrill, 1980). Body asymmetries in structure and alignment should be noted as well as tendencies to maintain specific postures.

Body composition is important in physical and motor fitness. Rimmer, cited by Sherrill (1981, p. 437), found that obesity characterized 30.2-59.6% of 363 SVH institutionalized mentally retarded persons. Standard skinfold calipers were used to estimate this dimension of fitness. Berg and Isaksson (1970) reported protocol for assessing body composition of the cerebral palsied as have several other Scandinavians.

Some of the fitness tests developed specifically for MR populations like those of Hayden (1964, 1968) and Johnson and Londeree (1976) are appropriate for SVH students. Many of the items, however, are based on skills such as long jumping, throwing, and running that profoundly handicapped persons do not usually demonstrate. Sherrill (1981, pp. 172-175) reviews these tests.

To determine *fundamental motor skills and patterns,* the various developmental scales reviewed by Jansma (1980) are sufficient in initial assessment stages. To develop behavioral objectives and instructional protocol, however, information must be gathered about the quality of the movement pattern (i.e., precisely what and where help is needed). The I CAN curriculum materials (Wessel, 1979) for the SVH provide excellent diagnostic assessment instruments for this purpose. Sherrill (1981) also provides illustrative checklists for this purpose, as well as illustrated sheets depicting developmental stages in the evolution of running, throwing, and jumping. Videotape and cinematographical techniques further enhance the probability of obtaining data sensitive enough to show change in SVH performance from one annual program review to the next.

To determine *skills in aquatics, dance, and individual and group games and sports,* adaptive behavior scales for readiness and game participation (Sherrill, 1981) are appropriate. Additionally, checklists developed in task analysis format such as those in swimming (Sherrill, 1981), in music and rhythms (Sherrill, 1979), and in various simple games (Wehman, 1977) facilitate the gathering of practical information needed for daily lesson planning. Some of the new Special Olympics materials (1981) developed specifically for moderately and SVH retarded students also offer excellent checklists.

To assess *associative cognitive and social learnings,* the teacher should observe play in several structured and nonstructured settings. Sherrill (1981) provides checklists for classifying SVH students into developmental play stages. The refined checklists and protocol described by Higginbotham, Baker, and Neill (1980) also are excellent. The Uzgiris and Hunt Scales of Sensorimotor Development (1975) provide six ordinal scales for assessing persons in Piaget's sensorimotor stage of intelligence. The discussion of this instrument by Fieber (1977) is excellent and reinforces the concept that early motor and cognitive behaviors cannot and should not be assessed separately.

Because body image and/or concept is among the first cognitive constructs to be developed in SVH children, it too may be assessed by the physical educator, although few existing instruments appear to be appropriate for SVH persons. Portions of Ayres' test of sensory integration (Ayres, 1980) may be the best measure of body image in the SVH.

In summary, some assessment should be done in relation to each of the physical education long-range goals. Data gathering should be a continuous process that is interwoven with teaching rather than a task which is completed before intervention.

Developmental Teaching

A number of curriculum models and/or teaching approaches are evolving to guide physical education for SVH students. Among these are the data-based curriculum of Dunn (1980) in cooperation with the staff of the Teaching Research Infant and Child Center in Monmouth, OR (Fredericks, 1980) and Wessel's I CAN materials (1979). Some materials, although originally intended for therapists, are easily used by adapted physical education specialists who have strong backgrounds in kinesiology and neurology. Among these are the works of Ayres (1972, 1980), Bobath (1966), and Galka and Fraser (1980). One of the few special education curriculum texts which includes physical education is that by Mori and Masters (1980). Three of this book's 13 chapters pertain to physical education. It seems essential that adapted physical educators assimilate the content of these and other works and continue to shape new curriculum models specifically for the SVH.

This writer recommends two distinctly different SVH developmental teaching approaches: National Association of Sports for Cerebral Palsy (NASCP) programming and language-arts-movement programming (LAMP), both of which are described in the remainder of this paper. Both rely heavily on task analysis (i.e., careful progression from simple to complex in presentation of new activities) and on joyous, humanizing, maximal involvement of the *whole* child. Both have been influenced greatly by long talks with SVH handicapped adults who have shared with me childhood experiences which added particular meaning to their lives as well as their present aspirations.

NASCP Programming

The National Association of Sports for Cerebral Palsy was organized in 1978, primarily to meet the needs of adults who could not compete equitably in activities of the National Wheelchair Athletic Association and the National Wheelchair Basketball Association. Since that time, NASCP has promoted international, national, regional, and local sports training and competition for persons of all ages. Its activities are not limited to the cerebral palsied but also include persons with conditions such as muscular dystrophy, multiple sclerosis, and arthrogryposis. The classification and rules guide manual (NASCP, 1980) describes numerous individual and team sports in which persons engage.

The motto of NASCP is "Sports by ability . . . not by disability." The NASCP classification system permits persons of like abilities to train and compete together. This system has much potential for revolutionizing public school physical education for the handicapped, at least in urban areas where sufficient numbers of persons of like abilities are in the same school. Most importantly, the NASCP approach stresses the right of every human being to participate in sports and to engage in risk-taking activities if he or she choses. No longer do handicapped persons want physicians, therapists, and teachers to make these decisions for them. No longer do they want to perpetuate the myth that competition is not good for cerebral palsied persons. They want to be exposed to as many leisure-time choices as possible and to the skills needed for vigorous sports competition.

NASCP uses eight classifications based on functional profiles in organizing its classifications. This paper is delimited to Classes I and II which include the most severely involved persons—those who are nonambulatory, quadriplegic, and often nonverbal.

Tables 1 and 2 describe the functional ability of persons in these classes and the sports in which they have demonstrated success. In so doing, they offer guidelines for age-appropriate physical education programming for secondary school students.

Table 1
NASCP Class I

Functional Profile
Severe quadriplegic/triplegic-wheelchair, using electric wheelchair, more spasticity present
Cannot push a manual wheelchair with arms or legs at all
Does not have manual ability to grasp softball or shotput
Has approximately 25% range of normal motion

Physical Education Activities
1. Distance throw with 5-oz beanbag
2. Precision throw at 8 concentric circular rings comprising floor target
   (a) 5-oz beanbag
   (b) Club—1 lb, 14 in. long
3. Bocce ball—individual or team
4. Bowling—closed/chute division with assistance, must be able to bowl each ball within 60 sec
5. Archery—30 arrows at 18 m distance
   May use mechanical release
   Must be able to shoot 6 arrows in 5 min
6. Wheelchair soccer—of 9 persons on team, 2 may be Class I
7. Slalom—race against time in obstacle course demarcated by traffic cones
8. Swimming—may wear support devices
   Freestyle 25 m
   Backstroke 25 m
9. Table tennis—21 points
10. Target rifle shooting—3 rounds of 10 shots each
    Target 10 m from firing line

Table 1, continued

11. Track—20-m electric chair dash
12. Weight lifting—bench press with lifter in supine position on horizontal bench (Universal weight machine)
13. Horseback riding
    Novice—for riders requiring a leader and 2 sidewalkers and/or backrider
    May be asked to perform at a walk, circles at the walk, reverses, and halt

Table 2
NASCP Class II

Functional Profile
Severe quadriplegic-wheelchair—normally propels wheelchair with legs, more athetosis present
Normally wheelchair bound, cannot ambulate without assistance or extreme difficulty
Has approximately 40% range of normal motion

Physical Education Activities
1. Field events for *upper extremity skill*
   (a) Club—1 lb, 14 in. long
   (b) Shotput—4 lb shot
   (c) Discus—regulation women's 7-in. diameter
   (d) Team bocce ball
2. Field events for *lower extremity skill*
   (a) Distance kick—12 in. Voit playground ball
   (b) Medicine ball thrust—6-lb ball
3. Bowling—closed/chute division with assistance. Must be able to bowl each ball within 60 sec
4. Archery—paired with Class I, 30 arrows at 18 m distance
5. Tricycling—1500-m race
6. Wheelchair soccer—of 9 team members, 2 may be Class II
7. Slalom—race against time in obstacle course demarcated by traffic cones
8. Swimming—may wear support devices
   Freestyle—25 m
   Backstroke—25 m
9. Table tennis—21 points
10. Target rifle shooting—3 rounds of 10 shots each
    Target 20 m from firing line
11. Track for *upper extremities propulsion*—20-m dash
12. Track for *foot propulsion*—60, 200, & 400 m
13. Weight lifting—bench press with lifter in supine position on horizontal bench (Universal weight machine)
14. Horseback riding

Ideas for teaching and coaching these activities are presented in a training guide written primarily by CP athletes themselves (NASCP, 1980). This and the classification and rules guide manual are available from United Cerebral Palsy Associations, Inc., 66 East 34th St., New York, NY 10016. NASCP also publishes a newsletter, *Sportsline*.

National Cerebral Palsy games are held every 2 years. At the third national games, held in Rhode Island during August 1981, approximately 500 athletes competed. Craig Huber, executive director of NASCP, indicates that approximately 25% of these persons were in Classes I and II (i.e., very severely handicapped). Opportunities also exist for these athletes to engage in international competition. Huber reports that Denmark, Holland, and England are far ahead of the US in facilitating sports involvement for SVH persons.

Language-Arts-Movement Programming

An equally exciting, but very different, SVH physical education model is integrated language-arts-movement activities which might be conceptualized as movement education or dance, depending on the age range of the learners. *Creative Arts for the Severely Handicapped* (Sherrill, 1979) is an outgrowth of this involvement which began in the 1970s as work with severely mentally retarded and deaf-blind persons and continued in cooperation with a new national organization founded in 1975. This organization is the National Committee Arts for the Handicapped (NCAH), 1825 Connecticut Ave. NW, Suite 418, Washington, DC 20009. During the 3-year period of 1978-80, NCAH implemented a federally funded special project on arts programming for the severely handicapped. The Texas Woman's University (TWU), in collaboration with a private school for SVH children, served as one of its three model sites. The purpose was to adapt arts (dance, music, drama, and visual arts) to the needs of the SVH. Pre- and posttest data were collected, and findings revealed that adaptive behaviors of SVH children were changed significantly by arts programming.

The arts programming at the TWU model site was heaviest in dance and/or movement; most of the staff implementing the program were graduate students preparing to be adapted physical education specialists. This interdisciplinary involvement supports the belief that physical education programming *for all students* should be one-third sports and games, one-third dance, and one-third aquatics. For SVH young children the emphasis should be on dance and aquatics (i.e., learning control of one's own body before being taught object control like ball handling).

Dance for the handicapped should not be confused with dance therapy, which is a well developed profession in its own right similar to occupational and physical therapy. The aim in teaching dance is physical education, NOT THERAPY! For persons wishing to know more about dance for SVH handicapped, an excellent film entitled "A Very Special Dance" is available for rent or purchase through AAHPERD Publication Sales, PO Box 870, Lanham, MD 20801.

Two principles should guide movement education with young SVH children: (a) movement—whether repetitious for range of motion outcomes or exploratory for sensorimotor learning—should be accompanied by singing, chanting, or music and (b) language and movement training should be integrated to help SVH children move from the sensorimotor to the preoperational stages of cognitive functioning. To implement these principles, the LAMP model relies heavily on Orff-Schulwerk (Bitcon, 1976) and the Van Dijk Coactive Movement pedagogy (Sternberg, Battle, & Hill, 1980; Van Dijk, 1965). Orff-Schulwerk was developed by a German named Carl Orff in the early 1900s and is now used throughout the world. It is a combination of music, drama, and movement which can be used to teach imitation skills to the very SVH or to promote movement improvisation and creativity in the less SVH. The best source of information in this country is a book by Bitcon (1976). The Van Dijk Coactive Movement Pedagogy originated in Holland in the 1960s and is used in deaf-blind programs throughout the world. Following are examples of both pedagogies.

Orff-Schulwerk Pedagogy. In Orff-Schulwerk the teacher always chants or sings. When the children are verbal, it involves their chanting back in rondo form as they move. "Peek A Boo, I see you," is Orff-Schulwerk in its simplest form. Bitcon (1976, pp. 34-41) offers the following Orff sensorimotor activities for nonverbal SVH children.

(a) The teacher passes an unbreakable mirror around a circle of 3 or 4 SVH children. As each child holds the mirror, the teacher chants:

> Look, look
> Look come see
> Can you find
> A face for me?

Responses of the children vary from licking, dropping, clutching, and polishing the mirror. Later they begin to point to parts of the face as the chant changes to:

> Look, look
> Look come see
> Can you find
> A nose for me?

Children with language chant with the teacher; others can be taught gesture or sign similar to that in action songs.

(b) To teach introductory ball handling, every child has a ball and a box, bucket, or basket. All perform in unison as the teacher chants:

> Put the ball in the bucket
> Dear_____, Dear_____
> Put the ball in the bucket
> Dear_____, Dear_____
>
> Take the ball from the bucket
> Dear_____, Dear_____
> Take the ball from the bucket
> Dear_____, Dear_____

(c) To teach feet and leg awareness, the children move from their wheelchairs in unison to a chant like:

> Stamp one foot
> Keep the other still
> Stamp both feet
> And move at will

or

> Danny and his dragon
> Did a dance one day
> They stomped and shuffled—
> It didn't matter which way.

Orff-Schulwerk, like all pedagogy, has numerous progressions from easy through difficult (i.e., some activities that even gifted children might enjoy). In addition to using words as accompaniment, it stresses rhythm instruments for children with sufficient coordination. For the others, gloves or socks with bells sewed into them are used. Even small movements that make noise (music) give SVH children a feeling of competence and control, thereby reinforcing them to want to move more.

Van Dijk Pedagogy. The Van Dijk Coactive Movement Teaching Model consists of six stages: (a) resonance behavior; (b) coactive movements; (c) nonrepresentational reference; (d) deferred motor imitation; (e) natural gesture; and (f) language. Its primary purpose is to teach language (i.e., to develop communication skills), but movement is always the method used.

Resonance Behavior

This is passively guided movement designed to achieve such objectives as (a) beginning development of body scheme and image; (b) beginning building of anticipatory behavior; and (c) beginning building of self-help skills. The bodies of the teacher and child move as one, closely touching, in activities such as rolling, seat-scooting, creeping, knee-walking, or walking across the mat. Initially for seat-scooting or creeping, the child may be placed between the teacher's legs.

These activities are done in a variety of environments: on mats, waterbeds, moon walks, trampolines, on floors with carpets of various textures, in grass, or even in wading pools. The teacher talks/sings/hums/whistles throughout the coactive movement; the same words/phrases should be used repeatedly with movement sequences. The child remains in this stage until the teacher senses some following and anticipating of movement. Any attempt by the child to assist or participate in the movement is rewarded.

Coactive Movements

In this stage the child and teacher cooperatively move together with the distance between their two bodies gradually increasing. In the beginning the procedure is very structured, using the same movement patterns as in the resonance stage. The emphasis is on teaching the child to imitate.

As the child grasps the idea of imitation, more and more activities are introduced: walking through tall grass, running down a hill, climbing over a fence, splashing through a wading pool, or exploring play equipment. Van Dijk emphasizes bench routines, during which the child imitates different ways of sitting, scooting, and eventually walking. Practice in sequencing begins in this stage, also. The teacher demonstrates increasingly longer chains of familiar actions and the child imitates.

Imitation of arm positions, leg positions, and different body positions is stressed. In accordance with the known progression from easy to difficult, bilateral movements are introduced first, then unilateral, and last crosslateral. To minimize balance problems, the children first imitate movements from a sitting or kneeling position.

Moving the body in relation to objects (chairs, tables, boxes, ladders, hulahoops, cage balls) also is introduced in this stage. Teachers initiate simple imitation games in relation to objects such as "peek-a-boo" and "where did I hide the ball?"

Nonrepresentational Reference

This stage overlaps stages 2 and 4 in time and teaching in that it emphasizes recognizing body parts and learning pointing behaviors. It is a stage that prepares for more advanced imitations.

Body image activities include: (a) rubbing body parts in a meaningful situation such as dressing or bathing; (b) pointing to a body part with a touch; and (c) pointing without a touch. When children are learning parts of the face and other nonvisible body parts, they use a mirror. From pointing to one's own body parts, the imitation moves to pointing to someone else's body parts, to those of an animal, to those of a doll, and finally to those in a picture. Other body awareness activities are imitated such as tracing around a body, painting and marking on body parts with shaving foam, soap suds, or other textures, and decorating body parts with stickers and ribbons.

Deferred Motor Imitation

This stage uses traditional perceptual-motor activities. Students imitate from memory with increasing spaces of time between teacher demonstration and student imitation. Some of the purposes are: (a) to create generalized imitative behaviors; (b) to teach/reinforce motor planning; and (c) to refine body perception. Increasing emphasis is placed on fine motor coordinations and hand/finger imitations with nonverbal children beginning to learn finger positions for the manual alphabet. In teaching children to generalize imitative behaviors, it is important to let them create their own movement and have others imitate. Orff-Schulwerk chants use this concept as well.

Natural Gesture

Gesturing is the beginning of true representational communication. Van Dijk (1965) emphasizes that a gesture representing an action is more meaningful than one describing an appearance; thus, a ball should be represented by the throwing action rather than circling the fingers.

Many physical educators withdraw when the SVH child reaches this stage, leaving further work to the classroom teacher and speech therapist. A growing number, however, are incorporating gesture, pantomime, and sign into dance and movement education.

Language

In this stage the focus is usually on total communication. Physical educators who wish to work with nonverbal SVH children should be competent in the use of total communication.

Summary

Psychomotor development with SVH children must teach language concurrently. It should be multidisciplinary/interdisciplinary/transdisciplinary. The LAMP approach to SVH physical education should result in leisure time competencies for rich, full living and good self-concept. The NASCP approach should help SVH students to derive the many values inherent in sports participation and games socialization.

References

AYRES, A.J. *Sensory integration and learning disorders.* Los Angeles: Western Psychological Services, 1972.

AYRES, A.J. *Southern California sensory integration test manual* (rev. ed.). Los Angeles: Western Psychological Services, 1980.

BERG, K., & Isaksson, B. Effect of physical activation and of improved nutrition on the body composition of school children with cerebral palsy. *Acta Paedriatrica Scandinavica,* 1970, **204,** 28.

BITCON, C. *The clinical and educational use of Orff-Schulwerk.* Santa Ana, CA: Rosha Press, 1976.

BLECK, E.E. Locomotor progress in cerebral palsy. *Developmental Medicine and Child Neurology,* 1975, **17,** 18-24.

BOBATH, K. *The motor deficit in patients with cerebral palsy.* Suffolk, England: Wm. Heinemann, 1966.

BUSCAGLIA, L. *The disabled and their parents: A counseling approach.* Thorofare, NJ: Charles B. Slack, 1975.

CAPUTE, A., Accardo, P., Vining, E., Rubenstein, J., Walcher, J., Harryman, S., & Ross, A. Primitive reflex profile—a pilot study. *Physical Therapy,* 1978, **58,** 1061-1065.

DUNN, J., Morehouse, J., Fredericks, H.D., Baldwin, V., Blair, F., & Moore, W. *A data based gymnasium: A systematic approach to physical education for the handicapped.* Monmouth, OR: Instructional Development, 1980.

FIEBER, N. Cognitive skills. In N.G. Haring (Ed.), *Developing effective individualized education programs for severely handicapped children and youth.* Columbus, OH: Special Press, 1977.

FREDERICKS, H.D. et al. *The teaching research curriculum for moderately and severely handicapped: Gross and fine motor skills.* Springfield, IL: Charles C. Thomas, 1980.

GALKA, G., & Fraser, B. *Gross motor management of severely multiply impaired students: Curriculum model.* Baltimore: University Park Press, 1980.

HAYDEN, F. *Physical fitness for the mentally retarded.* Ontario: Toronto Association for Retarded Citizens, 1964.

HAYDEN, F. The nature of physical performance in the trainable retarded. In G. Jervis (Ed.), *Expanding concepts in mental retardation.* Springfield, IL: Charles C. Thomas, 1968.

HIGGINBOTHAM, D., Baker, B., & Neill, R. Assessing the social participation and cognitive play abilities of hearing-impaired preschoolers. *Volta Review,* 1980, **82**(5), 261-271.

JANSMA, P. Psychomotor domain tests for the severely and profoundly handicapped. *Journal of Association for Severely Handicapped,* 1980, **5**(4), 368-381.

JOHNSON, L., & Londeree, B. *Motor fitness testing manual for the moderately mentally retarded.* Washington, DC: AAHPER, 1976.

MILANI-COMPARETTI, A., & Gidoni, E.A. Routine developmental examination in normal and retarded children. *Developmental Medicine and Child Neurology,* 1967, **9**, 631-638.

MOLNAR, G. Analysis of motor disorder in retarded infants and young children. *American Journal of Mental Deficiency,* 1978, **83**(3), 213-222.

MORI, A., & Masters, L. *Teaching the severely mentally retarded.* Germantown, MD: Aspens System, 1980.

NATIONAL Association of Sports for Cerebral Palsy. *A training guide to all aspects of cerebral palsy sports.* New York: United Cerebral Palsy Associations, 1980.

NATIONAL Association of Sports for Cerebral Palsy. *Classification and sports rules manual.* New York: United Cerebral Palsy Associations, 1980.

PART II: Implementation of Part B of the Education for All Handicapped Children Act of 1975, *Federal Register,* 1977, 424-478.

SHERRILL, C. (Ed.). *Creative arts for the severely handicapped* (2nd ed.). Springfield, IL: Charles C. Thomas, 1979.

SHERRILL, C. Posture training as a means of normalization. *Mental Retardation,* 1980, **18**, 135-138.

SHERRILL, C. *Adapted physical education and recreation: A multidisciplinary approach* (2nd ed.). Dubuque, IA: Wm. C. Brown, 1981.

SPECIAL Olympics, Inc. *Track and field sports skills instructional program.* Washington, DC: Joseph P. Kennedy, Jr., Foundation, 1981.

STERNBERG, L., Battle, C., & Hill, J. Prelanguage communication programming for the severely and profoundly handicapped. *Journal of Association for Severely Handicapped,* 1980, **5**(3), 224-233.

UZGIRIS, I.C., & Hunt, J. *Assessment in infancy: Ordinal scales of psychological development.* Urbana: University of Illinois Press, 1975.

VAN DIJK, J. Motor development in the education of deaf/blind children. *Proceedings of the conference on the deaf/blind,* Refones, Denmark. Boston: Perkins School for the Blind, 1965.

WEHMAN, P. *Helping the mentally retarded acquire play skills.* Springfield, IL: Charles C. Thomas, 1977.

WESSEL, J. *I CAN implementation guide: Teaching physical education and associated learning skills to the severely handicapped.* Northbrook, IL: Hubbard Scientific, 1979.

How to Include Blind Children in Vigorous Public School Physical Education

Charles Buell
US Association for Blind Athletes

US law states that visually impaired children are to be included in all courses at public schools which are feasible for them. Throughout the country thousands of legally blind children are being included in vigorous physical education in the public schools, but perhaps twice as many are not receiving any meaningful physical education.

Parents and educators often overprotect blind children, that is, children who have one-tenth or less normal vision. But overprotective attitudes may actually be detrimental to a blind child's development. Nearly 150 years of experience has confirmed Dr. Samuel Gridley Howe's belief that "Bumps and scratches affect only the bark, and do not injure the system like the rust of inaction." We have no evidence to indicate that blind children have more accidents than do their sighted peers, and very few eye conditions are endangered by vigorous physical activity.

It is important that visually impaired persons have as much, if not more, physical exercise as those who have normal vision. Blind people need more energy to accomplish the same activities of sighted individuals because they have to work harder to attain the same goals. The only way any person can gain physical fitness is to participate in vigorous exercise and for this reason, many blind children are being mainstreamed into public school vigorous physical education programs. This chapter will describe how to facilitate a blind child's participation in physical education classes.

Class Assignment and Teaching Modifications

Many public schools assign blind children to adapted physical education classes in which they are treated the same as severely handicapped individuals. Under most such conditions, they cannot possibly develop physical fitness.

In large secondary schools, sightless girls and boys should be permitted to select units, rather than being assigned to a single class. Thus, they might choose dancing, swimming, gymnastics, wrestling, weight training, or other physical conditioning activities.

Only minor changes need to be made when a visually impaired child enrolls in a public school physical education class. The amount of help these children need will vary a great deal. It is most important to remember that three-fourths of the legally blind children have useful vision, and thus are easier to integrate into normal activities. It will be helpful to most partially seeing children to be stationed near the instructor and to receive other visual cues; for example, you might use a brightly colored ball for ballgames.

For students who are sightless or have very little vision, it helps to assign a "buddy." Buddies give assistance only when a blind child does not understand the verbal instructions of the teacher, demonstrating the movement and permitting the blind child to feel their bodies in motion. In some cases, it is better for the buddy to move the sightless child's body parts through the exercise. Buddies may be selected from the top performers in the class. A teacher will find that many children usually volunteer to be buddies, especially if the teacher has nurtured the attitude that the sightless child belongs in the class. Teachers should give clear verbal descriptions of what they expect the whole class to do and need not spend additional time with a sightless child.

Activity Program in Mainstreaming

A number of physical activities need little or no modification for visually impaired children to participate whereas other activities may need to be altered. At no time, however, should an activity be modified to the point where sighted children become uncomfortable with it. Most blind individuals feel that the more an activity is modified, the less desirable it becomes.

Unmodified Activities

Several activities require little or no vision for participation. Teachers will find that an activity may need to be modified for one visually impaired child and not for another. How much vision a child has and how well he or she uses it is an important factor in determining whether modification of an activity is necessary.

Wrestling is one activity which requires no vision and so no changes are needed. If sightless wrestlers wish to start from the "touch" position, the rule book gives them this privilege. Each year, over 500 boys who are visually impaired compete in interscholastic and intercollegiate wrestling, and about 25 boys who have little or no vision annually place in state high school championships.

Judo and karate need little modification, even for sightless individuals. Most tumbling and gymnastic activities also require little or no modification; blind gymnasts have won letters at both high school and college levels. Visually impaired students can perform on the trampoline, particularly when they are coached with verbal instructions.

Swimming, weight lifting, and calisthenics need no modification for sightless participants. Dancing and other rhythmical movement also fit well into a mainstreaming program.

Blind students are easily included in races which are run in pairs. For example, a three-legged race can be fun for everyone, and the sack race also presents no problem for blind children. Relays in which students run in pairs are ideal for a mainstreamed class. Running the relays on oblong mats makes it easier for blind children to determine the turning point. Outdoors, the edge of a lawn can be used for the same purpose.

Activities Which Usually Require Modification

Ballgames usually need modification for visually impaired players. In football and flag football, sightless players perform best at the center and guard positions. A number of legally blind high school and college players have earned letters in football.

In kickball, a sightless player can place the ball on home plate, kick it, and run the bases with a sighted teammate. On defense, blind players are most useful as pitchers; they roll the ball toward the sound of the kickers' clapping hands.

In softball, a visually impaired student might bat from a tee and do physical fitness exercises between turns, such as rope jumping, squat-thrusts and running in place. In basketball, they can do exercises between free throws. A sightless child may serve for both teams in a game of volleyball.

Blind runners usually pair with a sighted partner in runs of a quarter mile or longer by holding or touching the partner's elbow. Harry Cordellos is one sightless runner who has used this method to place in the top one-third of the competition in more than 60 marathons, including the Boston Marathon. By stretching a sash cord 50-75 yards between two people, sprinting is made feasible for sightless individuals who touch the cord lightly during a dash. Less experienced totally blind sprinters slide a 5-inch section of hose along the cord.

Modifications of activities mentioned above are shown in a film, "Physical Education for Blind Children," Campbell Films, Saxton River, VT 05154.

Conclusion

It is feasible to include visually impaired children in programs of vigorous physical education in the public schools. Educators who are not following this practice need to change their attitudes, as thousands of legally blind children await the day when their problems will be more widely understood. If sighted children need participation, so do visually impaired boys and girls. They can't become physically fit by sitting or standing on the sidelines.

SECTION 3:
Recreation and Adapted Physical Activity

Today we recreation specialists are a part of a metamorphic process that has taken therapeutic recreation from the sterile, restricted confines of hospitals and institutions into viable, decentralized places where the handicapped can reach their full potential. As recreationists, we believe that recreation is a basic human need, especially for the handicapped. Some of our clients have physiological, psychological, and sociological limitations, but these provide an interesting challenge for us to supply a wide variety of activities and services. When we give our clients sensitive leadership, it is their gain — both therapeutic and pleasurable — as well as our own.

In this section the recreation leader will be allowed to travel back in time as John Nesbitt examines the origins of recreation for the disabled, and then brings us zooming forward to the present. Janet Pomeroy puts time in perspective by explaining her futuristic program in California — one that is in operation now! Compton, Witt, and Ellis' paper on assessment will help us to take the mystery out of determining which children and youth require specialized leisure services and what should be provided. Finally, Tague has presented timely information to help us utilize the potential of recreation for enhancing the quality of life among the elderly.

Recreation for Handicapped in the United States: A Historical Perspective

John A. Nesbitt
University of Iowa

Introductory Remarks

It is gratifying to express commendation of the International Federation for Adapted Physical Activity and the Organizing Committee of the III International Symposium on Adapted Physical Activity. Because it draws on the knowledge, insight, and experience of many countries, this conference is the most outstanding conference on adapted physical activity and special recreation held in the United States since 1968.

Throughout the 75-year history of the American organized play and recreation for handicapped movement there has been a continuing need to draw on international experience in addressing the recreation rights, needs, and aspirations of people who are disabled. Thus, this International Symposium is not only a major contribution to international exchange, it is also a major contribution to the introduction of ideas and information from abroad. American participants are indebted to those individuals who have come from other countries to share their knowledge.

I wish to commend the institutions and agencies that have lent their support to the III International Symposium, including the University of

New Orleans, the City of New Orleans, the New Orleans and Louisiana Offices for International Year for Disabled Persons, and the Louisiana State Department of Education and Special Education.

Finally, I wish to commend the participants in the III International Symposium for their support of this important international conference.

1981: 75th Anniversary

The year 1981 marked the 75th anniversary of the birth of both the American organized play and recreation movement and the organized play and recreation for special populations movement. The following brief description of the first 75 years of recreation for special populations is presented to provide the reader with a general overview of the evolution of the organized play and recreation for special populations movement in the United States. Further, problems and needs that exist at the present time in recreation for disabled persons are cited and recommendation is made for the further development of recreation for special populations over the next 25 years.

A Historical Sketch

This section will discuss briefly the following aspects of the recreation for special populations movement in the United States from 1900 to 1980: (1) organizing the special recreation movement; (2) representative innovations in institutional and community recreation service for special populations; (3) major actions at the national level, both governmental and nongovernmental; and (4) the literature of the field. Because of space limitations this cannot be considered more than a historical sketch.

1906-09

The Playground Association of America was formed in 1906 through the combined efforts of play leaders, recreation workers, physical educators, "Y" workers, youth leaders, institution workers serving the ill, delinquent, and disabled, philanthropists, educators, and community leaders. The PAA's purpose was to provide leadership for the nation in response to the enormous need for play and recreation opportunities for children and youth.

The PAA created its Committee on Play in Institutions during the first year of operation. The Committee was chaired successively from 1907 through 1910 by Sadie American, Hastings H. Hart, and Alexander Johnson. This committee conducted a survey of play and recreation services in institutions, organized sessions and papers at Annual Congresses of the PAA, and arranged for the publication of articles (Nesbitt, 1982).

One hundred and thirty institutions serving blind, deaf, deaf and dumb, delinquent, mentally ill, mentally retarded, and orphaned children responded to a PAA-CPI survey. Twenty-two of these institutions reported "an employee whose special duty it is to oversee the play of the children . . ." One-third of the 29 orphanages and the 25 reformatories responding "emphasized the necessity for a special director of play." In 1908 the Playground Association of America designated play in institutions as one of eight areas in its "Plan of Work for 1908" as follows: "3. An effort for the establishment of playgrounds in connection with institutions for children." Major figures in the establishment of the PAA such as Luther Halsey Gulick and Henry S. Curtis recognized the need for play and recreation for special populations and expressed the need to develop programs and services to meet those needs.

Support for play and recreation in institutions was expressed by leaders in institutional work and services to disabled work such as Rudolph R. Reeder, superintendent of the Orphan Asylum of the City of New York, Hastings-on-Hudson, NY; O.H. Burritt, principal of the Pennsylvania Institution for the Instruction of the Blind at Overbrook, PA; Clifford W. Beers, secretary of the National Committee for Mental Health; and Helen Keller.

The Appendix at the end of this chapter lists major publications from this period.

1910s

A "playground director" was employed in 1910 by the Sacramento Orphanage in a demonstration typical of the times. The "expense of the experiment" was borne by C.M. Goethe, a member of the Playground Association of America's Committee on Play in Institutions. Howard Bradstreet, secretary of the Park and Recreation Association of New York City, assisted in the provision of recreation service to the Colored Orphan Asylum, the Hebrew Orphan Asylum, the Home for Destitute Children, the Hospital for Crippled Children, and the Laura Franklin Hospital for Children. In 1913 the Van-Leuven Brown Hospital School for Crippled Boys and Girls of Detroit provided a camp which included a Boy Scout Troop of crippled boys and a Camp Fire group of crippled girls. The camp was located at Port Huron, MI, and included aquatics in the program.

In 1917 the American National Red Cross provided recreation services to ill and convalescent soldiers in hospitals and convalescent homes; the PAA created the War Camp Community Service program which included service to ill and convalescent soldiers.

In 1919 Delphone Dodge Ashbaugh was appointed Chair of the State Committee for the Michigan State Industrial Home for Girls. Mrs. Ashbaugh, who had served on the Detroit Recreation Commission, arranged employment of Beatrice Hunzicker, another Commission worker, to start a recreation program for the 400 girls at the home.

Major articles which appeared during the decade in *The Playground* included three articles which were published under the theme, "Play in Institutions: No Child Needs Play More Than the Child in an Institution." Other literature of this period is listed in the Appendix.

1920s

The Russell Sage Foundation performed a critical role in the founding and initial development of the Playground Association of America. The Foundation also provided technical and financial support to the PAA. The Foundation's Recreation Department was directed by Lee F. Hanmer, who also served as the first Field Secretary of the PAA. Play in institutions was among the concerns of the Russell Sage Foundation (Glenn, Brandt, & Andrews, 1947, Vol. 1, p. 350; Vol. 2, pp. 351-746).

From 1921 to 1926 the Russell Sage Foundation employed Robert K. Atkinson to carry out the following activities: to survey children's and adults' play and recreation programs in hospitals for mentally ill, reformatories, and other institutions; to conduct field service to 50 institutions, including the organization of demonstration programs; and to provide training institutes for institutional representatives of 125 institutions. He also provided training on recreation and physical education for "mental patients" and "subnormal children" at the Summer Institute for Institution Workers in Philadelphia, the New York Summer School of Physical Education held by New York State Department of Education at the Normal School in Cortland, and an extension course for workers at Kings Park and Central Islip State Hospitals.

The Russell Sage Foundation Recreation Department provided salary and staff support from 1921 to 1923 for Willem van der Wall, who conducted a series of studies and demonstrations in music at correctional institutions and institutions for the mentally ill. The work was performed under the auspices of the Committee for the Study of Music in Institutions for which Hanmer served as secretary. From 1923 to 1925 van der Wall released a series of reports on music in correctional institutions, music therapeutics in mental hospitals, psychotherpeutic value of music, and a systematic music program for mental hospitals. These led to the publication by the Russell Sage Foundation in 1936 of the 457-page *Music in Institutions,* the first "systematic presentation of aims, methods and cautions to be observed in the field of music in welfare work."

The Lincoln (IL) State School and Colony "Experiment" in forming a Department of Recreation and in its expanded recreation program was initiated in 1929. It led to the report in 1932 by Bertha Schlotter and

Margaret Svendsen entitled "An Experiment in Recreation with Mentally Retarded." The gains in theory and practice during this period are evident in the literature that appeared during the 1920s (see the Appendix).

1930s

The US Veterans Administration was created in 1930 with Recreational Therapy as one of the services provided. The PAA was now called the Playground and Recreation Association of America, and employed Erna K. Bunke in 1930 as Field Secretary for Play in Institutions with the PRAA Field Service. Bunke served thousands of recreation workers and hundreds of institutions through the training, consultation, demonstration, and technical assistance she provided. She held the Field Secretary position until 1935 when she was replaced by Jeanne H. Barnes, who served with similar energy. When Barnes joined the American National Red Cross in 1942 as part of the Red Cross's expansion of its World War II service, the Field Secretary position was not filled but the area was served by other staff and services of what had now become the National Recreation Association (changed from PRAA). The play in institutions area went without staffing until 1953 when Beatrice H. Hill was appointed Director of the NRA Consulting Service on Recreation for the Ill and Handicapped. She served in this capacity until 1960 when she founded Comeback, Inc., and was replaced by Morton Thompson, who served as director until 1965. After formation of the National Therapeutic Recreation Society interest area branch of the National Recreation and Park Association, Inc. (new name of the NRA), the following persons on the NRPA staff served successively for the disabled and disadvantaged program: Ira Hutchison, David C. Park, and Yvonne Washinton. The position included service as secretary for the NTRS (Nesbitt, 1982).

Community or special recreation programs that developed during the 1930s included the Recreation Center for the Adult Physically Handicapped in New York City (1935) which was directed by S.S. Lifson. In 1937 the Recreation Department of Akron, OH, provided a recreation service to shut-in and homebound handicapped children. The program was supported cooperatively by the Akron Recreation Department and the Board of Education. Consult the Appendix for books and major reports published during this decade.

1940s

From 1941 to 1945 the recreation service of the American National Red Cross was expanded to 1,800 Red Cross recreation workers providing service to ill, convalescent, and disabled soldiers in World War II military hospitals and clinics. In 1945 the US Veterans Administration designated the Recreation Service as one of the functions of the US VA Hospital Special Services Division along with Canteen, Chaplaincy, Library, and Voluntary Services. The Joseph P. Kennedy, Jr., Foundation was created in 1946; ultimately the Foundation's Special Olympics, Let's Play to Grow, Arts Festival, training, research, and other branches would involve over one million participants and volunteers annually on a national and international basis and would have enormous influence on creating positive attitudes toward full community participation by persons who are mentally retarded.

Goodwill Industries of Dayton, OH, provided a recreation program for its clients. Local agencies assisting included the Dayton Recreation Department, YMCA, Public Library, and American Red Cross. The Jefferson County, KY, Play and Recreation Board provided a recreation service to children with cerebral palsy at four Louisville schools.

In 1949 the Hospital Recreation Section of the American Recreation Society was formed. Related subsequent organizational developments were the founding in 1952 of the National Association of Recreation Therapists and the formation of the Recreation Therapy Section of the Recreation Division of the American Association for Health, Physical Education, and Recreation. The books and articles listed in the appendix are suggestive of the material that was published during the 1940s.

1950s

The San Francisco Recreation Center for the Handicapped was founded in 1950 by Janet Pomeroy. Other developments during the decade include the following. The Boston Recreation Department initiated a summer recreation program for the mentally retarded called Pleasure Island which was expanded to a year-round recreation program. New York's *Herald Tribune* Fresh Air Fund Camp Hidden Valley offered a program of camping for the handicapped and nonhandicapped together, as an integrated program. The US President's Committee on Employment of the Handicapped and the Morris Morganstern Foundation conducted the first national arts program for artists who are handicapped. International Handicapped Net, Inc., was founded by handicapped amateur radio operators; membership would grow to 2,500. Handi-cap Horizons, Inc., of Indianapolis conducted its first tour to Chicago. In the years to follow, Handi-cap Horizons groups would visit Western Europe, the British Isles, the Middle East, and New Zealand.

One thousand full-time recreation workers were employed in the US Veterans Administration. The 52 Association, Inc., in New York was founded to provide a 41-acre Sports and Recreation Center for disabled veterans providing swimming, boating, skiing, bicycling, and wheelchair sports.

In 1953 the Council for the Advancement of Hospitals Recreation (CAHR) was formed and was composed of the ARS Hospital Recreation Section, the AAHPER Recreation Therapy Section, and the National Association of Recreation Therapists. In 1954 the Council adopted Basic Concepts of Hospital Recreation and in 1956 established National Voluntary Registration for Hospital Recreation Personnel. *Recreation for the Ill and Handicapped* was published in 1957 by the National Association of Recreation Therapists; the publication was succeeded in 1967 by the *Therapeutic Recreation Journal* published by the National Recreation and Park Association (NTRS branch). Other books and major guides of this period are given in the Appendix.

1960s

Major organizational developments during the decade included the founding in 1960 of Comeback, Inc., the first nonprofit national organization serving the recreation needs of disabled persons; the convergence of various individuals and groups in the formation of the National Therapeutic Recreation Society interest area "branch" within the National Recreation and Park Association, Inc., in 1966; and the dissolution of both the National Association of Recreation Therapists and Comeback, Inc.,

In 1960 the Detroit Metropolitan Activities Club was started with 100 physically handicapped members whose ages ranged from 18 to 72. The Hospital Recreation Section of the American Recreation Society published *Recreation in Treatment Centers* in 1962; subsequently it was published by the NTRS-NRPA under the title *Therapeutic Recreation Annual*.

The US Office of Vocational Rehabilitation initiated support of recreation for handicapped through grants for training of master's-level specialists in recreation for the ill and handicapped, issued some 25 grants for research and demonstration in recreation for handicapped and related projects, and supported the Information Center on Recreation for the Handicapped conducted by Southern Illinois University.

In 1967 the Physical Education and Recreation for Handicapped Children Section of the Mental Retardation Act Amendments provided for training, research, and the US Secretary of Health, Education, and Welfare National Advisory Committee on Physical Education and Recreation for Handicapped Children; the PER program was assigned to the US Office of Education, Bureau of Education for the Handicapped, for administration. Subsequently, during the 1969-81 period, some 50 colleges, universities, youth agencies, rehabilitation services, etc., received grants for training, research, and special projects which totaled as much as $3 million per year.

The Appendix will acquaint you with books published during the decade.

1970s

Since the 1950s and 1960s increasing emphasis had been on community settlement of people who were emotionally impaired and mentally retarded—in contrast to the earlier practice of institutionalization. There was an increase in the community settlement orientation of recreation service in institutions and an expansion of recreation services for special populations by community parks, recreation, and arts. Section 504, the Civil Rights Act for the Handicapped, resulted in the creation of physical accessibility to many recreation areas and buildings. Recreation service was included in the Education for Handicapped Act and Regulation, opening up recreational opportunities for many handicapped children and youth attending regular schools. In 1977 the disabled consumer oriented White House Conference for Handicapped Individuals gave major attention to recreation, arts, sports, and leisure in the lives of disabled.

During the 1970s the National Therapeutic Recreation Society branch of the NRPA was active in working with national governmental and nongovernmental organizations to advance guidelines and standards for training, personnel, and services. The inservice training vehicle of regional conferences was initiated in the Midwest Symposiums on Therapeutic Recreation and, under the auspices of the NRPA, was expanded to other regions such as Mid-Atlantic and New England. The roster of professional membership in the NTRS-NRPA, Inc., was as high as 2,000 during the decade. Professional registration, initiated by the Council for the Advancement of Hospital Recreation in 1956, numbered 4,000 of which 2,000 were current.

The Physical Education and Recreation Service program of the US Special Education Program funded a series of grants for major curriculum development and program development projects. Working from the base created by the 1960 Comeback, Inc., Therapeutic Recreation Curriculum Conference, the program funded formal curriculum development conferences, field demonstration and evaluation of therapeutic recreation curricula at the 2-year, 4-year, master's and doctoral levels as well as career education for handicapped in recreation service. These were conducted by universities such as Temple University, University of Illinois, University of Kentucky, and University of Maryland. The Special Education PER Program also made grants for program development and training to agencies such as the American Camping Association, the American Foundation for the Blind, the Boy Scouts of America, and the YMCA of the USA. Grants also were made to conduct training in community or special recreation for disabled persons to schools such as Indiana University and the University of Iowa as well as to the state of New Jersey.

Organizational development included the formation of the International Federation for Adapted Physical Activity in 1973, the establishment of the National Consortium on Physical Education and Recreation for Handicapped, Inc., in 1975, and the founding of Special Recreation, Inc., in 1978. A series of books on recreation for disadvantaged and therapeutic recreation was published during the 1970s and examples are listed in the Appendix.

1980s

International activity in recreation for the handicapped received attention starting in the early 1980s. Rehabilitation International sponsored a seminar on recreation for the handicapped at its 14th World Congress and created a Commission on Sports, Recreation, and Leisure. Special Recreation, Inc., established an International Center on Special Recreation. The International Council on Health, Physical Education, and Recreation expanded recreation for the handicapped activities and sponsored an international seminar on special recreation at its 24th World Congress in the Philippines.

The Vocational Rehabilitation and Independent Living Rehabilitation Act administered by the US Rehabilitation Services Administration provided $3 million for demonstration of special recreation projects for disabled persons. Project MAY—Mainstreaming Activities for Youth—was initiated as a cooperative undertaking by national youth service agencies such as YMCA, YWCA, Boy Scouts, Girl Scouts, 4-H, Boys Clubs, and Jewish Settlements, among others, reflecting the society-wide effort to bring disabled Americans into the mainstream of American life.

General Problems and Needs

Some general pervasive problems and needs in recreation for disabled persons should be addressed (Nesbitt, 1978). Six of these are described below.

Negative Attitudes

Negative attitudes are pervasive. The general public as well as helping professionals harbor negative attitudes which preclude equal opportunity in recreation for disabled persons. *Action:* Need continues for national and international programs such as the United Nations International Year for Disabled Persons. All persons concerned about the disabled must put "creating positive attitudes" as a priority item on their work agendas.

Serving the Unserved and Underserved

During the 1970s it was estimated that only 10% of the disabled population was receiving recreation services; 90% were without it. The pattern has been to focus reports, evaluations, planning, and public demonstrations, for example, on those who are served rather than on disabled persons who are *not* served. *Action:* We need to go outside the existing institutions and outside the existing programs to reach the unserved and underserved by providing recreation service to disabled persons, children, youth, adults, and seniors.

Program Initiation, Expansion, and Improvement

Over the last 20 years many important programs have been started in sports, arts, and recreation for the disabled, but in every instance, in terms of age levels and category of disability only limited proportions of particular age levels or particular disability groups are being served. *Action:* We need to initiate new recreation programs and services for disabled persons. We should also improve many current programs and services in terms of increased inservice training of professionals and volunteers, increased facilities, better accessability, increased transportation services, and so on. Finally, we need to expand existing services to provide for greater participation.

Low Priority for Recreation for Disabled

Historically, recreation has experienced low priority among medical and rehabilitation services because those groups wanted recreation services to do the job. Public park and recreation services have given disabled persons a low priority based on the intention of serving the largest number at the least cost and the presumption that medically oriented services should serve disabled persons. *Action:* Both medical services and recreation services need to give appropriate priority to providing recreation for the disabled.

Advocacy for Recreation for Disabled

Historically very few individuals — disabled consumers, family, and professionals — have advocated the recreation needs of disabled persons at the local, state, national, or international levels. *Action:* Individuals, organizations and groups need to advocate the recreation needs of disabled persons at the local, state, national, and international levels.

International Cooperation and Technical Assistance

International activity in rehabilitation of the disabled has been significant, but recreation for the disabled has been a very small part of this activity. International cooperation and technical assistance in recreation has been limited, providing little opportunity for recreation for disabled persons' cooperation or technical assistance. *Action:* We need significant development in international recreation for disabled cooperation and technical assistance which can be fostered through individual support of organizations such as the International Federation for Adapted Physical Activity, the International Council for Health, Physical Education, and Recreation, Rehabilitation International, the World Leisure and Recreation Association, and the International Center on Special Recreation sponsored by Special Recreation, Inc.

The International Dimension

The American play and recreation movement is indebted to internationalism. Henry S. Curtis reported in 1916 "If we ask ourselves whence this movement and why it has developed as it has, the sources and reasons are fairly evident. The play movement in this country apparently owes its beginnings to an inspiration from Germany." (pp. 6-7)

The international organization with the oldest program service in special recreation for the disabled is the World Bureau of the Boy Scouts. The World Association of Girl Guides also includes disabled children in its program.

National programs that have provided technical assistance internationally bear mention. Starting in the 1950s, England's Stoke Mandeville Hospital program in sports for disabled, directed by Sir Ludwin Guttman, now deceased, conducted a program of technical assistance that facilitated major advances in sports for disabled persons throughout the world. In the 1960s Comeback, Inc., under the direction of Beatrice H. Hill, worked with Rehabilitation International and the World Rehabilitation Fund in disseminating to 60 nations the concept of recreation as an integral part of total rehabilitation.

The organized American recreation movement supported the establishment of the World Leisure and Recreation Association which in the 1950s sponsored the publication of a pamphlet on hospital recreation. The pamphlet was distributed internationally.

Since the mid-1970s the International Council for Health, Physical Education, and Recreation has sponsored an interest area in recreation for the handicapped including educational sessions at international conferences on handicap recreation. ICHPER urged UNESCO to include equal opportunity for disabled persons in the UNESCO Charter of Sport and Physical Education. ICHPER activity was highlighted by the sponsorship of a 2-day International Seminar on Special Recreation at ICHPER's 24th World Congress in Manila during July 1981 (Nesbitt, 1980).

The International Federation on Adapted Physical Activity, through its publications and Third Symposium, is a significant development and all possible encouragement and support should be provided to this organization through individual membership, purchase of its publications, and participation in its meetings. Over the span of 75 years international attention to special recreation for disabled persons has been limited. But the activity is increasing. Rehabilitation International in 1980 created a Commission on Sport, Recreation, and Leisure as a fifth program area along with the medical, social, educational, and vocational· rehabilitation program areas.

In 1980 Special Recreation, Inc., established an International Center on Special Recreation, which has: provided technical information and public education materials to organizations in 75 countries; published an international model directory on recreation for disabled persons; sponsored a series of papers; and recommended to various international organizations such as UNESCO how they might enhance the development of special recreation for disabled persons worldwide.

Although some activity exists at the international level in special recreation for disabled persons, this report should not create the impression that the activity level is adequate. The activity is not adequate. A review of the international exchange, cooperation, and technical assistance that has taken place in other fields such as rehabilitation medicine, social work, rehabilitation counseling, occupational therapy, physical therapy, and so on demonstrates just how limited international activity has been in recreation for disabled persons during post-World War II to 1981.

Because of the importance of international exchange to the creation of the play and recreation movement in the United States, it behooves American professionals to consider means to pass on to other nations what has been learned since 1906 and to continue to learn from them as well. These are the benefits of international exchange. One way of effecting international exchange immediately in special recreation, that is, sharing what one country has learned and observing their programs, would be for organizations at the appropriate level to award to each outgoing national branch or affiliate president, to each outgoing state president, and to each outgoing therapeutic or recreation section chair a foreign trip with all expenses paid. Each traveling officer could write an article providing one means of sharing experiences, new insights, and new convictions that were gained. International programs and projects would flow from this travel experience by leaders. What better way to refill the international exchange reservoir that brought the play movement to the United States?

We live in a world made very small by technology—a world also made very dangerous by technology. The real solution to the problems caused by a world made very small and very dangerous is for all nations and all people to live harmoniously in a spirit of international peace and goodwill. Modern professionals such as physical educators and recreation workers can render a small part of the international reconciliation and understanding that is necessary to create good relations worldwide.

References

CURTIS, H. *The practical conduct of play*. New York: MacMillan, 1916.

GLENN, J., Brandt, L., & Andrews, F. *Russell Sage Foundation* (Vols. 1 & 2). New York: Russell Sage Foundation, 1947.

NATIONAL Recreation Association. *Recreation 1930-39*. (Formerly the Playground and Recreation Association of America.)

NATIONAL Recreation Association. *Recreation and Parks and Recreation, 1960-69*. (Formerly National Park and Recreation.)

NESBITT, J. *National Institute on Special Recreation*. Iowa City: University of Iowa Recreation Education Program, 1978. (Available through ERIC.)

NESBITT, J. Special recreation for disabled persons gains acceptance in world rehabilitation movement. *Special Recreation Advocate,* 1980, **3**, 49 pp.

NESBITT, J. *Pioneers in special recreation*. Iowa City: Larc Press, 1982.

PLAYGROUND Association of America. *The Playground, 1910 to 1920*. (The association's name was later changed to Playground and Recreation Association of America.)

SCHLOTER, B., & Svendsen, M. *An experiment in recreation with the mentally retarded*. Illinois: State Department of Welfare, 1932. (Rev. 1951; rep. 1956.)

Appendix

This section lists literature from each period chronologically. Works cited in the text are given in the reference section which follows.

1906-09

1908 Playground Association of America. Report of the Committee on Play in Institutions. *Proceedings of the Second Annual Playground Congress and Yearbook, 1908.*

1908 Playground Association of America. Session on play in institutions, H.H. Hart, M.D., Chairman, Tentative report of the Committee (on Play in Institutions), discussion by F.H. Nibecker, discussion by Mrs. C.F. Weller. *Yearbook of the Playground Association of America, 1908-09.*

1908 Playground Association of America. Syllabus Five, Section X. Playgrounds for institutions. *A normal course in play for professional directors from the tentative report of the Committee on Play of the Playground Association of America, 1908.*

1909 Raymond Campbell of New Orleans, the one legged boy who has a record 4'-4½" in the high jump, and 7'-2" in the standing broad jump. *The Playground,* 1909. (The article stated, "Mr. Lombard, the director in charge of athletics reports that Master Campbell has become a leader among the boys, and exerts a splendid influence over them for fair play and gentlemanly conduct in the games.")

1910s

1911 Reeder, R.R. Play in institutions. *The Playground.*

1911 Burritt, O.H. Recreation in a school for the blind (Overbrook). *The Playground.*

1913 Beers, C. The need and value of play, recreation and diversional occupations among the insane. *The Playground.*

1915 Curtis, H.S. Play for institutions, orphan asylums. *The Playground.*

1916 Gulick. L.H. The need of play in institutions. *The Playground.*

1916 Hall, H.J., & Buck, M.M.C. *Handicrafts for the handicapped.*

1916 Wrightson, H.A. *Games and exercises for mental defective.*

1917 Miller, S., Jr. Recreation and prison reform. *The Playground.*

1917 Van-Leuven Hospital for Crippled Children. Recreation for crippled children. *The Playground.*

1919 Boyd, N.L. *Hospital and bedside games.*

1920s

1920 Brush, F.L. *Recreational therapy in convalescence and allied subnormal health conditions.*

1922 Atkinson, R.K. Recreation activities in institutions. *National Conference of Social Work proceedings.*

1923 Children's play in hospitals. *The Playground.*

1923 Atkinson, R.K. *Play for children in institutions.* Russell Sage Foundation.

1924 Atkinson, R.K. Reformative value of recreation. *Schools for adults in prisons.* US Bureau of Education.

1925 Van der Wall, W., Johnstone, E.R., Wannamaker, C., Moodie, E.S., & Arne, R.E. Recreation for the unadjusted; papers. *The Playground.*

1925 Dodds, S. *Work-and-play treatment at Longcliff* (Logansport, IN, State Hospital).

1925 Johnstone, E.R. Recreation for the feeble-minded. *American Physical Education Review.*
1925 Pangburn, W. A health clinic that prescribes recreation. *The Playground.*
1925 Moodie, E.S. Physical education at New Jersey State Hospital at Morris Plains, N.J. (mentally ill). *American Physical Education Review.*
1926 Whitten, M.S., and Whitten, H. *Pastimes for sick children.*
1927 Speakman, M.T. *Recreation for blind children.* US Children's Bureau, Bureau of Publication.

1930s

1934 Rathbone, J.L. *Corrective physical education.*
1936 Trowbridge, C.R. *Feeling better? Amusements and occupations for convalescents.*
1936 Davis, J.E. *Principles and practices of recreational therapy.*
1936 Van der Wall, W. *Music in institutions.*
1938 Davis, J.E. *Play and mental health: Principles and practices for teachers.*
1939 Rogerson, C.H. *Play therapy in childhood.*
1939 Stafford, G.T. *Sports for the handicapped.*

1940s

1942 Menninger, K.A. Recreation and morale. *Bulletin of the Menninger Clinic.*
1943 Davis, J.E. Recreation as an aid to community life of the mental hospital. *Occupational Therapy and Rehabilitation.*
1944 Schulack, N.R. Occupational-recreational programs in neuropsychiatric sections of army station hospitals. *War Medicine.*
1944 Andriola, J.P. Release of aggression through play therapy for ten year old patients. *Psychoanalytic Review.*
1945 Ickes, M. *Pastimes for the patient.*
1947 Axline, V.M. *Play therapy, the inner dynamic of childhood.*
1949 American Theater Wing. *Recreation is fun: A handbook on hospital recreation and entertainment.*

1950s

1950 Jackson, L., & Todd, K.M. *Child treatment and therapy of play.*
1952 Davis, J.W. *Clinical application of recreational therapy.*
1952 Hill, B.H. *Starting a recreation program in civilian hospital.*
1953 Williams, A. *Recreation for the aging.*
1954 Girl Scouts of America. *Working with the handicapped.*
1955 American National Red Cross. *Swimming for the handicapped.*

1955 Hunt, V.V. *Recreation for the handicapped.*
1957 Boy Scouts of America. *Scouting with handicapped boys.*
1959 Rathbone, J.L., & Lucas, C. *Recreation in total rehabilitation.*

1960s

1960 Chapman, F.M. *Recreation activities for the handicapped.*
1961 Carlson, B.W., & Gingland, D.R. *Play activities for the retarded child.*
1962 Lucas, C. *Recreation activity development for the aging in homes, hospitals and nursing homes.*
1964 Pomeroy, J. *Recreation for the physically handicapped.*
1965 Robbins, F., & Robbins, J. *Educational rhythmics for mentally handicapped children.*
1965 Gingland, D.R., & Stiles, W.E. *Music activities for retarded children.*
1966 Case, M. *Recreation for blind adults.*
1967 Merrill, T. *Activities for the aged and infirm. A handbook for the untrained worker.*
1968 Carlson, B.W., & Gingland, D.R. *Recreation for retarded teenagers and young adults.*

1970s

1970 Nesbitt, J., Brown, P., & Murphy, J. *Recreation and leisure service for the disadvantaged.*
1972 Frye, V., & Peters, M. *Therapeutic recreation: Its theory, philosophy and practice.*
1973 Kraus, R.G. *Therapeutic recreation service: Principles and practices.*
1973 Stein, T., & Sessoms, D. *Recreation and special populations.*
1974 Avedon, E.M. *Therapeutic recreation service: An applied behavioral science approach.*
1974 Overs, R.P., O'Connor, E., & Demarco, B. *Avocational activities for the handicapped: A handbook for avocational counseling.*
1974 Shivers, J., & Fait, H. *Therapeutic and adapted recreation service.*
1976 O'Morrow, G. *Therapeutic recreation: A helping profession.*
1978 Gunn, S., & Peterson, C. *Therapeutic recreation program design.*
1978 Nesbitt, J.A. *New concepts and new processes in special recreation.*

Recreation Unlimited: Responding to Persons with Severe Disabilities

Janet Pomeroy
Recreation Center for Handicapped, Inc.

Persons with disabilities have always been among us, but until recent years, we as a society have not been very aware of them. Many of them lived in institutions, out of our sight. Those who lived with their families usually stayed at home and were known only to their immediate neighbors. Any recreation they did enjoy was provided by their families or by the institutions. Some who were mildly disabled and who could "keep up" could be found in community recreation programs, although they were seldom identified as disabled.

Today all of this has changed. Disabled individuals are no longer being sent to institutions and those formerly institutionalized are being returned to their communities. Their needs, including the need for recreation, are now the responsibility of their communities.

The experience of the Recreation Center for the Handicapped, Inc., in San Francisco, CA, has exploded many myths concerning persons with disabilities and has demonstrated that programming for them is limited only by the imagination and convictions of the recreation providers.

Early History

In 1950, as a volunteer worker in a school for severely disabled children, I saw the need for a recreation program. I was greatly inspired to develop a program myself when I saw these children sitting idle at lunch and recess periods with no one to help them. Most had never been to park playgrounds or recreation centers, and no community recreation programs would include severely disabled youngsters.

With no funds, but a large amount of determination, I started a program of my own. When I saw the tremendous improvement in these children through participation in enjoyable activities, I was greatly encouraged and gratified, and decided this would be my career. I saw children improve in their speech so that they could be in a play; great improvement in physical coordination and mobilization was common. Children who could not use their hands learned to paint, sketch, and work in pottery with their toes. I discovered that recreation activities of all types could serve as a stimulus for these children for greater learning, improved mental and physical health, and for greater self-realization and social development.

From seeing this, I began to realize the tremendous role that recreation can play in developing a child's potential. With my limited knowledge of severe disabilities, then, and my lack of professional training and experience at that time, I believed strongly that these persons had a right to participate in recreational activities the same as all children, and that programs should be *provided by the community—in the community*. I entered Junior College and continued my volunteer work with the goal of earning a degree in recreation.

The Beginning

While I was a sophomore in college, a foundation heard of the program I had started at the school and offered a small grant-in-aid to expand the concept of community recreation for the disabled. I then approached the San Francisco Recreation and Park Department for a facility. Eventually, we were given one room in a large, old building that formerly had been used as a restaurant and had been sitting empty for 12 years. We started with six teens and young adults, 3 days each week, using volunteers for staff. The building, heat, gas, and lighting were given to us for $1 per year.

Within 3 months, 45 children and adults were enrolled, with many more requests to participate in the program. The grant expired after 2 years, but the apparent need to continue was so great that it was decided to incorporate, form a Board of Directors, and attempt to gain support from the community.

Development of Community Support

For 12 years, the Center was supported through voluntary contributions raised by the staff and Board of Directors. These funds were raised primarily from various service clubs, men and women's fraternal associations, and fund-raising events such as rummage sales, fashion shows, teas, luncheons, horse shows, and letter appeals. Eventually, through a community study of needs assessment of disabled individuals involving local health and human services agencies, and some political support from state legislators, the Recreation and Park Department agreed to contract services from the Center for serving severely disabled people.

Philosophy of the Center

Since its inception, the basic philosophy of the Center has remained consistent. That is, that recreation for all persons is a need and a right; that as citizens and taxpayers, persons with disabilities are entitled to their share of community-based (year-round) recreation opportunities (not just summer camping). They are also entitled to participate in all aspects of community life and to have identical privileges and responsibilities. Disabled individuals are more *like* others than different from them with the same basic needs, interests, and desires. They have a right to select and share in the planning and evaluation of their own recreation programs. Even for the severely disabled, and insofar as possible, there should be an atmosphere of freedom—freedom of choice, freedom to express oneself in spite of severe limitations. Recreation is viewed as a developmental mode, a vehicle to assist people with disabilities to reach their potentials.

In conducting community-based recreation programs for all ages and types of disabled individuals and groups, the Center has continued to operate by the basic philosophy standards and principles of general community recreation which are: personal fulfillments; democratic human relations; leisure skills and interests; health and fitness; creative expression and esthetic appreciation. Specific objectives are based on interests, desires, and needs of individual participants, which will help them to progress toward greater degrees of intellectual advancement. In addition, leaders take into account the lack of previous opportunities for social relationships and for recreation programs in general. Programs conducted in the least restrictive environment have always had a major goal of preparing disabled people for eventual integration into total community life.

Growth and Development of the Center

Through the experiences of the Center we have discovered a key to unlocking the potentials of disabled individuals and have shown the community the ability side of its disabled citizens. The Center has demonstrated that the range of programming opportunities is limited only by the creativity and resourcefulness of recreation staff who serve them.

Holding consistently to the philosophy previously mentioned, the Center has received sufficient community support to keep pace with the growing demands for service. The program has evolved from the staff's direct experience in working with the disabled participants. *In effect, the disabled themselves have been the teachers by expressing and demonstrating their needs and potentials.* With a basic background in recreation, the staff has needed only to be interested, alert, and flexible to work with disabled participants and to have a perception of their individual differences and abilities. Moreover, the Center's willingness to provide the essential support services required to meet the needs of individuals with severe disabilities is a most significant factor.

During the almost 30 years of providing recreation services to disabled people, the Center has become keenly aware of one important difference between the needs of most of the severely disabled and those of nondisabled individuals, a difference that has strongly influenced the direction that programming has taken. Some disabled children and teens attend school, but many do not. A few disabled adults attend workshops, but the vast majority have been judged to lack the feasibility for work training or job experience. Their days are filled with emptiness and recreation has been seen as the only possible outlet for their energies. Parents, social agencies, and the disabled themselves are increasingly turning to recreation programs, either as a point of entry for disabled people into the community service system, or for fulfillment of their full range of social, emotional, physical, and intellectual needs.

Needs Influencing the Direction of the Program

As the Center's experience in meeting the recreational needs of disabled people grew, so, too, did an acute awareness of the other unmet needs of disabled people. As needs were identified, services were expanded to fulfill them. As each new service was added, the need for additional support services was apparent. Several examples of this phenomenon are highlighted below.

Transportation

It was first necessary to solve the practical problem of making the program accessible to all individuals, including the bedfast and multidisabled. While the Center originally started its program with taxi-cab service and volunteer drivers, it soon became apparent that a more economical and permanent type of transportation would have to be provided for those initially enrolled, and to serve the many other individuals already on a long waiting list.

Specially equipped buses, maxi-vans, and station wagons were added over a period of 30 years, donated by various groups and individuals. Vehicles are painted white and bear the Center's name and address, the Center logo, and the donor's name; they have created a great deal of publicity and community awareness for the Center and have become symbolic of services to the disabled. Because of the Center's expertise in the provision of specialized transportation, many San Francisco community agencies serving the disabled have requested that the Center provide transportation services for their constituents. At present, the Center is providing transportation for nine other agencies on a contractual basis including day care centers, schools, rehabilitation workshops, senior centers, and others.

Social Services

As the provision of transportation and open eligibility made the program easily accessible and available, it soon became apparent that there were large gaps in other services for these persons at the community level. These observations led to the inclusion of social services as a necessary part of the program offered. Two social workers have now been employed to serve as liaison between the Center and the community agencies and to provide case-work services to Center participants and their families. This includes intake procedures, home visits, information and referrals, coordination with Center program staff, and evaluations. Disabled participants and their families are helped to find the nonrecreational services they need, and, in turn, the social agencies have provided specialized services to the Center such as case conferences, screening, and case management of Center participants, as needed.

Day Care

The Day Care program was established when the Medical Director of the Child Development Center at Children's Hospital in San Francisco identified 200 children not accepted in schools because they were too severely disabled, and had not acquired self-help skills. Many had been placed on long lists for admission into already overcrowded state institutions. Parents faced with the 24-hour-a-day care of such children were desperate for some type of service. When the problem came to the Center's attention, it was decided to explore possibilities of starting a program for these children. A series of meetings was held with the Medical Director of the hospital and parents, and ultimately it was decided that the Center would undertake the program as a pilot project. Parents agreed to pay a nominal fee which would help toward the cost of transportation. Because of the limited funds, staff and transportation, only 12 children were enrolled 3 days each week. However, there were so many requests for admission that the Center ultimately expanded the program to 6 days each week.

In addition to mental retardation, many of these children were severely handicapped and emotionally disturbed. Some were cerebral palsied with visual handicaps; some were partially sighted, and others were totally blind. Other handicaps, combined with mental retardation, included: deaf and hard of hearing, epilepsy, brain tumors, Down's syndrome, emotionally disturbed, neurologically handicapped, microcephaly and multiple congenital hyperactivity, short attention span, distractibility, and sensitivity to noises. Many were in wheelchairs, some were on crutches, and a large number were confined to their cribs or beds. Most of these children required custodial care, such as toileting and feeding.

Community support for the program was obtained through television stories describing the need for the program and through special fund-raising events. Some financial support was obtained through the State Department of Social Services. Later, financial assistance was given by the San Francisco Recreation and Park Department. Many volunteers responded to the Center's request for help in working with the children and others donated equipment and supplies such as cribs, clothing, and food.

Over a period of 17 years, approximately 1,500 multidisabled children have been enrolled. Over half of these children, originally diagnosed as persons who would never be eligible for school programs, improved sufficiently in physical, social, emotional and self-help skills, and general maturation to be accepted in city schools for the disabled or in special classes in regular schools. In dramatic instances, some were accepted in regular classes in regular schools. With the passage of federal legislation, the Education of All Handicapped Children's Act (PL 94-142) which guarantees all disabled children access to a free, appropriate education, the focus of the Day Care program has changed from children to adults.

Nutrition

Because many of the families with disabled children or adults were in lower income brackets, the need for nutritional support became apparent. Hot breakfasts, lunches, and dinners were initiated when it was recognized that hunger or poor nutrition contributed to the erratic behavior of some of the children and adults, and depressed their ability to function effectively.

The food program created the need for a full-time chef and other staff for the daily preparation and serving of well-balanced meals. Now, as part of the nutritional program, cooking classes are held for children and adults, where they learn the fundamentals of cooking, basic nutrition, and grocery shopping. Such skills are essential if our participants are to realize their full potential and live independently in the community.

Deinstitutionalization of Disabled Individuals

The change in public policy leading to the closing of state institutions and returning disabled individuals into communities had a significant impact on the City of San Francisco and subsequently on the direction of the Center's program. Some 293 Board and Care group homes were established to accommodate the constantly increasing numbers of persons who were returning to the community from state institutions. This sudden influx created an urgent need for recreation and day activity programs for these persons. Hundreds were referred to the Center, and a long waiting list was soon accumulated. Although the Center was the only agency in the community that had the necessary space to expand its program, funds were needed for additional staff and transportation. Ultimately, the Community Mental Health Services responded to this need and agreed to purchase recreation services from the Center on a contractual basis through the state legislated Short-Doyle Act. Currently, the Center is serving approximately 1,000 *previously institutionalized* retarded and disabled young adults and seniors, but still has a long waiting list of persons in need of our services.

Outreach Programming

With continued growth in enrollment, the staff began to realize the need for a new facility, but also with the recognition that no building would ever be large enough, and that the expansion of some programs would have to be made by a more extensive use of community resources.

Satellite or outreach programming was the immediate solution to part of this problem. The concept for outreach grew out of an increasing need to serve severely disabled and mentally retarded persons who were confined to their homes on a permanent, long-term, or temporary basis.

The dynamic response to outreach programs was beyond all expectations and clearly showed the need for future expansion. Today, the Outreach programs serve over 900 individuals. The programs offer the following services:

- One-to-one visits for those who cannot leave their homes due to the severity of their disability, their inability to socially interact in a group, or their fear of going out.

- Small travel groups for physically disabled seniors, mobile severely retarded who are in transition to a group situation, and the mentally ill who live in Board and Care Homes.
- An infant stimulation program for developmentally delayed or severely disabled children from the day of birth until progress makes a day care placement possible.
- A group socialization program for seniors in 18 Housing Authority apartment complexes.
- Socialization and resocialization programs for the elderly in 17 small residential care homes.
- Four mainstreaming programs for disabled school children. These programs are made possible with the cooperation of the San Francisco Unified School District and the Municipal Recreation and Park Department. All programs are conducted after school; some are in recreation and park playground facilities, and others are at the school site. The primary purpose of these programs is to integrate the children into recreational activities with the nondisabled child.
- A pilot mainstreaming program for mentally ill/mentally retarded adults recently returned from state institutions. The primary purpose of the program is to teach self-help and independent living skills through socialization programs within a community setting.

Outreach programming points to a new direction in the search for ways to integrate and to expand services to large and small groups who can best — or only — be served in their neighborhoods and homes; and provides an excellent vehicle for mainstreaming the disabled with nondisabled. Such outreach programs also stimulate and maximize interagency cooperation in meeting the needs of disabled citizens in a community setting.

Design and Construction of New Facilities

While the Outreach program was expanding, three large, new buildings were being designed and constructed, not only to serve the participants more adequately but to allow for increasing enrollment. These new facilities, located in a heavily wooded 5½-acre site, are designed to meet the needs of severely disabled persons in the least restrictive environment. The main Recreation Center building is single story, with corridors and doorways wide enough to accommodate wheelchairs. The facility includes rooms designed for day care recreational activities, staff offices, and related facilities. A large swimming pool complex has a pool with a special ramp for wheelchairs and gurneys, designed so the water can be kept at a comfortable 80 to 90° for therapeutic swimming.

A newly constructed gymnasium has a large playing space vaulted by a skylight. Modular gymnastic apparatus has been assembled and special mats are available. Portable basketball units can be lowered or raised for the beginning player in wheelchairs. A physical fitness room provides muscle-building and stamina training.

The Day Camp is adjacent to the Center in a triangular plot of open space, surrounded by eucalyptus trees and native bushes; a nearby play area has swings, climbing equipment, and slides. The camp site has eight separate units for campers which are equipped with campfire circles, picnic tables, and barbecues. The site also has a wooden stage and a tent-enclosed table provides protection from wind for arts and crafts projects.

Summary of the Center's Response to Needs

The Center's program today represents a dynamic response to the needs of disabled persons. The Center is the primary provider of socialization programs for the adult mentally retarded who have spent many years in institutions, and is a major factor in their successful adjustment to community living. A Day Care program serves profoundly retarded, multi-disabled young adults who would otherwise vegetate in their homes or require hospitalization. A preschool program is provided for severely disabled infants and children ranging from 1 to 3 years of age. A wide range of recreation and leisure-time activities also are provided for children and teens enrolled in school, for school graduates, for physically disabled adults, and for senior citizens. In addition, a cooperative program with the San Francisco Community College District provides adult education instructors in specialized fields.

Through the Center's policy of designing programs to meet the demonstrated needs of the disabled, the components of the current range of programming have developed naturally. Recreation activities are selected and structured in the Day Care program to promote the developmental needs of the adults through recreation and social interaction. In the other programs, recreation activities are designed to supplement and reinforce other life experiences of the participants. These programs inevitably are broad and varied because the life experiences of most of our participants have been extremely limited due to the multiplicity and severity of their disabilities.

The educational component is not the traditional academic model, but a purposeful technique for structuring activities to help participants gain the basic social, physical, and intellectual skills that are necessary if they are to gain maximal benefits from recreation and leisure-time pursuits. Although nutrition itself may not be considered recreation, meal times, barbecues, picnics, etc., provide an invaluable social experience for the participants and contribute to their overall well-being.

The recreation agency is frequently the first, and often the only agency, with which retarded and disabled people become involved. They bring with them a variety of problems and needs that are not the responsibility of recreation. However, recreation personnel can work closely with social agencies in helping participants and their families to find the services they need. In turn, these agencies can provide valuable consultation services to the recreation staff, to the mutual benefit of the disabled.

Future Plans to Respond to Trends—Projected Expansion of Programs for the Elderly

National statistics show that the adult population is increasing very rapidly and it is estimated that by the year 2010, there will be 40 million elderly people in the United States. The current and future needs for this population, as outlined by the Administration on Aging, will be the establishment of multipurpose centers that will provide, through a comprehensive and coordinated system, for social services, nutrition, transportation, outreach information and referral, homemaker services, and others.

These needs can only be fulfilled through cooperation among all community agencies and organizations in advocacy, identification, political involvement, coordination of services, and the provision of recreation and socialization programs.

In order to continue to meet these needs, the Center has developed a 20-year plan, part of which calls for the construction of a day care multipurpose center for the aging. The program will emphasize socialization activities which will develop self-help skills, improve physical functioning, enhance self-esteem, and promote new interests. Activities will include physical fitness, swimming, gymnastics, cooking, cultural arts and hobbies, music, dance, parties, and excursions into the community.

Expansion of Services for the Mentally Ill and Mentally Retarded

The mentally ill/mentally retarded is a growing population due to better assessment and identification, and because of patients' release from state institutions. A recent State of California survey indicates that some 240 mentally ill/mentally retarded are ready to return to the San Francisco community to live in board and care homes, provided they can be assured of recreation and socialization programs that will include them 5 days each week.

The Center plans to construct a day care facility for the mentally ill/mentally retarded where they will have access to the swimming pool, gymnasium, and programs for socialization and nutrition at the Center. Here, they will be taught the basics of self-help and independent living skills such as cooking, personal grooming, adult education as needed, and socialization skills. Leisure education related skills will also be an integral part of the program to facilitate the participants' independent leisure functioning.

Continued Mainstreaming of Severely Disabled Children and Adults

One of the primary goals of the Center has been that of (mainstreaming) integration of the severely disabled into community-based programs with the nondisabled citizen. This has required a specially designed program of education, training of staff, and shared resources to provide a continuum of services to the disabled population.

Because the Center has facilities such as the swimming pool, gymnasium, and a large recreation center building, the staff has encouraged "reverse mainstreaming" of the nondisabled population. For example, parents of nondisabled children and parents of disabled children are taught how to swim and how to teach their children to swim. These programs are conducted several times each week for groups of disabled and nondisabled children and parents. In addition, a "Kindergym" program for disabled and nondisabled children is conducted in the gymnasium on a weekly basis. This is also a parent-participation program in which children learn gross motor and social skills as they explore their environment, meet new friends, and enjoy diverse, colorful play equipment.

Future Funding

Although there has been widespread discussion at top administrative levels of massive budget-cutting across the whole spectrum of government programs we hope that the Center will be able to continue its "public-private" partnership approach which has been very successful. This concept is one whereby federal funds can be used to purchase recreation, day care, and social rehabilitation services from public and private agencies on a contractual basis. In California, this type of financing for children and adults is subsidized through a contractual arrangement with city and county Social Services Departments, which administer the federal funds. The Center holds four contracts that are covered by federal funds. One contract provides 75% federal funds and requires 25% local matching funds. The San Francisco Recreation and Park Department provides the 25% matching funds, which generates $3 for every $1 required from local sources.

The Center will continue to raise a large portion of its budget through private resources from a large group of donors who assist the Center financially. These include foundations, men and women's fraternal associations, service clubs, the Parents' Auxiliary, and individuals. Recently, corporations in San Francisco have come together to determine how they can help nonprofit agencies if the government cuts back on support of social programs. Some corporations, such as Levi Strauss, have organized "Community Involvement Teams" composed of employees interested in developing creative ways of raising funds for nonprofit agencies. This team currently is exploring ways and means of raising funds for the Center.

One creative approach that is being used by both public and private agencies is called marketing. This method involves selling one specific aspect of the program, such as "adopt a park" or "adopt an animal in the zoo," and in the case of the Center, "mainstreaming severely disabled school children with nondisabled children in recreation programs in the community."

Experiences of the Center have shown that providing adequate funding must be a continual process. Diversification seems to be the key. The process includes education of the public advocacy at local, state, and national levels, working with the legislative process, lobbying at various governmental levels, and developing expertise in grantsmanship.

Need for Education and Training of Persons in Recreation in Developing Countries

Through its 30 years of service, the Center is recognized nationally and internationally as a pioneer and a model in developing recreation, education, socialization, and health care programs for the severely disabled of all races and creeds. It has shared its expertise nationally and internationally through lectures, workshops, conferences, seminars, and films, and through voluminous written materials.

Because the Center is partially supported through federal funds, governmental agencies at all levels are aware of its programs and use its facilities as a resource for information and referrals. As a result, individuals and groups from around the world visit the Center almost daily. On a yearly basis, a minimum of 25 college and university students spend a semester at the Center in an intensive internship which is required for their undergraduate or graduate degrees.

As a result of the national significance of the Center's program, demand on the Center for use as a training laboratory has grown beyond all expectations. In order to meet these demands, the Center is planning to build an educational training and conference facility with dormitories for semester or weekend housing for students, recreators, educators, and others. In the past, many students from various parts of the United States and abroad have made inquiries about training and education at the Center, but have found that the cost of motels and hotels was prohibitive and they were therefore unable to pursue training opportunities.

The recreation profession greatly needs individuals from a variety of ethnic backgrounds to better serve the total needs of the community. The availability of education and training at the conference site would encourage these individuals to enter the profession and to develop expertise in this area.

The Center also has plans to develop and publish a wide variety of handbooks for initiating and implementing recreation programs for the disabled and to disseminate these materials nationally and internationally. In addition, some of the current staff of the Center will be serving as international consultants. These are staff members who plan to take a leave of absence for a year or more to travel, lecture, and assist wherever they are needed.

Conclusions

In providing community recreation programs for multidisabled children and adults, professional recreators must look at "recreation unlimited." Recreation must play a much broader role in serving these persons than the traditional role of supplementing and enriching lives that are already filled with normal experiences.

The broader role of permitting the needs, interests, and abilities of disabled persons to determine program design and scope can be accomplished. In addition, recreation can become a point of entry into the community service system. Advantages for providing this kind of service under one agency, using many community resources, includes elimination of labeling disabled individuals to determine the agency in which they should be served, and most important, it keeps the "misfits" from falling into the cracks. In many communities, it also has the advantage of providing the most economical use of professional personnel and resources.

Serving persons with multidisabilities and those who have been institutionalized for long periods of time means getting involved in transportation, liaison with community agencies, nutrition, developmental needs of children, and educational aspects essential for them to gain maximal benefits from recreation and leisure-time pursuits.

Each community must identify the needs of its special population and examine the resources to meet those needs. Every community has the potential of starting or expanding programs. The key is commitment to the rights of disabled individuals, recognition of their needs, and determination to provide services to meet those needs. Begin small, with a focus on quality programs, not on numbers. Only through quality programs will disabled individuals be able to reach their potentials and take their place in the mainstream of society.

Development and Validation of a Leisure Diagnostic Battery for Handicapped Children and Youth[1]

David M. Compton
University of Missouri-Columbia

Peter A. Witt and Gary D. Ellis
North Texas State University

Need for Assessment of Leisure Functioning

In recent years we have been giving increased attention to the leisure portion of our lives. In earlier times our perception of leisure was limited to the number of free hours left over after work, but now it is often associated with our feelings toward our free time and with our approach to life in general. "Leisure," it has been stated, "is the opportunity for personal growth and advancement; it is the seed bed of cultural development; it is the opportunity for coming close to the purpose and meaning of life . . . [it is] the feeling one gets when in the process of learning, or expressing, or creating" (Witt & Groom, 1979).

---

[1]This paper was prepared pursuant grant G007902257, Office for Special Education, United States Department of Education. The opinions expressed do not necessarily reflect the position or policy of the US Department of Education, North Texas State University, or the University of Missouri-Columbia, and no official endorsement by the party should be inferred. Dr. Witt served as project director, Dr. Compton served as associate project director, and Mr. Ellis served as project coordinator. Instrumentation and reports are available from the Division of Recreation and Leisure Studies, North Texas State University.

This emerging view is to consider leisure as a state of mind. Thus, leisure is an experience that can occur at any time during any activity, and the key determinant of whether an experience is leisure is in the mind of the beholder. Leisure researchers such as Iso-Ahola (1980), Neulinger (1974), and Mannel (1980) have gone so far as to specify certain conditions that would be necessary for an individual to view a particular experience as leisure. These conditions include: (a) a sense of freedom, (b) intrinsic motivation, and (c) a feeling of competence.

In order to fully grasp this new perception of leisure, it is necessary to examine play, playfulness, and recreation as they relate to leisure. These concepts have often been used to describe different aspects of the leisure experience. Play, playfulness, and recreation can be thought of as activities and approaches which lead to pleasurable, recreative, leisure state of mind outcomes. In this sense, the nature of an activity—whether it qualifies as play or recreation—is dependent on the outcomes of the experience. An assessment of an individual's functioning in leisure, therefore, should be focused on outcomes of activities as well as motivational and situational antecedents which lead to these outcomes.

The term "leisure functioning" may be used to describe the behavior and perceptions of individuals relative to their ability to use play and recreation to attain leisure and the concomitant benefits associated with leisure. Adequate leisure functioning, therefore, would provide the individual with such benefits as positive self-concept; enhanced personal learning ability; mental health; creativity; and physical, emotional, and social growth and development. It is also important to recognize, however, that deficits in leisure functioning may not only preclude the development or occurrence of these benefits, but may in themselves create such undesirable consequences as drug abuse, vandalism, depression, and feelings of isolation (Iso-Ahola, 1980).

The impact of leisure on the life of the individual has made assessment of leisure functioning an important need. Through assessment, it becomes possible to identify deficiencies in leisure functioning and to take remedial action in deficient areas. In this manner, individuals may obtain optimal benefits from their leisure experiences. The need for assessment instruments for this purpose was made particularly evident by the passage of Public Law 94-142. That law requires that an assessment of leisure functioning be a part of an overall individualized education plan (IEP) of handicapped students. In response to that requirement, and to the need for means of assessment in that area, the Leisure Diagnostic Battery was developed.

Background of the Leisure Diagnostic Battery

The Leisure Diagnostic Battery was created under the auspices of the United States Department of Education/Office of Special Education,

Division of Innovation and Development. It addresses the need created by PL 94-142 for the assessment of recreation and leisure functioning as a part of the handicapped student's overall individualized educational plan (IEP). The LDB is also useful in institutional and community recreation settings where assessment of leisure functioning is desired. The goals of LDB development project include the production of the Battery, a user's manual, and an IEP guide. The purposes of the LDB are fourfold:

(1) To enable the assessment of individuals' current level of leisure functioning

(2) To determine areas where improvement of current leisure functioning is needed

(3) To determine via post assessment the impact of offered services on leisure functioning

(4) To facilitate research on the structure of leisure functioning to enable a better understanding of the value, purpose, and outcomes of leisure experiences.

Unique Conceptual Structure of the Leisure Diagnostic Battery

The LDB provides an innovative approach to the assessment of leisure functioning. One area of innovation is the multidimensional nature of the proposed battery. Unlike other leisure assessment instruments, the battery covers a wide range of components that reflect a variety of facets of leisure functioning. This is consistent with the approaches advocated in the leisure education literature which have included a variety of components in the overall leisure education process. For example, Mundy and Odum (1979) delineate five leisure education components: leisure awareness, self-awareness, decision-making, leisure skills, and social interaction. Gunn and Peterson (1978) suggest four components with slight differences from Mundy and Odum's components. Their system includes: (1) developing an awareness of leisure values and attitudes; (2) developing social interaction skills; (3) developing leisure activity skills; and (4) developing knowledge of leisure resources.

The LDB includes all the above components in some form, consisting of traditional areas of social and psychomotor skills, decision-making, knowledge of opportunities, and leisure attitudes. In addition, further theoretical definition has been given to the component areas so that emphasis in several additional areas emerge and are highlighted as critical for overall leisure functioning. For example, the LDB has three components which investigate the "attributions" respondents make concerning their freedom to act, intrinsic motivation, and competence. The battery also includes two components which look at the style of an individual's involvement in leisure, that is, depth of involvement and playfulness. Finally, the LDB determines the ability of an individual to satisfy basic needs via leisure involvements.

A second innovative aspect of the LDB is its use of attribution theory as a theoretical basis for some of the components. This theory suggests that one of the critical determining factors in achieving optimal leisure functioning is the individuals' judgments or attributions about their freedom to act, source of motivation, and degree of competence.

Iso-Ahola (1980) has described the importance of an attributional approach for understanding and interpreting leisure behavior and as a means for improving leisure functioning. Attribution theory is based on the concept that it is not necessarily the "fact" or reality of an individual's freedom to act, for example, but persons' *perception* of their freedom to act that will make the greatest impact on leisure functioning and satisfaction. Persons who ascribe to themselves control over their own decisions and who ascribe the cause of their behavior to internal as opposed to external sources will thus strengthen their overall adjustment.

A third innovative aspect of the proposed battery is the inclusion of scales dealing with the "style" of an individual's leisure involvements. Thus, the work of Lieberman (1977) has been used to construct a measure of an individual's playfulness and Csikszentmihalyi's (1955) concept of flow has been used to develop a scale to measure the depth of an individual's involvement in leisure experiences. Although both of these areas are difficult to conceptualize, their inclusion in the battery adds an important dimension to our understanding of leisure functioning. Inclusion of variables dealing with style suggest that it is not only *what* you do that determines if you are satisfied, but ultimately the *way* you participate that determines the satisfaction, adjustive and functional outcomes of leisure involvement. That is, the more you show characteristics of spontaneity, joy, and a sense of humor, the more qualities such as adjustment, learning, and creativity will be enhanced. In a like manner, the elements that characterize depth of involvement such as focusing of attention and richer perception will greatly determine psychological, cognitive, and behavioral outcomes.

A final innovative aspect of the LDB is reflected in one scale of the battery which focuses on the degree to which an individual can satisfy basic needs for achieving optimal arousal (Ellis, 1973), relaxation, catharsis, compensation, and dissipation of excess random energy via leisure involvements. Thus, the scale looks at the outcomes of leisure experiences and the adjustive potential accruing to the individual as a result of leisure involvement.

Components and Structure of the Leisure Diagnostic Battery

The LDB has eight components. These components are based on eight factors which impact upon leisure functioning and are described in Table 1. The Leisure Diagnostic Battery includes instruments which assess the general areas of leisure functioning.

Based on this framework, two versions of the LDB have been developed. Version A is designed for use with 9- to 15-year-old youth who have "normal" cognitive functioning. It has been used with the orthopedically impaired, deaf, asthmatic, and students in public schools. Version B, on the other hand, is designed for use with 9- to 15-year-old educable mentally retarded individuals. Version B has been applied to mentally retarded individuals in institutional as well as community settings.

The major differences between versions A and B are their response formats and the administrative procedures. Version A is completed by the client who reads an item and indicates, on a three-point scale, the extent to which that item describes or "sounds like" the client. Version B is

Table 1
Characteristics of the Leisure Diagnostic Battery

Components	Purpose
Leisure preferences	To determine relative strength of preference in five domains of leisure activities and to assess preferred modes of involvement
Playfulness	To determine an individual's existing degree of playfulness/spontaneity
Knowledge of leisure opportunities	To determine an individual's knowledge of leisure opportunities
Leisure barriers	To determine problems that an individual encounters when trying to participate in activities during free time
Depth of involvement in leisure	To determine the degree of involvement that an individual is able to achieve during leisure activity experiences
Leisure needs	To determine the degree of ability an individual has to meet certain needs via leisure experiences
Perceived competence	To determine the degree of competence or ability individuals perceive themselves as possessing
Leisure perceived control	To determine whether individuals believe events in their lives to be under their own control (internal locus of control) or are a result of fate or luck or powerful others (external locus of control)

somewhat different. All items from version A are reworded to form questions. These questions are read to the client who may respond with either a "yes" or "no." A version A item might, for example, be "I am a good player." The version B counterpart is "Are you a good player?" Because of the question-and-answer dialog, version B requires individual, one-to-one administration.

Two scales are exceptions to the above discussion of response formats. These are the Knowledge of Leisure Opportunities Test and the Leisure Preferences Inventory. Both of these are consistent with the system of wording items on the two scales, that is, version A involves statements whereas version B involves questions. The administration procedure and response formats, however, are very different. The "knowledge" test on version A is a multiple-choice instrument with one "correct" answer and three distractors for each question. The version A "preferences" scale involves a forced choice between preferred domains of activities and between different preferred styles of participation. For version B, response formats are multiple choice, but pictures are used on each of these scales to hold client interest and to facilitate the making of choices.

The LDB Process

These instruments form the basis for the overall "LDB process" of assessment through remediation. As shown in Figure 1, that process begins with assessment of "freedom to." Five scales are involved in this phase of the process. These include the Perceived Leisure Competence Scale, the Perceived Leisure Control Scale, the Leisure Needs Scale, the Playfulness Scale and the Depth of Involvement in Leisure Experiences Scale. All items are summed across these five scales to obtain a "freedom to" or a "perceived freedom" score.

The second phase of the LDB process, the "assessment follow-up," involves the identification of sources of barriers prohibiting a sense of "freedom from." Two scales are included in the LDB for this purpose. The Knowledge of Leisure Alternatives Test is intended to provide users with an indication of the client's degree of awareness of leisure opportunities in his or her environment. The lack of awareness of these alternatives is thought to be a major barrier to a state of "freedom from." The Barriers to Involvement in Leisure Scale is the second instrument measuring a "freedom from" element. That scale is intended to measure individuals' general perceptions of various personal and environmental barriers to their leisure activities. Included on the scale are items dealing with such constraints as architectural barriers, financial barriers, time barriers, and transportation barriers. Both the Knowledge of Leisure Opportunities Test and the Barriers to Leisure Involvement Scale are considered to be major inhibitors of perceived freedom (feeling "freedom to").

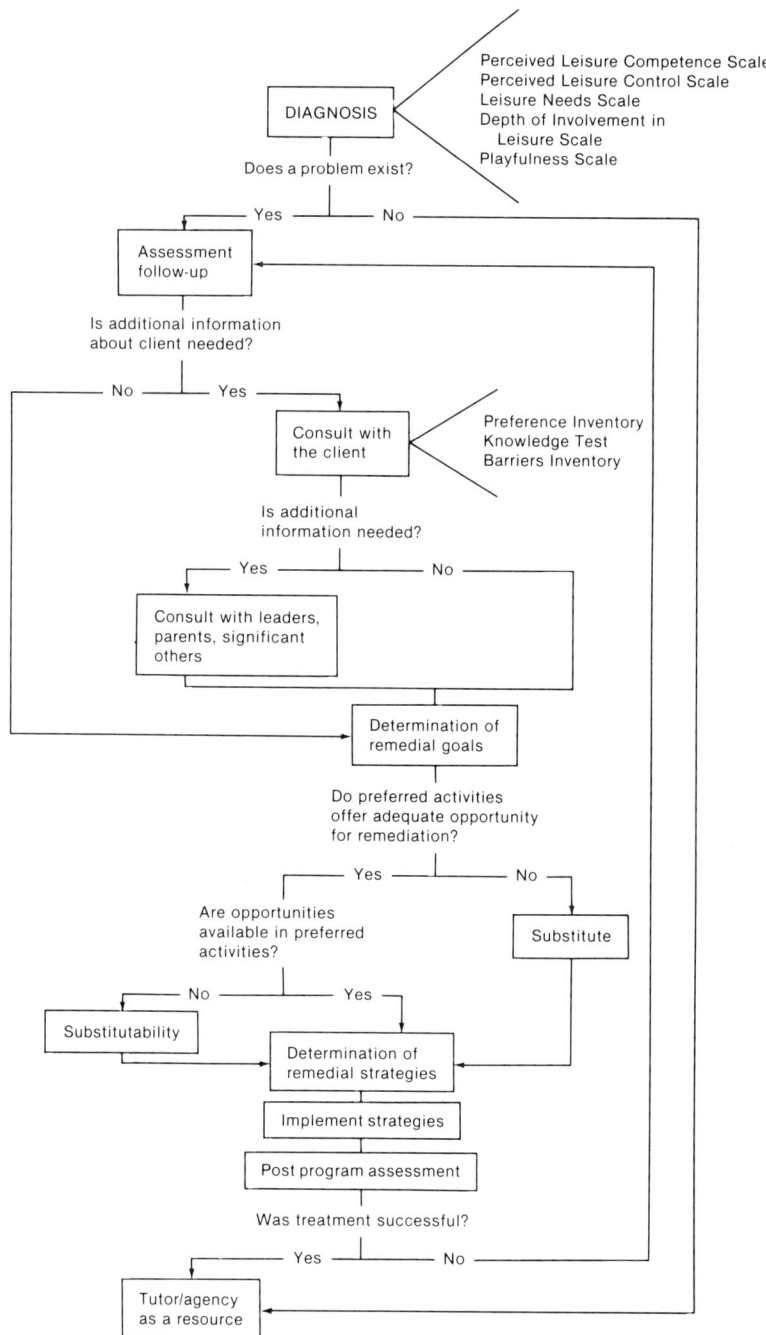

Figure 1 — The LDB process.

The reader should note that the LDB process does not assume that the "knowledge" and "barriers" instruments provide a comprehensive assessment of "freedom from" constraints to leisure. In fact, numerous other problems may be present. The individual's psychomotor skills may be inadequate, and the social skills may be poor. A prohibitive cultural barrier may be present. Each of these is an area in which active barriers may be prohibiting feelings of "freedom to." Relative to the LDB process, leaders may choose to follow-up with assessments in any of several areas following an initial diagnosis of limited perceived freedom. These assessments may take the form of formal testing or informal consultations with the client or significant others in the client's life. This consultation phase is the third phase of the LDB process.

The fourth and fifth phases involve the delineation of remedial objectives and the implementation of remedial efforts associated with those objectives. This is a rather complex process which relies heavily upon attribution theory as a means for remediating deficiencies. Briefly, the approach is individualized, focusing on the nature and content of interactions between the client and the leader. In this approach, activities serve only as the mediums within which these interactions take place. The process thereby becomes sort of an unobtrusive approach to counseling. The process is far removed from and shows much greater promise than traditional approaches which involve activity analysis and establish the activity as the central aspect of remediation. This process is discussed in-depth in the *Leisure Diagnostic Battery Remediation Guide* (1982).

The sixth and final step of the remediation process is the post-treatment assessment. This step is needed to determine the effectiveness of the remediation strategies in enhancing the client's leisure functioning. As suggested by Figure 1, the step involves the remediation of the primary diagnosis instruments and repeating the LDB process for identified deficiencies. If the same deficiencies are identified in the second administration of the scales, the leader may conclude that remedial efforts were ineffective. If, on the other hand, deficiencies are identified in new areas, the leader will know that either new problems have emerged in the process or that, for this individual, problems are aligned in hierarchical fashion with the removal of one barrier simply leading to the emergence of the next. Each of these possibilities has implications to the development of remediation objectives and strategies.

Development of the LDB

Scale development within each LDB component area followed a very meticulous process. A comprehensive review of literature relative to each component was conducted. This review enabled the project staff to delineate subcategories or domains of each concept to be assessed. Identified domains to be included in the playfulness component, for example, were cognitive spontaneity, physical spontaneity, social spontaneity, manifest joy, and sense of humor (Lieberman, 1977). Domains of perceived competence, similarly, included cognitive competence, physical competence, social competence, and physical competence (Harter, 1979). Based on this review of literature, a conceptual paper describing the rationale and structure underlying each LDB scale was developed. This paper is available upon request from North Texas State University, Division of Recreation and Leisure Studies. The domains identified for inclusion on each scale are included in the Appendix.

The identified domains of each concept formed a content outline for each scale. Scale items were developed from this outline. In the initial phase of development, an attempt was made to maintain balance within each scale by constructing an equal number of items to represent each domain. In latter rounds of testing, this principle was relaxed a bit in order to maximize homogeneity of the items. Although conceptual domains within scales of the final version in some cases may be unequally weighted in terms of numbers of items, all key areas are represented in some way on each scale.

Several rounds of testing were used in the process of refining the LDB and its individual components. Included were 9- to 15-year-old individuals in the following samples:

- 72 participants in the City of Dallas, TX, summer playground program;
- 192 individuals with orthopedic impairments from several public schools throughout the country;
- 292 mentally retarded individuals from several school and institutional sites throughout the country;
- 206 students of public schools throughout the country;
- 182 mentally retarded individuals from public schools and institutions throughout the country;
- 200 students from public schools in Columbia, MO; and
- 104 mentally retarded students from public schools in Columbia and St. Louis.

In addition, data were collected from 72 9- to 14-year-old students from the Oklahoma School for the Deaf. Each of these rounds of testing contributed to the refinement of the conceptualization, to item analysis, and to the examination of reliability and validity.

Item analysis was used extensively to refine the instrumentation. Factor analysis, inter-item correlations, item-total correlations and multiple correlations of each item with all other items on each scale were used to select items for inclusion on the final instruments and to identify ambiguous items which were detracting from the measurement. An item was considered to be contributing to the measurement if it loaded highly in a significant or meaningful factor, if it correlated highly with other items, if its item-total correlation was greater than .2, and if the multiple correlation was moderate. Using these criteria, it was possible to develop reliable scales of about 20 items each from an original pool of approximately twice as many items per scale.

Many significant contributions to understanding the conceptualization of the LDB were derived from the scale development process. Data analysis repeatedly provided evidence of validity in the interrelationships of scales measuring "freedom to" in the initial diagnosis and of the scales measuring constraints to freedom ("freedom from") in the assessment follow-up. Validity was also evident in the lack of relationship between the LDB and demographic and social desirability variables. Alpha reliabilities ranged from .86 to .96 for version A and from .71 to .90 for version B in the final round of testing (see Table 2). These results assisted in the conceptualization and operationalization of remedial strategies and they contributed greatly to the refinement of the instrumentation. In addition, they targeted specific areas for refining and upgrading the LDB instruments and the remediation process.

The LDB: Implications for Service

The LDB may usher in a new era in therapeutic recreation, special education, and other disciplines which focus on the needs of handicapped children and youth. With the demand on all professionals to become

Table 2
Alpha Reliabilities of the LDB

Scale	Version A	Version B
Perceived freedom	.96	.90
Perceived leisure competence	.89	.73
Perceived leisure control	.88	.68
Leisure needs	.90	.77
Depth of involvement in leisure experiences	.88	.71
Playfulness	.90	.75
Barriers to leisure opportunities	.86	.76
Knowledge of leisure opportunities	.90	.83
Preferences subscales		
Active/passive style	.57	.63
Group/individual style	.71	.66
Risk/nonrisk style	.57	.67

more accountable for the services they provide, it is apparent that the role of assessment will increase in the future. Several implications for services to handicapped children and youth are evident.

First, it is apparent that the dawn of an era of valid and reliable instrumentation by which assessment of leisure functioning can be conducted is upon us. The LDB may represent the beginning of an era in which a number of instruments will be developed which should produce corroborative evidence regarding leisure functioning of handicapped individuals. This instrumentation will greatly assist the profession in the conduct of precise and well founded diagnoses of deficiencies in leisure functioning.

Second, a new role appears to be emerging which will have great importance on the therapeutic recreation field—the diagnostician. With available instrumentation, it is necessary to begin to prepare competent diagnosticians who are well schooled in tests and measurement as well as critical competencies, for example, learning theories, social psychology of leisure behavior, and prescriptive programming. The diagnostician will serve a critical role in the overall rehabilitation, education, or developmental process. With precise analyses of leisure functioning and clear interpretations of its meaning, the therapist, educator, or facilitator should be in a better position to affect the positive development in leisure functioning of the child.

Third, no longer will imprecise inventories or checklists serve as the cornerstone of judgment by therapists, clinicians, or educators. Precise and calculated testing coupled with systematic observations will replace unfounded judgments as the bases for treatment or educational design.

Fourth, the application of instrumentation and the collection of data will allow the profession to develop a body of knowledge on leisure functioning which can be interpreted in a narrative or criterion referenced sense. These data will serve as corroborative evidence that certain intervention techniques and strategies used by the therapist or educator clearly affect the level of leisure functioning of the handicapped individual. Through precise studies under laboratory conditions (as well as longitudinal studies), we may be in a position to assess leisure functioning of the individual to once and for all lay to rest notions that leisure does not really matter.

The Status of Leisure Assessment: An Assessment

The LDB represents a certain amount of conceptual and practical progress toward the development of appropriate and usable assessment materials. What remains, of course, is for an enlightened cadre of workers to take the developed materials and begin to use them in a variety of practical situations. This will lead to upgrading of professional status, improvement of services to clients, and a better perception of our purpose and mission.

The assessment process represents a new frontier because being successful requires that we know what we are trying to accomplish and what leisure really means. As usual, recreation services for the handicapped are at the forefront of helping us conceptualize the basic meaning of our field and finding methods of translating philosophy into action. A comprehensive approach to assessment of leisure functioning will help us to better understand the leisure needs of handicapped children and youth and to better plan services and program for meeting delineated needs. Janet Pomeroy, Founder and Director of the San Francisco Recreation Center for the Handicapped, has documented that the handicapped have come out of hiding. It is time now that assessment efforts be less shadowy and more enlightened. It will move us closer to seeing the light at the end of the tunnel in terms of the promise of full opportunity, equal access, and realization of our leisure potential.

References

BLOOM, B.S., & Krathwohl, D.R. *Taxonomy of educational objectives. Handbook 1: Cognitive domain.* New York: Longmans, 1956.

BREGHA, F. Leisure and freedom re-examined. In T. Goodale and P. Witt (Eds.), *Recreation and leisure: Issues in an era of change.* State College, PA: Venture, 1980.

COMPTON, D.M. Facilitating leisure behavior. In C.R. Edginton, D.M. Compton, & C.J. Hanson (Eds.), *Recreation and leisure programming.* Philadelphia: Saunders College, 1980.

CSIKZENTMIHALYI, M. *Beyond boredom and anxiety.* San Francisco: Jossey-Bass, 1955.

DECI, E. *Intrinsic motivation.* New York: Plenum, 1975.

ELLIS, G., et al. *Leisure Diagnostic Battery Remediation Guide.* Denton, TX: Leisure Diagnostic Battery Project, 1979.

ELLIS, M.J. *Why people play.* Englewood Cliffs, NJ: Prentice-Hall, 1973. Fishbein, M., & Ajzen, I. *Belief, attitude, intention and behavior: An introduction to theory and research.* Reading, MA: Addison-Wesley, 1975.

FISHBEIN, M., & Ajzen, J. *Belief, attitude, intention and behavior: An introduction to theory and research.* Reading, MA: Addison-Wesley, 1975.

GUNN, S.C., & Peterson, C.A. *Therapeutic recreation program design: Principles and procedures.* Englewood Cliffs, NJ: Prentice-Hall, 1978.

HARTER, S. *Perceived Competence Scale for Children.* University of Denver, 1979.

ISO-AHOLA, S.E. *The social psychology of leisure and recreation.* Dubuque, IA: William C. Brown Publishing, 1980.

KERLINGER, F.N. *Foundations of behavioral research* (2nd ed.). New York: Holt, Rinehart and Winston, 1973.

LIEBERMAN, J.N. *Playfulness: Its relationship to imagination and creativity.* Brooklyn: Academic Press, 1977.

MANNEL, R.C. Social psychological techniques and strategies for studying leisure experiences. In S.E. Iso-Ahola (Ed.), *Social psychological perspectives on leisure and recreation.* Springfield, IL: Charles C. Thomas, 1980.

MUNDY, J., & Odum, L. *Leisure education: Theory and practice.* New York: Wiley, 1979.

NEULINGER, J. *The psychology of leisure.* Springfield, IL: Charles C. Thomas, 1974.

OVERS, R.D., Taylor, S., & Adkins, C. *Avocational counseling in Milwaukee.* Milwaukee: Milwaukee Curative Workshops, 1974.

ROTTER, J.B. Generalized expectancies for internal versus external control of reinforcement. *Psychological Monograph,* 1966, **80**(1; whole no. 609).

WITT, P.A., & Goodale, T. Barriers to leisure and stage of family lifestyle. *Leisure Sciences,* 1981, **4**, 29-50.

WITT, P.A., & Groom, R. Dangers and problems associated with current approaches to developing leisure interest finders. *Therapeutic Recreation Journal,* 1979, **13**, 19-31.

Appendix
Components, Purposes, and Domains of the LDB

Scale	Purpose	Domains
1. Scales measuring "freedom to"		
Perceived freedom	To enable the assessment of clients' perceived freedom ("freedom to") in leisure.	A scale score is obtained by summing across all items of scales measuring "freedom to."
Perceived leisure competence	To enable the assessment of clients' perceptions of their degree of personal competence in recreation and leisure endeavors.	1. Cognitive competence 2. Social competence 3. Physical competence 4. General competence
Perceived leisure control	To enable the assessment of clients' degree of internality, or the extent to which they control events and outcomes in their leisure experiences.	Each item is designed to reflect the presence or absence of an internal stable tendency for attributions.

Leisure needs	To enable the assessment of clients' abilities to satisfy intrinsic needs via recreation and leisure experiences.	1. Relaxation 2. Surplus energy 3. Compensation 4. Catharsis 5. Optimal arousal 6. Gregariousness 7. Status 8. Creative expression 9. Skill development 10. Self image
Depth of involvement in leisure experiences	To enable the assessment of the extent to which individuals become absorbed, or achieve "flow" during activities.	Each item reflects an element of Csikzentmihalyi's "flow" concept (1955): 1. Centering of attention 2. Merging of action and awareness 3. Loss of self consciousness 4. Perception of control over self and environment 5. Noncontradictory demands for action with immediate feedback 6. The absence of a need for external rewards
Playfulness	To enable the assessment of clients' degree of playfulness.	Based on Lieberman's (1975) work with the playfulness concept: 1. Cognitive spontaneity 2. Physical spontaneity 3. Social spontaneity 4. Manifest joy 5. Sense of humor

2. Scales measuring "freedom from" barriers to leisure

Barriers to leisure involvement	To enable the identification of problems clients encounter when trying to select or participate in recreation and leisure experiences.	1. Communication barriers 2. Social skills barriers 3. Decision making barriers 4. Desire/interest barriers 5. Time barriers 6. Financial barriers 7. Lack of opportunities barriers 8. Lack of ability barriers 9. Mental barriers 10. Accessibility barriers

Knowledge of leisure opportunities	To enable the determination of individuals' knowledge of specific information concerning leisure opportunities.	1. Who can participate 2. What the activities are 3. Where opportunities are present 4. When opportunities occur 5. How much cost is involved in various activities

3. Scale used in the remediation process

Leisure preferences scale	To enable the determination of individuals' preferred leisure activities and their preferred style of participation.	1. Sports 2. Arts & crafts 3. Mental & linguistics 4. Nature 5. Music & drama 6. Active/passive style preference 7. Group/individual style preference 8. Risk/nonrisk style preference

The Effects of Increased Recreation Opportunities on Life Satisfaction and Physical/Mental Health of the Elderly—A Reconnaissance Evaluation

Jean Tague
Texas Woman's University

Why Is Research on Recreation for the Elderly Important?

During the past decades a marked increase in interest has been shown for problems of the aged in the United States. In part, this concern for the latter part of the lifespan can be attributed to the noticeable increase in the number of elderly people in our population. In 1900 approximately three million persons were 65 years of age or over, and in 1978 the population had risen to 22 million. It has been estimated that this number will reach 30 million by 1990 and 46 million by the year 2025 (Butler & Lewis, 1977).

The social and economic changes that have accompanied industrialization have also brought changes in the status of older people. Aging workers usually are retired at a fixed age under the rules of a formal retirement system. They are financially dependent on social security, old-age assistance, pension funds, or personal income from other sources. A relatively small number of people receive income from the latter source (Samuelson, 1978). Changing economic patterns, differing family characteristics, population shifts, the individual's health status, copious amount of free time, and many other factors have created numerous problems for older people. Of these, leisure has become one of the major problems facing the aged in the Twentieth Century.

The impact of tomorrow's "grayed" society is of concern to many gerontologists. Most feel that the consequences of the sheer numbers of older persons will affect our entire cultural life and that the current public policies in housing, medical care, pensions, crime control, employment, consumer protection, health and social services, and recreation will have to be drastically revised. If professional recreators are to plan appropriate and adequate services for the elderly, they must identify and address the knowledge gaps in the effects of recreation on the elderly.

What Do We Know?

Many researchers have examined life satisfaction of the elderly. In an attempt to determine variables that affect perceived life satisfaction and the extent to which these variables are associated with the satisfaction, researchers have concentrated on a number of areas. Those most commonly studied are health, socioeconomic status, income and financial status, fear and crime, isolation, activity, and social contacts (Lemon, Bengtson, & Peterson, 1972). At best, the evidence supporting any one of these variables studied as important to life satisfaction is mixed. A positive relationship may be found in one research effort, but the same variable may be found to have no relationship in another study. It is unclear which type of variables are associated with and/or predict life satisfaction among the elderly.

In the area of activity, numerous studies have been completed using different populations and different measures of activity. One of the earliest studies (Havighurst, 1961) identified two theories of successful aging. The "activity theory" was defined as one in which the older person maintains, as long as possible, the activities and attitudes of middle age. The "disengagement theory" describes the older person as deserving and accepting a process of disengagement from active life. Both theories have stimulated a great deal of research. Although the studies of activity and life satisfaction provide varying evidence, in general the findings reveal that lack of social interaction and activity are clearly related to lower expressed satisfaction with life, low morale, and lower contentment, thus supporting the activity/engagement theory. Tobin and Neugarten (1961) obtained evidence that social interaction was positively associated with life satisfaction. This was substantiated by Graney (1975). A positive relationship between increased frequency of participation in leisure activities and life satisfaction was found by Palmore (1968), DeCarlo (1974), and Peppers (1973). Bley, Goodman, Dye, and Harle (1972) found a significant association between the erratic use of leisure and low morale, satisfaction, and adjustment.

Toseland and Sykes (1977), in a study of participation in a senior citizen center, found that the activity level, financial status, and health were important predictors of life satisfaction in older persons. Activity level was by far the best predictor of life satisfaction. However, this study also revealed that senior citizen center participation was not a predictor of life satisfaction. There was no correlation between a respondent's life satisfaction score and frequency of center attendance. Thompson (1973) found that participation in clubs and organizations is an antecedent to one's perception of health and morale. However, differences appear to exist between urban and nonurban populations. For nonurban samples, organizational participation and church-related activities are consistently associated with well-being (Edwards & Klemmack, 1973; Palmore & Luikart, 1972; Pihiblad & Adams, 1972; Pihiblad & McNamara, 1965). For urban populations this relationship appears not to hold (Bull & Aucoin, 1975; Lemon, Bengtson, & Peterson, 1972). It was also demonstrated that participation in voluntary associations has a much weaker relationship to well-being when controls of health and income level are introduced (Bull & Aucoin, 1975; Cutler, 1973; Edwards & Klemmack, 1973).

Tobin and Neugarten (1961) obtained evidence supporting the prediction that with advancing age activities become more important in predicting life satisfaction. Markides and Martin (1979) found that activity was a strong positive predictor of life satisfaction for both sexes. Cumming and Henry's (1961) study of age-related activity patterns in women found little change over the lifespan because their roles did not change as radically as men's. Recent studies by Fox (1977) and Jaslow (1976) found women who worked were more active after retirement than their non-working peers.

From the data of Lemon and associates (1972) the correlation between informal activities and well-being became significant when people in poorer health were not included. This is not the case, however, for the data of Bultena and Oyler (1971).

Another area of investigation is that of leisure choices and needs. London, Crandall, and Seals (1977) observed that interpersonal involvement, such as developing a close friendship, was one of the three basic dimensions of leisure needs. Ritchi (1975) found that social opportunities were the most important determinant of leisure participation. Ragheb and Griffith (Note 1) found that leisure satisfaction obtained from leisure choices contributed much more than leisure participation to the life satisfaction of older persons.

In researching the institutionalized aged, Quilitch (1974) found that the regular provision of planned group activity (bingo) considerably increased the activity of residents in a geriatric ward.

Jenkins, Felce, Lunt, and Powell (1977) found that the level of engagement in activity of the residents of two homes for the elderly increased substantially when the experimenter provided simple recreation materials and interacted with the residents while they used them. These findings were also confirmed by McClannahan and Risley (1975).

While the majority of studies concentrated on the relationship between the frequency of participation in activities and life satisfaction, other researchers were starting to investigate the quality of the activity experience. Lowenthal and Haven (1968) provided evidence that showed that the quality or type of interaction, not the quantity, was the more important predictor of life satisfaction of the aged. Where the activities are meaningful and promote self-evaluation, morale is strongly affected (Maddox & Eisdorfer, 1962; Phillips, 1969; Saltz, 1971). Ray (1979) also found that the quality of activity one pursues may be more important than the quantity. Ragheb and Griffith (Note 1) conducted a study to determine the relationship between leisure participation/leisure satisfaction/life satisfaction. They found that (1) the higher the frequency of participation in leisure activities the higher the life satisfaction; (2) the more the leisure participation the higher the leisure satisfaction; (3) the greater the leisure satisfaction the greater the life satisfaction; (4) with the exception of the physiological component, the younger the individual the higher the satisfaction elicited from the six components of leisure (physiological, psychological, educational, environmental, outdoor, and social); and (5) the more the leisure satisfaction gained from each of the six components the higher the life satisfaction. These findings support the activity/engagement theory and suggest that leisure satisfaction and leisure participation play a definite role in life satisfaction, and point out the importance of providing leisure opportunities that carry the potential of leisure satisfaction.

Other studies tended to counter the activity theory in part or to provide total support for the disengagement theory. Ray (1979) found little evidence to indicate the positive impact of activity breadth on life satisfaction. Neither the number of activities nor frequency of participation was significant to high life satisfaction. Lemon, Bengtson, and Peterson (1972) did not find a positive correlation between the frequency of participation in activities and life satisfaction. Rosow (1963) indicated that older people found their greatest sense of life satisfaction from being with family (80%) and from work (70%) rather than from recreation (37%) or visiting with neighbors (35%).

Empirical research suggests that the social and psychological concomitants of aging are influenced by lifestyle patterns established earlier in the life cycle (Maddox, 1963). From this perspective, then, the variables of morale, social participation, and health are indicative of the way persons spent their earlier lives rather than a result of the aging process as such (Simpson & McKinney, 1966). Thus, a causal relationship of activity to life satisfaction is suggested, but not conclusively established.

Research related to physical activity shows that the levels of participation are positively associated with psychological attitudes (Davis, 1967; Kreitler & Kreitler, 1970). Studies of the effects of a variety of exercise, jogging, walking, and aquatics programs have reported improvements in range of motion and muscle strength (Agate, 1965), and decreases in work pulse, both postexercise diastolic and systolic blood pressure and blood lactate concentration, and significant changes in physical work capacity, percentage of body fat, vital capacity, and oxygen transport capacity (Barry, Steinmetz, Page, & Rodahl, 1966; deVries, 1971; Daykin, 1967). Allen (1965) suggested that after completing an exercise program the subjects slept better and were able to perform more self-care functions. Spirduso (1975) indicated that lifestyle of physical activity may play a more dominant role in determining reaction and movement time speed than age. The results of this study strongly suggest vigorous sports participation as a significant function in retarding the onset of aging. In general, exercise programs have distinct and well documented physiological, biochemical, and psychological effects (Ismail & Young, 1977).

Who Knows?

Most research on activity and the aged has been produced by persons in the fields of sociology, psychology, and physical education; some studies also have been completed by psychiatrists and other medical doctors. Reports of the research appear primarily in the various publications of gerontology and geriatrics. Research related specifically to recreation and written by recreationists is contained, for the most part, in unpublished theses and dissertations, symposium papers, and other ephemeral works.

While articles that describe recreation programs for the elderly appear in recreation journals, few reports of pure research are found in these publications. A limited number of reports of research projects appear in the *Journal of Leisure Research;* however, this publication is not widely read by practitioners in the field of recreation, with the result that recreation practitioners are generally unaware of results of research related to activity and the elderly.

What Next?

Knowledge relative to the quality of leisure participation in relation to life satisfaction is lacking. Lowenthal and Haven (1968), as well as

Rosow (1963), have criticized the literature on activity and well-being for neglecting to consider the quality of the activity and the intimacy of interaction. Recreation researchers should take special note of this void in the literature. All recreation experiences have, as a minimum, three major components: an activity component, a social setting component, and a biophysical environment component. Recreation researchers need to address the areas of activity and intimacy with regard to which of these is measured, which controlled, and which assumed.

Another major gap in research results from the absence of longitudinal studies. A number of authors have suggested that the lesser well-being of persons with lower activity, as found in cross-sectional studies, may reflect life-long personality characteristics that cannot be influenced by an increase or decline in activity as is implied (Rose, 1964; Rosow, 1963). Lowenthal and Haven (1968) found a difference of only 12% in the number of persons classified as having high morale (at time two) between those showing increased versus decreased social interaction. Maddox (1963) found some increase in well-being for those people showing extreme increases in activity over 3 years but slight net changes for those who showed an extreme decline in activity. Moderate correlations were found by Graney (1975) for a small sample over 4 years. More substantial associations were found by Bultena (1969) and Havighurst, Neugarten, and Tobin (1968) for retrospective reports of change in activity; but the validity of such reports is subject to question.

Ray (1979) also addresses the problem of the quality of activities one pursues, suggesting that a rigid categorization of activity types may not be an appropriate method of predicting life satisfaction. He suggests that a method of looking at the experience of activities and the relevance to the individual might be more appropriate.

The concept of leisure satisfaction has only recently become evident in the literature; thus, knowledge of the concept remains limited. A review of the literature revealed a limited number of studies which dealt directly with leisure satisfaction. This research used tests having undocumented reliability and/or validity (London, Crandall, & Seals, 1977; McIntyre, 1972; Milwaukee Avocational Satisfaction Questionnaire: Part I, 1977; Orthner, 1975; Winters, 1973). Beard and Ragheb (1980) have outlined studies needed to provide data on some unanswered questions related to their Leisure Satisfaction Scale (LSS):

(1) What is the relationship between age and satisfaction derived from leisure activities for each of the "need areas?" Are there periods or stages of one's lifetime when the satisfaction of social or physical need, etc., is of more importance than in other periods?

(2) Do the types of needs filled by leisure activities vary from male to female participants?

(3) How does income and educational level relate to leisure satisfaction?

(4) Does marital status have implications for the value of leisure activity?

(5) What are the roles of leisure activities in satisfying the needs associated with an individual's retirement from employment?

The authors have stated that only the content and construct validity of the LSS have been addressed and these only partially. The relationships between the LSS and other traits remain to be explored (Beard & Ragheb, 1980).

Markides and Martin (1979), who developed an Activity Index to measure formal and informal activity, also have identified an area for future research: research into the intervening role of informal versus formal activity measures.

The research completed by Maddox (1963) and Simpson and McKinney (1966) demonstrates that the "early learning" theory must be taken into consideration when planning for recreation for the elderly. The fact that persons' social behavior and participation in the older years is influenced to a high degree by their social behavior and participation in the earlier part of their lives suggests that the recreational interests, needs, and participation of the elderly will have to be periodically re-examined. Each new generation will have had different "early life" experiences and will bring into their retirement years interests, needs, and participation patterns that are unlike those of the persons who retired during the previous decade.

Based on a review of the literature, the following areas have been identified in which further research needs to be completed relative to recreational opportunities and life satisfaction of the aged:

- Institutionalized aged, homebound aged, rural aged, blue-collar and lower socioeconomic persons need to be studied relative to leisure and life satisfaction.
- Additional studies should be undertaken in which the "activities" can clearly be identified as recreational.
- Additional work needs to be done to determine the types of activities that are most satisfying to older persons.
- Those factors which motivate older persons to participate in recreational activities need to be identified and analyzed.
- The effects of leisure education on the recreation participation of the elderly needs to be examined.

- The potential of day care and outreach programs for the elderly needs to be identified.

Other topics that need to be researched include:

- Types of recreation facilities preferred by older people.
- Longitudinal analysis of the effects of physical activity on aging.
- Effects of physical activity on long-term institutionalized geriatrics.
- Longitudinal studies of the relationship of participation in voluntary associations to life satisfaction, including an assessment of life satisfaction before and after joining voluntary associations.

Summary and Recommendations

It would appear that, while a great deal of research has been completed on "activity" as it relates to life satisfaction and physical/mental health of the elderly, very little pure research has been produced in which "recreational activities/opportunities" have been studied. Many knowledge gaps remain and research is needed if agencies are to meet the future recreational needs of the aged.

The research that has been produced has been accomplished for the most part by persons other than recreationists and has been published in journals other than those of the field of recreation. The results of the research show that a causal relationship of activity to life satisfaction is suggested, but not conclusively established. The research on exercise programs and other physical activity programs have distinct and well documented physiological, biochemical, and psychological effects.

It is recommended that funding be made available to two or three Departments of Recreation and Leisure Studies housed at major universities to develop and carry out specific research topics related to recreation and the elderly. If possible, one or more longitudinal studies should be funded. A small task force of educators with expertise in the field of aging could establish a priority list of topics. As funds became available, topics from this list would be researched. It would be important to publish the results of such research in the publications of the National Recreation and Park Association and to present the results at national and regional conferences of this organization. It is equally important that current research be made available to practitioners through the HCRS Information Exchange, specifically through *Notifications* and *Share* and through the various publications of the American Association for Health, Physical Education and Recreation. Reciprocally, publication of recreation research in gerontology and health journals would make persons in other fields more aware of the contributions of recreation to the life satisfaction of the elderly. It is critical that all practitioners who work with the elderly be apprised of current information produced by this research.

Reference Note

1. Ragheb, M.G., & Griffith, C.A. *The contribution of leisure participation and leisure satisfaction to life satisfaction of older persons.* Manuscript submitted for publication, 1980.

References

AGATE, M. Case studies of preventative and remedial exercise to improve functional capacity of the well aging. *Gerontologist,* 1965, **5**, 30.

ALLEN, J. The use of isometric exercises in a geriatric treatment program. *Geriatrics,* 1965, **20**, 346-347.

BARRY, A.J., Steinmetz, R., Page, H.F., & Rodahl, K. The effects of physical conditioning on older individuals. II. Motor performance and cognitive function. *Journal of Gerontology,* 1966, **21**, 192-199.

BEARD, J.G., & Ragheb, M.G. Measuring leisure satisfaction. *Journal of Leisure Research,* 1980, **12**, 20-33.

BLEY, N.B., Goodman, M., Dye, D., & Harle, B. Characteristics of aged participants in age-segregated leisure program. *Gerontologist,* 1972, **12**, 368-370.

BULL, C.N., & Aucoin, J.B. Voluntary association participation and life satisfaction: A replication note. *Journal of Gerontology,* 1975, **30**, 73-76.

BULTENA, G. Life continuity and morale in old age. *Gerontologist,* 1969, **9**, 251-253.

BULTENA, G., & Oyler, R. Effects of health on disengagement and morale. *Aging and Human Development,* 1971, **12**, 142-148.

BUTLER, R.N., & Lewis, M.I. *Aging and mental health: Positive psychosocial approaches* (2nd ed.). St. Louis: C.V. Mosby, 1977.

CLARK, B.A., Wade, M.G., Massey, B.H., & Van Dyke, R. Response of institutionalized geriatric mental patients to a twelve-week program of regular physical activity. *Journal of Gerontology,* 1975, **30**, 565-573.

CUMMING, E., & Henry, W. *Growing old.* New York: Basic Books, 1961.

CUTLER, S. Volunteer association participation and life satisfaction: A cautionary research note. *Journal of Gerontology,* 1973, **28**, 96-100.

DAVIS, R.W. Activity therapy in a geriatric setting. *Journal of American Geriatrics Society,* 1967, **15**, 1144-1152.

DAYKIN, H.P. The application of isometrics in geriatric treatment. *American Corrective Therapy Journal,* 1967, **21**, 203-205.

DECARLO, T.J. Recreation participation patterns and successful aging. *Journal of Gerontology,* 1974, **29**, 416-422.

DEVRIES, H.A. Exercise intensity threshold for improvement of cardiovascular respiratory function in older men. *Geriatrics,* 1971, **26**, 94-101.

EDWARDS, J.N., & Klemmack, D.L. Correlates of life satisfaction: A re-examination. *Journal of Gerontology,* 1973, **28**, 497-502.

FOX, J.H. Effects of retirement and former work life on women's adaptations in old age. *Journal of Gerontology,* 1977, **32**, 196-202.

GRANEY, M.J. Happiness and social participation in aging. *Journal of Gerontology,* 1975, **30**, 701-706.

HAVIGHURST, R.J. Successful aging. *Gerontologist,* 1961, **1**, 8-12.

HAVIGHURST, R., Neugarten, B., & Tobin, S. Disengagement and patterns of aging. In B.N. Newgarten (Ed.), *Middle age and aging.* Chicago: University of Chicago Press, 1968.

ISMAIL, A.H., & Young, R.J. Effect of chronic exercise on the multivariate relationships between selected biochemical and personality variables. *Multivariate Behavioral Research,* 1977, **12**, 49-67.

JASLOW, P. Employment, retirement and morale among older women. *Journal of Gerontology,* 1976, **31**, 212-218.

JENKINS, J., Felce, D., Lunt, B., & Powell, L. Increasing engagement in activity of residents in old people's homes by providing recreation materials. *Behavior Research and Therapy,* 1977, **15**, 429-434.

KREITLER, H., & Kreitler, S. Movement and again: A psychological approach. In E. Jokl (Ed.), *Physical activity and aging. Vol. 4., Medicine and sport.* Baltimore: University Park Press, 1970.

LEMON, B.W., Bengtson, V.L., & Peterson, J.A. An exploration of the activity theory of aging: Activity types and life satisfaction among in-movers to a retirement community. *Journal of Gerontology,* 1972, **72**, 511-523.

LONDON, M. Crandall, R., & Seals, G. The contribution of job and leisure satisfaction to quality of life. *Journal of Applied Psychology,* 1977, **62**, 328-334.

LOWENTHAL, M., & Haven, C. Interaction and adaptation: Intimacy as a critical variable. In B. Neugarten (Ed.), *Middle age and aging.* Chicago: University of Chicago Press, 1968.

MADDOX, G. Activity and morale: A longitudinal study of selected elderly subjects. *Social Forces,* 1963, **42**, 195-204.

MADDOX, G.I., & Eisdorfer, D. Some correlates of activity and morale among the elderly. *Social Forces,* 1962, **40**, 254-280.

MARKIDES, K.S., & Martin, H.W. A causal model of life satisfaction among the elderly. *Journal of Gerontology,* 1979, **34**, 86-93.

MCCLANNAHAN, L.E., & Risley, T.R. Activities and materials for severely disabled patients. *Nursing Homes,* December 1974-January 1975.

MCINTYRE, F. Motivator-hygiene comparison of work and leisure satisfaction. Unpublished doctoral dissertation, Case Western Reserve, 1972.

MILWAUKEE Avocational Satisfaction Questionnaire: Part I. In A. Epperson, P.A. Witt, & G. Hitzhusen, *Leisure counseling: An aspect of leisure education.* Springfield, IL: Charles C. Thomas, 1977.

ORTHNER, D. Leisure activity patterns and marital satisfaction over the marital career. *Journal of Marriage and the Family,* 1975, **37,** 91-102.

PALMORE, E.B. The effects of aging on activities and attitudes. *Gerontologist,* 1968, **8,** 259-263.

PALMORE, E., & Kivett, V. Change in life satisfaction: A longitudinal study of persons aged 46-70. *Journal of Gerontology,* 1977, **32,** 311-316.

PALMORE, E., & Luikart, C. Health and social factors related to life satisfaction. *Journal of Health and Social Behavior,* 1972, **18,** 68-80.

PEPPERS, L.G. Leisure activity and adjustment to the retirement process (Doctoral dissertation, Oklahoma State University, 1973). *Dissertation Abstracts,* 1973, **35,** 6825A, Ord. No. 75-8858.

PHILLIPS, D.L. Social class, social participation and happiness: A consideration of "interactive opportunities" and "investment." *The Sociological Quarterly,* 1969, **10,** 3-21.

PIHIBLAD, C., & Adams, D. Widowhood, social participation and life satisfaction. *Aging and Human Development,* 1972, **3,** 323-330.

PIHIBLAD, C.T., & McNamara, R.L. Social adjustment of elderly people in three small towns. In H. Rose and W. Peterson (Eds.), *Older people and their social world.* Philadelphia: F.A. Davis, 1965.

QUILITCH, H.R. Purposeful activity increased on a geriatric ward through programmed recreation. *Journal of American Geriatrics Society,* 1974, **22,** 226-229.

RAGHEB, M.G., & Beard, J.G. Leisure satisfaction: Concept, theory, and measurement. In S. Iso-Ahola (Ed.), *Social psychological perspectives on leisure and recreation.* Springfield, IL: Charles C. Thomas, 1980.

RAY, R.O. The LSI—Form A as applied to older adults: Technical note on scoring patterns. *Journal of American Geriatrics Society,* 1979, **27,** 418-420.

RITCHI, J.R. On the derivation of leisure activity types—A perceptual mapping approach. *Journal of Leisure Research,* 1975, **7,** 128-140.

ROSE, A. A current theoretical issue in social gerontology. *Gerontologist,* 1964, **4,** 46-50.

ROSOW, I. Adjustment of the normal aged. In R. Williams (Ed.), *Processes of aging* (vol. 2). New York: Atherton Press, 1963.

ROSOW, I. *Social integration of the aged.* New York: Free Press, 1967.

SALTZ, R. Aging persons as child-care workers in a foster grandparent program: Psychosocial efforts and work performance. *Aging and Human Development,* 1971, **2,** 314-340.

SAMUELSON, R.J. Aging America—Who will shoulder the growing burden? *National Journal,* 1978 (October), 18-24.

SIMPSON, I.H., & McKinney, J.C. (Eds.) *Social aspects of aging.* Durham, NC: Duke University Press, 1966.

SPIRDUSO, W.W. Reaction and movement time as a function of age and physical activity level. *Journal of Gerontology,* 1975, **30,** 435-440.

THOMPSON, G. Work versus leisure roles: An investigation of morale among employed and retired men. *Journal of Gerontology,* 1973, **28,** 339-344.

TOBIN, S.S., & Neugarten, B.L. Life satisfaction and social interaction in aging. *Journal of Gerontology,* 1961, **16,** 344-346.

TOSELAND, M., & Sykes, J. Senior citizens center participation and other correlates of life satisfaction. *The Gerontologist,* 1977, **17,** 235-241.

TOSELAND, R., & Rasch, J. Factors contributing to older person's satisfaction with their communities. *The Gerontologist,* 1978, **4,** 395-401.

WINTERS, R. Relationship between job satisfaction and leisure satisfaction. (Doctoral dissertation, State University of New York at Buffalo, 1973). *Dissertation Abstracts International,* 1973, **34,** 3077 A-3078A.

SECTION 4:
Theory and Research in Motor Development

Understanding movement is basic to understanding humans. Nearly all human behavior can be traced to movement. Because adapted physical activity relies on movement, it was not surprising that many speakers at the Symposium addressed theoretical and research considerations related to movement. Jean Pyfer shares her observations of factors affecting motor development and causing delays. After reading her article, many of your questions about developmental topics, including reflex inhibition, vestibular functioning, and ocular control, will be answered. In a similar style, Walter Davis will guide us through an approach to perceptual-motor learning that balances the development of the child with environmental events.

In their articles dealing with generalization, first Fait and then Auxter ask us to look at our training programs with a skeptical eye. Are we using appropriate measurement tests? Are our training programs working? When the handicapped learn our programs, can they use the learned skills in the world of work or the world of leisure?

Stein concludes the section with an engineering feat. He helps us to understand how to build a bridge over bad programs, apathy, and irrelevance, by using information from research and clearer conceptualization.

Factors Affecting Motor Development Delays

Jean Pyfer
Texas Woman's University

The developmentally delayed child is that youngster who fails to demonstrate normal cognitive and psychomotor milestones of growth. These are the children who for some reason do not mature neurologically to the point where they can function as efficiently as their normal peers. I do not mean to imply that all developmentally delayed children cannot mature neurologically, rather, experience has taught us that these children, if left to their own timetables, will not progress through all stages of sequential development. Those who miss but a few steps will, in later life, demonstrate very subtle motor delays. Those who fail to develop major sequential developmental building blocks will evidence a large number of movement inabilities. Fortunately, a growing body of research suggests these children can mature and function efficiently if their delays are recognized early and if appropriate intervention strategies are initiated. Ability to assess accurately and facilitate development of the delayed child has improved dramatically during the last decade.

For the last 15 years I have worked with developmentally delayed children who were labeled as trainable or educable mentally retarded, learning-disabled, emotionally disturbed, hyperactive, or just clumsy. The first 5 of those years I spent trying to improve children's motor functioning levels by applying learning theories that were plentiful in the 1960s. After failing in most cases to produce significant changes, I turned to observing children's developmental patterns and attempted to conceptualize a model of the hierarchical sequences through which they progressed as they grew and matured. It took 2 years to design a model that seemed to reflect normal stages through which children need to pass in order to perform motor patterns efficiently. That tentative model is shown in Figure 1.

We have spent the last 8 years testing and observing developmentally delayed children in trying to determine which sensory input systems affect integration and output levels of performance, and how perceptual-motor integration delays affect motor output performance.

To help assess the model we completed a study in 1977 that analyzed the motor performance of 262 learning-disabled children (Pyfer & Alley, Note 1). After statistically analyzing test results from the Lincoln Oseretsky Motor Development Scale, Fiorentino Reflex Test, Purdue Perceptual Motor Survey, Frostig Developmental Vision Test, vestibular and tactile portions of the Southern California Battery of Sensory Integration Tests, and refractive and orthoptic visual test results plus extensive medical, family, and educational histories, we found that the children demonstrated three clearly distinct motor profiles. Twenty-six of the children performed at or above normal standards on all of the perceptual-motor tests. Seventeen of the children exhibited motor performance 2 to 3 years below peer expectations on all tests; that is, their motor performance profiles were depressed in all areas tested. The remaining 210 subjects exhibited a very jagged motor profile. They matched or exceeded age standards on some categories of performance, but failed to achieve normative standards in other areas. In that study we identified a number of performances that grouped together in predictable factors for each group. We are in the process of replicating that study now with data from an additional 150 children. The outstanding fact we learned from the 1977 study was that children's motor development patterns evolve in a consistent pattern but the profile of one developmentally delayed child will not necessarily match that of all children with delays. For that reason, it is necessary for us to observe each child individually and draw conclusions about where developmentally that child is functioning. My intent in this chapter is to share my research findings and observations from the last 10 years. I will discuss characteristic motor development patterns, sensory and neurological components that contribute to motor function, behaviors that characterize specific sensory and neurological delays, and evidence to support these observations.

Motor Output	Running, jumping, hopping	Skipping, galloping, throwing	Catching, kicking, writing
Perceptual-Motor Integration	Laterality Directionality Bilaterial integration		Body image Visual tracking Spatial awareness
Sensory Input	Reflexes Vestibular Kinetheses		Tactile Refractive vision Orthoptic vision

Figure 1—Stages necessary for efficient motor performance.

Characteristic Developmental Patterns of the Young Child

During the first year of life a child is a reactive agent. That is, automatic, built-in, reactions to stimuli dictate the child's movement responses. A series of reflexes enables children to lift their heads, balance on all fours, grasp objects, and turn their heads toward an outstretched hand. At this time the physical control of the child's movement is centered in the lower portions of the central nervous system (CNS). Reflex arcs are mediated at the spinal cord, brain stem, and midbrain levels. Children are able to lift their heads, roll over, sit, and eventually stand only if environmental demands and neurological integrity permits the stimulus-response to occur.

By the end of the first year cortical control is beginning to develop. The child, though somewhat nearsighted, can use both eyes in unison and eventually can visually track moving objects with ease. The auditory system has matured, and the child can grasp and release objects at will, can stand and, in most cases, can walk. These functions are possible only if the CNS has been stimulated enough to permit development of motor pathways from the spinal cord through the cortical level.

During the ages of 1 to 4 years the ability to walk, run, and jump develops and matures. By age 4 years the brain is 90% of adult weight and the shaping of the cerebral cortex is complete. Mylination of nerve fibers connecting the cerebral cortex to the cerebellum enables the child to begin to progress from jerky, staccato movement patterns to more fluid, rhythmical motions. Motor control develops in cephalo-caudal and proximo-distal directions; that is, control of the head precedes control of the trunk and legs, and control of the trunk precedes control of the arms, hands, and fingers. This directional progression must occur to enable the child to move about with ease and to use the hands with facility.

From ages 4 to 8 years movement capability is more closely related to physiological maturation than to chronological age. During ages 4 to 8 all basic locomotor skills mature from poorly integrated to finely coordinated patterns. Normally developing children become very competent during this time. They can separate head and trunk motion plus demonstrate enough body stability to work very capably and efficiently with their hands.

The careful observer can determine neurophysiological development normality by observing the child's movement during these years. The developmentally delayed child often demonstrates some fairly evident abnormal motor behaviors. For instance, it is not uncommon for these children to be described as awkward and clumsy. They trip and fall often, and do not judge accurately the location of moving projectiles. They often are unable to catch and throw efficiently. As a result of their ineptitude, they usually attempt to avoid playing with peers; instead, they seek out the companionship of younger children or adults. With careful observation, many of these abnormal patterns can be identified with and related directly to poorly developed sensory-motor systems. Once the underlying cause has been discovered, appropriate intervention can relieve or eliminate the dysfunctioning systems. In the next section I will discuss some sensory and neurological components that affect motor development.

Sensory and Neurological Components Affecting Motor Development

The predominating neuromuscular system during the first year of life is that which controls primitive reflexes. Primitive reflexes are automatic reactions that enable the child to lift the head, prop up on two hands, turn the face toward the extended hand, assume an all-fours position, and eventually crawl. Most of these reflexes are under muscle spindle control; that is, when a given set of muscle spindles are activated through stretch or contraction of adjacent muscle fibers, an electrical impulse is fired and projected over the sensory nerve to the spinal cord, brain stem, or midbrain where it synapses with a motor neuron. The impulse is then projected over the motor neuron to a muscle group, and once contact with the motor endplate is made, a muscle contraction results in an automatic movement.

Other primitive reflexes are under control of the labyrinthine portion of the inner ear. When a child moves his or her head against gravity, the labyrinthine is activated and a neuronal impulse is sent to a muscle group. The muscles, in turn, contract and cause movement. Should any of these primitive reflexes fail to develop at the proper time, the child is unable to demonstrate movement patterns expected at that age and also will be limited in further movement development. That is, children who cannot lift their heads will not learn to control head movement, which will limit their ability to sit, stand, and eventually walk.

Primitive reflex action tends to promote development of the neuromuscular system. As these pathways and muscles are used and developed, control of higher levels of the CNS is facilitated. As higher control levels are developed, the primitive reflexes are phased out, so to speak. We never actually lose the reflexes; they are simply layered over and suppressed by higher control centers. An example of cases in which primitive reflexes are not suppressed is cerebral palsy. All of us have observed the many extraneous movement of the individual with severe cerebral palsy involvement. What you are observing are primitive reflexes in action. The cerebral palsied individual's voluntary motor control center has been damaged, and as a result, primitive reflexes that are controlled by lower centers of the CNS are not suppressed. Presence of these primitive reflexes grossly limit the cerebral palsied individual's ability to control movement patterns. But not all individuals who demonstrate primitive reflexes are cerebral palsied. Some simply have developmental delays that interfere with advanced motor control.

Primitive reflexes that persist beyond the first year of life can be identified by checking a child in supine, prone, and all-fours positions. From a supine position, a 4-year-old child should be able to get into a flexed position such as wrapping the arms around the flexed knees, and hold that position for 4 or 5 seconds. The 5-year-old child should be able to hold that position for 10 seconds. From a prone position, the 4- or 5-year-old child should be able to lift and hold the upper trunk off the floor momentarily. By placing 5-year-old children on all-fours and pushing their heads down, we can watch for reactions in the upper limbs. Should the arms tend to flex, we know that the symmetrical tonic neck may not have phased out yet. Also, observe children as they move. A tendency to run or hop stiff-legged could be indication of primitive reflex persistence.

Children should begin to show equilibrium reflexes near the end of the first year of life. As their name suggests, equilibrium reactions affect our ability to maintain balance, particularly moving balance. During movement, as our center of gravity shifts over our base of support, equilibrium reflexes enable us to alter our posture in such a way that we are able to remain in an upright position. Equilibrium reflex development is necessary if a child is to control movement while running, jumping, hopping, and performing other active movement patterns. Most of these reactions also are activated by muscle spindles; however, mediation between the sensory impulse and the motor neuron occurs at the cortical level. The child who does not develop equilibrium reflexes is clumsy and tends to fall often. They also have difficulty with any agility movements requiring sudden shifts in direction.

A sensory system closely aligned with reflexes is the semicircular canal of the inner ear—what most people call the vestibular system. Sensory receptors in the semicircular canals react to rotary and linear motions of the head. The sensory impulses are sent over the eighth cranial nerve to the cerebellum and the brain stem. Impulses from the vestibular system to the brain stem make multisynaptic connections with nerves that lead down the spinal cord and affect equilibrium reactions, with motor nerves that control eye movement, and with nerves that lead to the somatosensory portion of the cerebral cortex. Vestibular input is necessary for static and dynamic balance development, eye tracking ability, and motor planning. Children who are slow to develop good vestibular functioning are delayed in all gross motor patterns requiring coordination of both sides of the body, ability to maintain held postures, eye-hand coordination, and fine motor control.

Vestibular development can be ascertained by observing a child's balance ability. A 3-year-old child who cannot walk a 10-foot line heel to toe or a 4-year-old who cannot maintain balance on a low balance beam may be experiencing vestibular delay. A 5-year-old should be able to stand on one foot with eyes open for 10 seconds and eyes closed for five seconds. The 6-year-old improves in ability to balance with eyes closed for 7 seconds. The 7-year-old should be able to balance on one foot, eyes open or closed, for 10 seconds. Any wide discrepancy between expected performance with eyes closed may be an indication that the vestibular system is not developing on schedule.

Vision, often thought to be the most important sensory input system for cognitive development, also plays a major role in motor function. Of primary importance to efficient movement is orthoptic vision—the ability to move the eyes in unison for good depth perception. Should the extra-ocular muscles that control movements of the eye not be equally balanced, one or both eyes will deviate from the intended direction. Imbalances of this sort almost always interfere with depth perception judgments; in turn, poor depth perception results in poor hand-eye and foot-eye coordination. To determine the efficiency of children's orthoptic vision, observe them while they are performing hand-eye or foot-eye coordination tasks. The child with orthoptic problems will demonstrate immature catching patterns, will miss a ball or strike it off-center when attempting to kick, will descend steps one at a time, and will often avoid climbing apparatus altogether.

Over the years I have been fascinated with the fact that children with reflex delays often demonstrate both vestibular delays and depth perception difficulties. The neurological literature along with some of our studies have clarified these relationships somewhat. In the first place, the vestibular portion of the inner ear develops during the first trimester of pregnancy. In a study we completed in 1978, we examined the pregnancy history and birth records of 108 children with motor delays (Marker, 1980) in looking for some clue as to why these children had delayed development. One important fact that surfaced was a significant portion of the mothers of these children were X-rayed during the first trimester of pregnancy. Possible fetal vestibular damage as a result of the X-ray might explain the children's later balance difficulties. Beyond that evidence we can look to the multisynaptic connections of the vestibular system with other neurons in the brain stem. Vestibular impulses sent down the spinal cord are known to override and alter reflex mediations at the lower levels, so it could be that if the vestibular signals are weak and/or poorly formed, primitive reflexes may be expressed rather than suppressed. Vestibular impulses sent to the extra-ocular muscles of the eyes facilitate positioning of the eyes in relation to the angle the head is held. Once again, inadequate or inappropriate vestibular signals could delay development of muscular control of the eyes.

Hand-eye coordination may be delayed in the child with vestibular dysfunction because of the difficulty with visual control; some neurological literature suggests, however, that as long as an individual has to consciously work on controlling balance (rather than having it automatically controlled by the vestibular system), the CNS does not have time to attend to fine motor control (Quiros & Schrager, 1979). The relationships between vestibular, reflex and visual-motor development is an area where a tremendous amount of solid research is needed.

The ability to determine internally where in space the limbs are located is known as kinesthesis or kinesthetic sense. When we move our limbs we activate kinesthetic receptors located primarily in the joints of the body. These impulses are sent to the somatosensory portion of the brain where spatial maps are then constructed. Tactile and vestibular impulses merge with the kinesthetic impulses in the somatosensory portion of the cerebrum. Together, these three sensory input systems program the voluntary motor control portion of the brain. Should either vestibular, kinesthetic, or tactile impulses fail to reach the somatosensory area, motor planning is severely impaired. Kinesthetic function is thought to be evidenced when a child attempts to move the arms into held positions, for instance, level with the shoulders, or when they attempt to perform tasks like "angels-in-the-snow." Inaccurate positionings often are indicators of delayed kinesthetic functioning. Hypotonia is also believed to be directly related to poor kinesthetic discrimination.

The tactile system enables us to determine where our bodies end and space begins and to discriminate between a variety of textures. We have worked with some hyperactive children who were unable to tolerate tactile stimuli. These individuals, known as "tactile defensive," exhibit a strong dislike for being touched or held and for having to remain seated for any length of time. Because tests for tactile defensiveness are limited in validity and reliability, I often depend more on observation and parent report rather than standardized test results. These children seldom initiate touch and physically withdraw when they are touched. Parents report that from the time the child was born, he or she squirmed when held, avoided some textures of food, and refused to sit still. We believe these children are not integrating tactile stimulation, probably because of a delay in development of the reticular system that overlies the brain stem and midbrain.

All of these neurological systems have a dramatic role in developing motor control. The relationships among and between the systems, though complex, are becoming increasingly clearer. As I have indicated, careful observation will usually help the teacher determine which sensory-motor areas are failing to develop normally. Once we determine where delays are occurring, we can select appropriate activities to facilitate neuromuscular development.

In working with a learning-disabled population, we have found that once you are successful in facilitating sensory input and perceptual-motor integration performance, those children not only will demonstrate normal motor output function, but will continue to develop further at the same rate and level as their peers (Broxterman & Stebbins, 1981; McLaughlin, 1980). Even adults have been found to respond favorably to a sensory-input stimulation program (Nobles, 1980). We have some evidence that children not provided with a specific intervention program will continue to perform below standard as they grow older (Lassman, 1981); that is, youngsters with sensory motor delays will not just outgrow the problem.

Our present studies are aimed at attempting to determine causative factors for motor development delays as well as to verify groupings of abnormal behavior patterns. Until we can pinpoint causes and eradicate those factors causing motor delays, the responsibility for promoting the growth and development of these children rests with those of us trained in motor development facilitation. If we have the needed skills and knowledge about developmental sequences, we can help developmentally delayed children gain mastery over their motor performance.

The observant professional can determine whether sensory systems and/or perceptual-motor integration processes have developed or whether maturational delays are interfering with motor function. Once the cause of the motor delay has been identified, we can intervene consistently with appropriate activities, persisting until a child shows improvement. Developmentally delayed children can grow and develop if they are provided a stimulating environment geared to their specific needs. Once they acquire the basic structures needed for more advanced movement patterns, they will develop higher functioning levels.

Reference Note

1. Pyfer, J.L., & Alley, G. *Sensory-perceptual-motor dysfunction of learning disabled children.* Presentation at First World Congress on Future Special Education, Stirling, Scotland, 1978.

References

BROXTERMAN, J., & Stebbins, A.L. The significance of visual training in the treatment of learning disabilities. *American Corrective Therapy Journal,* Sept.-Oct. 1981.

LASSMAN, S.L. *Follow-up study of untreated perceptual-motor dysfunctional children.* Unpublished master's thesis, University of Kansas, 1981.

MARKER, M.A. *Influence of perinatal factors on perceptual-motor function.* unpublished master's thesis, University of Kansas, 1980.

MCLAUGHLIN, E. Follow-up study on children remediated for perceptual-motor dysfunction at the University of Kansas perceptual-motor clinic. (University of Oregon, 1980.) *Microfische.*

NOBLES, L.B. The effects of vestibular stimulation on congenitally blind adults. (Eugene: University of Oregon, 1980.) *Microfische.*

QUIROS, J.B., & Schrager, O.L. *Neuropsychological fundamentals in learning disabilities.* San Rafael, CA: Academic Therapy Publications, 1979.

An Ecological Approach to Perceptual-Motor Learning

Walter E. Davis
Kent State University

It is recognized that perception and movement relate, but the exact nature of this relationship is little understood. Traditionally, the two systems have been considered as functionally separate entities tied by a linear, causal relationship. In this view, the senses serve as passive channels through which sense data (input) flows over the central nervous system to be compared with memory, integrated, organized, or in some other way processed in order to arrive at a percept. From this sensory-perceptual process, information is derived for directing or controlling action (output).

An alternative approach, however, holds that perception and action are functionally inseparable, that one process cannot be understood without implicating the other. This approach is an ecological one, as championed by James J. Gibson (1966; 1979) and his followers and is radically different from the traditional way of thinking. From this view, the relationship between perception and action is one of mutual compatibility and mutual constraint rather than linear causality. As a result of this belief, we need to reformulate many traditional concepts.

Presented here, from the ecological perspective, are three concepts regarding the relationship of perception and action. First, perception is redefined as a direct pickup of information rather than as a linear processing constructive procedure. Further, information is described in animal-relevant rather than animal-neutral terms. Second, following Gibson (1966) and Lee (1978), perceptual information required in the planning and the regulating of movement is reclassified. Third, a brief review of how the perceptual systems function in obtaining information for action is given, emphasizing the primacy of vision. Finally, by way of summary we consider ways of moving toward a reclassification of perceptual-motor deficits from an ecological perspective.

Redefinition of Perception

At issue is the central question of how humans gain knowledge of their world. Traditionally, it is held that the world is given only as punctate stimuli, a molecular level description as given by physics. For example, the predicates of visual perception often are given in terms of light intensities and wave lengths. Having reduced the world to particles, it is then necessary to "put it back together again" in order to arrive at a percept. This humpty-dumpty type of procedure is said to be performed by mental processes. Thus, the meaning of objects and events is provided by the mind, and consequently, people are considered logically separate from their environment. Perception, in this view, is a constructive process by which a percept is built up from smaller units. It is a chain of cause-and-effect relationships beginning with the world and ending in a percept (Fitch & Turvey, 1978).

By contrast, from an ecological perspective, perception is considered a process of directly obtaining meaning from one's environment. People are functionally inseparable from their environment. In explanations of perception, the objects and events in the environment are described in animal-relevant terms—that is, according to what they afford the animal, whether for good or for bad. Thus, for example, an object is said to be "reachable," "graspable," "throwable," etc. Such an object has meaning to the perceiver but this meaning cannot be part of either the perceiver alone or the object alone. Meaning is a property of both perceivers and their environment—the ecosystem. We shall return to this point later, but for now let us consider more carefully the variables for perception.

It is true that light is necessary for visual perception and can be described in terms of intensities and wavelengths, and that these variables relate to photosensitive cells located in the eye-neural system. However, such a description of the visual-sensory processes is at one level and a description of visually perceiving an apple (or other object) is at a different level. From an ecological perspective the two descriptions cannot relate causally (Shaw & Turvey, in press). There are not first photons, then wavelengths, then patterns of the light. These events occur simultaneously. Therefore, a description of the light as given by physics does not relate causally to the object which patterns light. Rather, physics provides the support for the functionally defined properties of the environment (Shaw & Bransford, 1977; Shaw & Turvey, in press). It is these functionally defined properties that are of primary concern here in our discussion of perception and following are examples of how information is extracted from the environment.

Again using visual perception as an example, we note that optical information[1] is information which is extracted from a "flowing ambient optic array" (Gibson, 1979). An array means having an arrangement and ambient means surrounding. The light which surrounds an observer is structured by the objects from which it reflects and thus contains information specific to those objects. Both the light, as a medium, and the object, as a source, are required for visual perception. To underscore these points, we recognize that in homogeneous darkness (i.e., without light) there is no visual perception; likewise, in homogeneous light, that is, in which light is not structured by objects, as in the case of heavy fog, there is also no visual perception.

Consider as examples of directly obtainable information ecological laws regarding visual detection of locomotion and object motion. For purposes of illustration one can imagine the walls of the room as the ambient optic array. As we locomote, the edges of our field of view will sweep over the array causing it to flow. As we move forward, the walls of the room move backward, that is, the optic array flows outward specifying approach. As we move backward, the inflow of the optic array specifies retreat. This is always the case, whether we sample the array from the front, side, or back and whether we move actively or passively. Those who have witnessed cinematography presented on 360-degree screens can attest to this fact. This procedure simulates visual information specifying locomotion.

Now consider object motion as distinct from locomotion. Whereas in locomotor activity the total optic array is transformed, in object motion only a part of the array is disrupted. For example, when an object moves across one's visual field, some background (optic array) is covered up (deleted) and reappears (is accreted) again. This partial disruption specifies not only the motion of the object but the direction of that motion. Deletion of part of the array occurs on the side toward which the

---

[1]The term information is not used to mean a message between a sender and a receiver as in the traditional usage. It is used, unfortunately, for lack of a better term. See Gibson (1979) for an elaboration of optical information.

object is moving and accretion occurs on the opposite side. If the rate of deletion is equal to accretion, then the object is moving exactly parallel with one's visual field. An asymetrical deletion and accretion specifies that the object is more or less moving toward or away from the observer; the degree depends on the ratio of deletion to accretion and the side on which they are occurring. Symmetrical contraction, equal accretion on all sides of the object, specifies that the object is moving directly away from the perceiver. On the other hand, symmetrical expansion of the object specifies an object coming toward the observer and the rate of expansion is specific to the time of collision (Lee, 1976). This information is used in catching and diving, and can be picked up at an early age (Schiff, 1965).

It is the case then that information (in Gibsonian terms) is available directly and specifies objects and events. It is not the case that this relevant information is so easily described as it might seem from the examples just given. The challenge for researchers in the area of perceptual motor ability in special populations is to describe the information attended to by persons with varying handicapping conditions as they act in their environment.

In preceding paragraphs, we have described some of the environmental properties in animal-functional terms. However, to complete the mutual compatibility picture we must also describe the activities of the animal in environment-functional terms. Although space here does not allow for an elaboration on this point, it is acknowledged, in an ecological approach that the specific capabilities and needs of the animal constrain those activities in which it engages, as well as the fact that the specific combination of the environmental properties provide constraints on what is afforded for animal activity. Perceptual information, then, not only is specific to the object or event and describable in perceiver-related terms, (i.e., affordances); perceptual information also is specific to the perceiver. Thus, for example, objects that afford grasping for an adult may not afford grasping for an infant. Further, an object cannot be described as graspable unless there is an animal which can be described as a grasper.

Although the specific environmental properties are a constraint on what information is available for the perceiver, it is also the case that the specific properties of the perceiver—its capabilities and needs—constrain what information is extracted. Therefore, the act of perception is a function of both the environment and the perceiver. The percept of graspability, then, is a property of both the *object* and the perceiver, a property of the ecosystem. This concept of mutual compatibility and mutual constraint between animal and its environment has been stressed because it underlies the ecological approach. This mutual compatibility concept also applies to the relationship between perception and action. From this perspective we describe in more detail how perceptual information constrains activities.

Reclassification of Information for Planning and Regulating Movement

Fundamental to an understanding of perception is an understanding of movement. Perception is that which is experienced in "the exploratory activity of looking around, getting around, and looking at things." (Gibson, 1979, p. 147) What we perceive constrains what we do and what we do constrains what we perceive. As Gibson well recognized, it is advantageous if not absolutely necessary for a person to move in order to improve perception and that perception in turn guides that movement. For example, in seeing that an opening affords passing through, one moves toward it; in approaching, more precise perceptual information as to the passability of the opening is gained and allows for guidance toward the opening; and as one passes through, one perceives that passing through is achieved. It is in this way that perception and action combine as functional effects determined by their complementary relationship (Shaw & Turvey, in press). In this sense, the perceptual information provides the context or the constraints for actions. As such, information may be classified as three types required in the planning and the regulating of movement (Lee, 1978).

Exteroceptive information is about the layout of the environment and about external objects and events described relative to the perceiver and is information for planning movement. *Proprioceptive information* is about the position, orientation, and movement of the body parts relative to the body and is information for controlling movement. A third type of information recognized by Gibson (1958) and formally described by Lee (1978) is *exproprioceptive information*. This is information about the position, orientation, and movement of the body as a whole, or parts of the body, relative to the environment. The distinction between proprioceptive and exproprioceptive information can easily be made by considering the flight of a bird against the wind. Information about the movements of the limbs is provided through the muscle and joint receptors, but does not specify total body movement in the relationship to the ground. The latter is exproprioceptive information which is obtained through the visual system. Such information is for both planning and controlling movement.

What is important to recognize in this reclassification is that it is *types of information* that are described rather than types of sensory receptors as in the classical view. For example, eyes and ears are generally considered as exteroceptors and the muscle-joint receptors are relegated as proprioceptors. It can be argued, as does Lee (1978) rather convincingly, that this latter classification is misleading. The perceptual systems as described by Gibson (1966) are capable of providing all types of information. Further, it is argued that vision is primary in providing all three types of information and thus is the most powerful in planning and in controlling movement. To bolster this claim, we shall consider each perceptual system and how it functions to pick up exteroceptive, proprioceptive, and exproprioceptive information.

Perceptual Systems in Planning and Controlling Movement

Although here each perceptual system is considered separately in its act of picking up information, it is important to recognize that the perceptual systems function not only solely but more often concurrently. The information obtained by the perceptual systems may be equivalent (redundant) or equivocal (contradictory). In most natural situations it is equivalent. However, under some circumstances, usually contrived, information from different systems does conflict.

The somatosensory system, unlike the other systems, has receptor cells over the entire body. Through active or exploratory touch an abundance of information is obtainable. This is especially true of the hands because they perform many different tasks and in so doing gather exteroceptive information about the shape and texture of objects that are manipulated. They also pick up proprioceptive information. Proprioceptive information also comes through the muscle and articular receptors which allow one to detect limb position in absence of vision.

The somatosensory system is also exproprioceptive as touch permits you to gather information about your relationship to the environment. The vestibular system is solely exproprioceptive. It registers both linear and rotary changes in movement (i.e., acceleration and deceleration) of the head during both passive and active conditions, but it is not sensitive to constant motion. The vestibular system is active in providing information for the control of balance; as will be demonstrated later, however, its role is not a dominant one. The vestibular system does function in cooperation with the visual system through reflex connections in coordinating movements of the eyes and head. Thus, when the joint, muscle, somatosensory and vestibular systems are taken together as the haptic system, it is trimodal—that is, it picks up all three types of information.

The auditory system is clearly trimodal. Exteroceptively, it functions to pick up information about the direction of an event, (i.e., where the sound is coming from), thus aiding orientation toward that event. Auditory exteroceptive information also helps to identify the nature of the event. When you speak, the auditory system picks up proprioceptive information allowing for the control of speech. Evidence to this fact is that congenitally deaf persons experience difficulty in acquiring voice control which will allow them to speak clearly.

The auditory system is also exproprioceptive as demonstrated by echo perception (Rice, 1967). Although the human auditory apparatus is not as effective a sonar system as the one found in some bats, humans, both blind and sighted, are capable of projecting their voices and receiving information about their location relative to the environment. Thus, as shown, the auditory system is trimodal.

With the exception of the auditory system in detecting verbal communication, the visual system is the most powerful exteroceptive sense (Lee, 1978). Information about the environment gathered through sight is indeed very rich, and few people would disagree. Lee (1978) argues that vision is the most powerful proprioceptive and exproprioceptive sense, as well. You can easily compare the visual and haptic systems in the pickup of proprioceptive information by stretching your arms forward and then touching your index fingers together with and without the use of vision.

Exproprioceptively, the superiority of the visual system in controlling movement is shown both experimentally and practically. Lee and his colleagues (Lee & Aronson, 1974; Lee & Lishman, 1975) cleverly devised experiments demonstrating the power of vision in controlling balance. They constructed a "swinging room" — a large, bottomless box suspended just above the floor. When the walls moved horizontally forward, the visual information specified to the subjects standing stationary in the room was that the subjects themselves were moving in the opposite direction. The illustration given earlier is recalled. Lee and Aronson (1974) placed infants in the room and when the walls moved backward the visual information specified to the subjects that they were falling forward. This promoted an unconscious compensatory adjustment in their stance. The children leaned backward and because they had in fact not been falling forward, they lost their balance and fell backward.

Even more dramatically, visual control was demonstrated with adults standing in the room (Lee & Lishman, 1975). The walls were oscillated horizontally for a distance of 6 mm. The subjects oscillated in conjunction with the room and did so without any conscious awareness. Thus, even though the vestibular, muscular, joint, and somatosensory systems provided information specifying stable upright standing, the visual system specified movement on which both infants and adults appeared to rely. These experiments demonstrate the primacy of visual information for controlling movement.

Practical experience tells one that during the learning of any motor skills, visual cues are superior to cues from other modalities. For example, when you first learn to dribble a basketball, vision is used primarily to guide the hands in controlling the bouncing ball. Indeed, in nearly all experiences of initially learning a motor skill, vision is the primary source of control.

All perceptual systems are important in acquiring information for movement activities. It would seem, however, from the evidence presented here, that vision is the most important. We would quickly point out, though, in particular with regard to perceptual-motor deficiency, that any perceptual system — haptic, auditory, or visual — is capable alone of picking up information necessary in the planning and the controlling of movement.

Summary

In the preceding pages we have described, albeit briefly, some of the important concepts in an ecological approach to perceptual-motor learning. By way of summary we consider, again briefly, how these concepts might begin to move us toward a reclassification of perceptual-motor deficits.

In the ecological approach, perception and action are processes of the ecosystem, that is, the animal-environment synergy. Likewise, deficiencies in perceptual-motor performance also are properties of the ecosystem and cannot be attributed to either the environment or the animal alone. The implication is that an understanding of a perceptual-motor deficit entails three descriptions, one of the animal in environment-related terms, one of the environment in animal-related terms, and one of the relationship between the two. Yet, in contrast, the traditional approach is to identify the deficit as if it were a property of the animal to the near total exclusion of environmental considerations. Thus, the traditional labels of learning-disabled, mentally retarded, cerebral palsied, etc., are attached to the individual regardless of the context under which these individuals function. Such an individual is seen as possessing these characteristics. Thus, one *is* learning-disabled. Instead, we suggest that one must conceptualize labeling as a process of describing the environmental circumstances under which the individual normally operates, the changing relationship between the individual and his or her environment, as well as a description of particular characteristics of the individual.

The practice of attaching categorical labels to the person is not surprising given the traditional approach to understanding perceptual-motor deficiencies, which is to do the analysis on the person. More specifically, in an attempt to locate the source of a deficit, search is conducted almost exclusively in parts of the central nervous system (e.g., Ayres, 1974; Geschwind, 1975). The traditional approach, then, is an attempt to tie overt behavior causally to specific anatomical sites within the nervous system. Such practices persist in the clinical fields in spite of the tremendous requirements, as amply pointed out by Grimm and Nashner (1979), which would seemingly thwart such a project.

> Appreciating that a stationary neurologic deficit represents what is 'left over' after compensation is completed, a second point is that the dimen-

sions of the deficit represent the best mix of systems, their redundancy and the limitations they impose on performance are necessary baseline studies before making a functional correlation between a lesion and motor disturbance. (Grimm & Nashner, 1979, p. 74)

From an ecological perspective, the role of the nervous system in the processes of perception and action takes on quite a different form. Activity at the level of neurons provides causal support for overt behavior but does not relate to that behavior in a linear causal manner. The nervous system is not seen as being solely responsible for the organization and control of perception and action (cf, Kelso & Tuller, 1981). Neural action is necessary for behavior to occur in a manner analogous to a telescope which allows one to see a distant star. The nervous system and telescope are the medium but in neither case is linear causality to be inferred.

The practice of classifying perceptual motor deficits in relation to the anatomical site of the lesion within the nervous system falls short in providing the proper understanding of the deficiency and has often led to confusion and conflict, as in the case of the classification schemes in cerebral palsies and apraxias (cf, Roy, 1978). Using the anatomical approach one has difficulty in explaining, for example, why, in what is called frontal apraxia (Geschwind, 1975), the patient is rarely able to perform habit skills (e.g., making the sign of the cross) at the clinician's request but is able to do so in the proper context (e.g., in a church).

From an ecological approach, the context of the movement must always be duly considered in a description of perceptual-motor performance. Or, perhaps it is more accurate to say that the several "nested" contexts, from the immediate environment to the community environment to the larger societal environment, all must be considered (see Bronfenbrenner, 1979, for an elaboration). Each context serves to constrain the other and together they provide constraints on perceptual motor performance. To reiterate, then, a description of the environments in terms of their functional relationship with the individual, a description of the individual relative to the environment, and a description of the relationship between individuals and their environment is required in order to fully describe perceptual motor deficits. Such a task is formidable, indeed, but is necessary if real advances in the theory and practice of perceptual-motor learning are to be made.

References

AYRES, A.J. *Sensory integration and learning disabilities.* Los Angeles: Western Psychological Services, 1974.

BRONFENBRENNER, U. *The ecology of human movement.* Cambridge, MA: Harvard University Press, 1979.

FITCH, H., & Turvey, M.T. On the control of activity: Some remarks from an ecological point of view. In D. Landers and R. Christina (Eds.), *Psychology of motor behavior and sport,* Champaign, IL: Human Kinetics Publishers, 1978.

GESCHWIND, N. The apraxias: Neural mechanisms of disorders of learned movements. *American Scientist,* 1975, **63,** 188-195.

GIBSON, J.J. Visually controlled locomotion and visual orientation in animals. *British Journal of Psychology,* 1958, **49,** 182-194.

GIBSON, J.J. *The senses considered as perceptual systems* Boston: Houghton-Mifflin, 1966.

GIBSON, J.J. *The ecological approach to visual perception.* Boston: Houghton-Mifflin, 1979.

GRIMM, R.J., & Nashner, L.M. Long loop dyscontrol. In E. Desmedt (Ed.), Cerebral control in man: Long loop mechanisms. *Progress in clinical neurophysiology,* 1979, **4,** 70-84.

KELSO, J.A., & Tuller, B. Towards a theory of apractic syndromes. *Brain and Language,* 1981, **12,** 224-245.

LEE, D.N. A theory of visual control of breaking based on information about time to collision. *Perception,* 1976, **5,** 437-459.

LEE, D.N. On the function of vision. In H. Pick and J. Saltzman (Eds.), *Modes of perceiving and processing information.* Hillsdale, NJ: Erlbaum Press, 1978.

LEE, D.N., & Aronson, E. Visual Proprioceptive control of standing in human infants. *Perception and Psychophysics,* 1974, **15,** 529-532.

LEE, D.N., & Lishman, J.R. Visual proprioceptive control of stance. *Journal of Human Movement Studies,* 1975, **1,** 87-95.

RICE, C.E. Human echo perception. *Science,* 1967, **155,** 656-664.

ROY, E.A. Apraxia: A new look at an old syndrome. *Journal of Human Movement Studies,* 1978, **4,** 191-210.

SCHIFF, W. Perception of impending collisions. *Psychological Monographs,* 1965, **79**(604), 1-26.

SHAW, R.E., & Bransford, J. Introduction: Psychological approaches to the problems of knowledge. In R.E. Shaw and J. Bransford (Eds.), *Perceiving, acting, and knowing: Toward an ecological psychology.* Hillsdale, NJ: Erlbaum Associates, 1977.

SHAW, R.E., & Turvey, M.T. Coalitions as models for ecosystems: A realistic perspective on perceptual organization. In M. Kubovy and J. Pomerantz (Eds.), *Perceptual organization,* Hillsdale, NJ: Erlbaum Associates, in press.

TURVEY, M.T., & Shaw, R.E. The primacy of perceiving: An ecological reformulation of perception for understanding memory. In L.G. Nilsson (Ed.), *Perspectives on memory research: Essays in honor of Uppsala University's 500 anniversary.* Hillsdale, NJ: Erlbaum Associates, 1979.

Evaluation of Motor Skills of the Handicapped: Theory and Practice

Hollis Fait
University of Connecticut

Today one of the pressing problems of physical education for handicapped children, besides the decrease in federal funding to programs for the handicapped, is the testing and evaluation of the motor skills of children with handicaps. Although the federal government now threatens the continued existence of many programs, it originally was instrumental in developing the concern about evaluation of motor skills of handicapped children. Congress passed PL 94-142 which requires the evaluation of all handicapped school children taking part in physical education to determine their present status and to measure their progress. This requirement focused professional attention on the selection and use of appropriate, valid tools for evaluation of motor skills.

Unfortunately, valid evaluation instruments were not immediately available and their number remains small today for several reasons. First, theoretical concepts of the nature of motor learning and evaluation of motor skills in physical education have not been clearly established. Second, as new knowledge has become available, many physical educators have not applied the information to their practices but have instead adhered to outmoded concepts. A third reason is the ready acceptance and application of invalidated theories of transfer of motor learning to academic skills and other motor skills.

Important to the understanding of the limitations and potentialities of evaluating motor skills is an accurate perception of the nature of the transfer. To examine the circumstances and to clarify how one acquired skill can be transferred to another skill, let us look at theories and studies in early 20th Century that cast some illumination on the subject. The three theories I would like for you to recall and reexamine with me are: generalization theory, identical elements theory, and Gestaltic theory.

The generalization theory was first suggested by Judd (1905). He concluded that general instructions were transferable because he had found that individuals could more easily hit a submerged target with an arrow when the refraction of light principle was explained to them. Judd believed that motor accuracy was due to unconscious transfer from previous tasks to present movement needs. Results of several studies (Norcross, 1921; Seashore and Bevelas, 1941; Seymore, 1956) reported in the years subsequent to Judd's work seem to substantiate the generalization theory, at least as a partial explanation of how training is transferred.

In contrast to generalization theory, Thorndike (1901) contended that transfer is possible only when elements of one task correspond exactly to those of a second. He considered these elements to consist of similar stimuli or responses that are identical. Subsequent research (Henry, 1949; Lindeburg, 1949; Nelson and Henry, 1956) gave support to the idea that transfer does occur readily when there are identical elements in the activity and the likeness is recognized by the performer.

The Gestaltic theory opposed the concept of specificity of transfer but did not refute the concept that transfer occurs through the discovery of piecemeal stimuli, causing specific responses of simple movements that are common to both skills. The Gestaltics felt that transfer occurred because of the presence of common patterns, configurations, or relationships. Credence was added to Gestaltic theory when Cratty (1962) discovered that practicing a small pattern of movements while blindfolded facilitated large-pattern learning of a similar pattern and that practice in reverse caused large-pattern learning to be impeded by small-pattern learning.

On the surface it appears that the three theories are in serious disagreement with one another, but actually they are not. Studies show unequivocally that transfer *does* occur by generalizing, identifying identical elements, and learning common patterns or relationships. Based on the overwhelming evidence, transfer of learning can be said to occur in all of these ways. Also note that in all of the situations cited above, cognition plays a very important part in the transfer. Generalization is an intellectual process, as are recognizing like elements and conceptualizing common patterns, configurations, and relationships.

In summary, transfer of acquired motor skills to another motor skill depends on (a) general factors underlying several tasks, (b) recognition of identical elements, and (c) understanding the total task as it relates to another total task. All of these factors involve a high level of cognition.

Transfer of learning cannot be expected to occur willy-nilly. Clearly, if we wish students to learn to hit a tennis ball, we do not teach them how to draw lines between dots—we teach them the strokes of tennis. If there is any transfer between the skills of connecting dots and hitting a tennis ball, it is so insignificant that no present-day research measuring device can determine it. The same point is true with respect to evaluation of motor skill. To determine how well a student can hit the tennis ball, we must use a test which evaluates that skill, not one which measures ability to draw lines between dots. This is especially true when we seek to determine improvement in a skill after a period of practice. So many tests of general motor ability fail to take into account the limitations of transfer, and perceptual motor ability tests, when they are used to measure improvement in motor ability, suffer the same problem. They do not provide overall measurement of motor ability as often claimed; rather, they offer information concerning the ability to perform a specific motor skill.

The best known of the perceptual motor tests used to measure motor skills are the Frostig's Developmental Test of Visual Perception, Purdue Perceptual-Motor Survey by Kephart and Roach, and Ayres' Southern California Sensory Integration Motor Tests. Part of Frostig's test purports to measure eye-hand coordination. Test items include drawing a line with a pencil between horizontal lines, between curved lines, and connecting dots or figures. Although these items do measure eye-hand coordination, it is only the specific kind of eye-hand coordination required to perform the items. One of Kephart's test items for measuring what he calls body image is the Kraus-Weber test, a test which really measures flexibility and strength in certain parts of the body. His test of balance and posture consists of walking a beam, hopping, and jumping. Again, the items of this test measure specific motor abilities and tell very little about the total motor ability.

The Lincoln-Oseretsky Motor Development Scale and the Bruininks-Oseretsky Test of Motor Proficiency are other tests used commonly for assessing motor ability, particularly of the mentally retarded. Both tests appear to provide an adequate procedure for determining the level of motor ability and could be used in identifying students who need special consideration in physical education classes. In the Bruininks-Oseretsky test (1978) it was found that the mean scores for the test of mentally retarded subjects were less than the mean scores of the nonretarded subjects at the .01 level of confidence, which is in agreement with numerous studies (Cratty, 1973; Rarick and Francis, 1960), indicating that mentally retarded individuals show less ability in motor performance than their nonretarded peers. Claims have been made that the Bruininks-Oseretsky (1978) test can be used in assessing the effectiveness of physical education programs; no evidence supports this contention, however. Because the transfer from one skill to the next is limited, the use of scores to evaluate the quality of a program could be viable only if the skills in the test were taught in the program, and no good program would concentrate on such a limited number of activities.

Some empirical evidence to support this observation is provided by a recent pilot study (Fait, Note 1) comparing test results on several skills after one of the skills had been taught (e.g., comparison of balance on one leg after the skill had been taught with balance in bouncing on a spring board without practice; also, catching a ball after instruction compared to bouncing a ball without practice). The results indicate no improvement in the skills that had not been taught whereas considerable improvement was noted in the skills that had been taught. Undeniably, such tests as the Bruininks-Oseretsky test and the perceptual-motor tests provide interesting information about perception and/or may identify low levels of motor skills. Most of these tests have been evaluated for construct validity based on the fact that those with low motor skills usually score lower on motor skill tests than those with more proficient motor skills. Consequently, the tests are useful as screening tools. But, for use as before-and-after tests to measure progress over a period of time in general motor performance, they have little value. Changes in the score will occur only by chance or with practice of the test items or other items of sufficient similarity to permit generalization by the learner.

Many of my former students who are practitioners have been terribly confused by their results using these tests in motor skill programs for the handicapped. They have set up pretests, provided good motor activity programs, retested, and compared the results; but they have found very little, if any, improvement. If the tests were valid, then the interpretation has to be that the program was poor. In case after case the programs were found not to be inferior; they did not, however, provide instruction in the activities that are items of the test. So, of course, the tests showed no improvement. For the most part, teaching the items of the test would result in a pretty sterile physical education program and would produce little gain in improving overall motor skill development of participants.

The foregoing discussion does not deny that underlying "ability traits" may exist (Fleishman, 1967) that are relatively enduring in nature and are not modified to any great extent by practice, such as speed of muscular contraction, force as related to muscle length (Note 2), and the quality of neuroresponses that affect the performance and learning of the many different kinds of motor skills. Therefore, it is quite possible that some individuals are able to learn and perform different motor tasks at a very high rate and level because they possess superior ability traits and not necessarily because the result of learning one skill is transferred to the learning of another skill.

Without valid tests of general motor ability, how can we evaluate motor ability? The answer is to measure specific motor skills that are the foundation of effective motor performance. Which motor skills are these? They are those that I call basic skills—those skills used most frequently and which are most important in the daily life functions and play of children. With this definition, the specific skills that constitute the basic ones will vary in different environments and may also be quite different from one child to the next. For example, in a lifestyle devoid of dancing and games that involve skipping and galloping, the skills of skipping and galloping would not be basic for children of that society. Walking and running are not basic skills for a paraplegic child confined to a wheelchair. For such a child, the skill of propelling would be basic whereas for others it would not.

A very effective measuring device for evaluating basic motor skills is the behavioral objective which presents the skill to be learned in terms that make possible easy determination of whether the skill has been accomplished. For example, a behavioral objective for a specific type of catch may be the chest pass of a large ball, executing the following: (a) take one step in direction of pass and shift weight forward with either foot, (b) place thumbs behind ball; emphasize wrist snap by bringing thumbs forward so they will face direction of pass after release of ball, (c) hold elbows comfortably at the sides and point fingers in direction of the throw, and (d) synchronize these movements so that the ball is propelled sharply forward.

The statement clearly establishes the basic skill to be measured and the results will indicate the degree of efficiency obtained as defined in the items of the statement. As you will note, the items describe the most effective way to make a chest pass based on the principles of movement. The results of the test will provide information only about the student's competence in making the correct movements of a chest pass. No other information about the eye-hand coordination required in other activities is sought or provided, nor does the test provide extensive information about the coordination of the arm in performing other skills. The *I CAN* Program developed by Janet Wessel and associates at Michigan State University is an excellent example of an instructional system for handicapped students that incorporates an evaluation system based on behavioral objectives.

Special motor skill tests that use the concept of behavioral objectives can be developed to evaluate the quality of performance in motor skills of every kind (Fait, 1978). In testing to determine how efficiently and effectively a student can make an overhand throw, teachers must give consideration to the components of the throw—the arm brought back behind the shoulder, a step made with the opposite foot as the throw is made, the elbow preceding the upper arm, the wrist snapped when the ball is released, etc. Such a test would provide information about the effectiveness of the specific movements of the throw; it does not provide much information about total coordination of the arm muscles in any other motor skill dissimilar to overhand throwing. Tests of this kind can, however, be used to tell a good deal about the motor ability of a student, especially if the skills to be tested are basic, that is, are used frequently in the student's everyday life. Skills such as walking, running, throwing, catching, striking, and kicking can be labeled as the basic skills of most children because of the frequency of use in their play and everyday activities.

In designing a test to evaluate the components of a skill such as the overhand throw, it is necessary to analyze the movements required to perform effectively. Analysis should be based on the principles of movement; for example, the use of various parts of the body to apply force over a long period of time.

In order to be able to teach and evaluate movement, teachers must know how the movement is most effectively performed and must consider the physical capacity of the individuals being tested. The overhand throw test, for example, might be modified for those under the age of 6 because children younger than that lack the maturity required to perform this skill in the most efficient way for the mature individual. The test would require further modification if it were to be used with orthopedically handicapped students.

In designing a test for evaluating a handicapped child's throw the tester needs to assess the child's limitations and potentialities. For example, if the individual is a partially paraplegic child, testers must consider his or her potential for movement in the arms. It may be found, for example, that the individual has flexion and extension of the fingers but has only flexion of the lower arm (the biceps are functional but not the triceps); in other words, grasp and release with the hands are possible and the forearm can be flexed. Throwing a ball in the usual way is impossible because the arm cannot be extended; however, a throw over the shoulder may be possible. Analysis of this means of throwing the ball produces these components in a good throw for this person: (a) good grasp of the object; (b) overextended wrist to start with; (c) sharp contraction of the biceps; (d) sharp extension of the wrist; and (e) release of the ball at the proper time so it is propelled in a straight line.

Remember that most skills are made up of many components so to keep a test at a practical length, it is necessary to exclude some of the components from consideration in the evaluation. Those few retained should be the ones most essential to efficient performance of the skill and the ones most frequently performed incorrectly. (For a battery of tests that evaluate basic motor skills using the procedure I have described, write to me at the University of Connecticut.)

I would like to leave you with this thought: It is time to discard that often repeated observation "It's a good theory but it won't work." If a theory won't work, it certainly isn't a good one! So it is with the theories about the motor skill evaluation. If a test developed to evaluate achievement in motor skills does not do this, we, as researchers and theoreticians, must reexamine the theoretical construct of the test. As practitioners, we should stop using the test and select an evaluation procedure that will provide us with valid information about the motor skill achievement of those whom we are evaluating. We cannot otherwise truly serve our handicapped students.

Reference Notes

1. Fait, H.F. *A pilot study to determine the feasibility of comparing practiced and non-practiced performance to determine amount of transfer of training.* University of Connecticut, unpublished manuscript, 1979.
2. Turvey, M. University of Connecticut, personal communication, 1981.

References

BRUININKS, R.H. *Bruininks-Oseretsky test: Examiners manual.* Circle Pines, MN: American Guidance Service, 1978.

CRATTY, B.J. Transfer of small-pattern practice to large pattern learning. *Research Quarterly*, 1962, **33**, 523-535.

CRATTY, B.J. *Movement behavior and motor learning* (3rd ed.). Philadelphia: Lea and Febiger, 1973.

FAIT, H.F. *Special physical education: Adapted, corrective, developmental* (4th ed.). Philadelphia: W.B. Saunders, 1978.

FLEISHMAN, E.A. *Learning and individual differences.* Columbus, OH: Charles E. Merrill Books, Inc., 1967.

HENRY, F.M. Increase in speed of movement by motivation and transfer of motivated improvement. *Research Quarterly*, 1949, **20**, 180-195.

JUDD, C.H. Movement and consciousness. *Psychological Review*, 1905, **7**, 199-226.

LINDEBURG, F.A. A study of the degree of transfer between quickening exercises and other coordinated movement. *Research Quarterly*, 1949, **20**, 180-195.

NELSON, C.A., & Henry, F.M. Age differences and interrelationships between skill and learning in gross motor performance. *Research Quarterly*, 1956, **27**, 162-175.

NORCROSS, W.H. Experiment on the transfer of training. *Journal of Comparative Psychology,* 1921, 313-363.

RARICK. L., & Francis, R.J. Motor characteristics of the mentally retarded. *Competitive research monograph* (No. 1, OE-35005). U.S. Office of Education, 1960.

SEASHORE, H.G., & Bavelas, A. The function of knowledge of results in Thorndike's line drawing experiment. *Psychological Review,* 1941, **48**, 153-164.

SEYMORE, W.D. Transfer of training in engineering skills. *Perceptual Motor Skills,* 1956, **7**, 235-237.

THORNDIKE, E.L., & Woodsworth, R.S. The influence of improvement in one mental function upon the efficiency of other functions. *Psychological Review.* 1901, **8**, 247-261.

Generalization of Motor Skills from Training to Natural Environments

David Auxter
Slippery Rock State College

Application of research results to education for the handicapped lacks the precision needed in helping those persons develop motor skills for self-sufficient living in natural community environments. With perfect fidelity to demonstration and research, experts can testify that all children are capable of learning. Experts know that for every type and combination of handicapping conditions, educational strategies and techniques have been developed, tested, and found productive. But for all of the investment in curriculum development, learning materials, and techniques for training teachers, a delivery system has not produced results which are sufficiently systematic, precise, or coherent enough to enable documentation of progress on skills toward self-sufficient living in natural community environments. And for good reason, because what we know is not systematized as methodology for direct service personnel to use in documenting which skills relating to self-sufficiency the student has learned.

The goal of professionals who develop motor skill instruction for the handicapped should be application for the best available behavioral and instructional technology. A well established principle of law in the US is that given two technologies of equivalent cost, the better technology should be used (Hoover, 1932). Professionals often disagree as to approaches for providing services to the handicapped, but litigation in the courts through expert testimony has identified technology that produces remarkable results. Consider the work of Gold (1975) who trained another person to teach a blind-deaf, physically handicapped, mentally retarded person with an IQ of 28 to assemble a complex Bendix bicycle brake in 20 trials. Bellemy (1976) testified in federal court on research that is equally impressive; he taught a mentally retarded person MA 3 to assemble a complex oscilloscope cam switch involving 77 steps. This type of technology defines the state of the art for conducting individualized programming for the handicapped. But incorporating the behavioral technology described by Gold and Bellemy into practice in applied settings is another matter. Results from research and demonstration have not been applied coherently for helping the handicapped develop motor skills bearing direct relationship to self-sufficiency (*Armstrong vs Kline,* 1979; *Fialkowski vs Pittenger,* 1976; *PARC vs Pennsylvania,* 1979; *PARC vs Pennsylvania,* 1981). Thus, we need to develop procedures and methodology which incorporate existing technology for individualized instruction into the educational delivery system to help the handicapped develop self-sufficient living.

Problem

Research on education for the handicapped should be directed toward development of behavior which facilitates self-sufficiency in the natural community. The requirement from governmental agencies in the US for documentation of each handicapped person's behavioral progress provides an invaluable research laboratory. Natural environments with community-based assessment and programming can be a setting for meaningful research on motor skill development of the handicapped. Clearly, an important need is for implementation research using as independent variable the measured learning of the handicapped for self-sufficient living. Motor skills acquired in training settings are of little value to the handicapped unless they can be generalized as functional skills in natural community environments. Baer, Wolf, and Risely (1968) indicate that generalization of skills and abilities must be programmed rather than expected. Therefore, in order to facilitate generalization of trained motor skills, we should attempt to match the skills of specific individuals with the demands of specific natural environments in which the skills will be used. The purpose of this study was to explore the development of procedures for generalizing the skills attained in training settings to natural environments.

Methodology

If we are to develop methods and procedures for teaching the handicapped to generalize motor skills contributing to self-sufficiency, we must experiment using diverse environments and populations. Therefore, we explored generalization methodology in special schools for the handicapped, institutions for the mentally retarded, intermediate care facilities for the mentally retarded, and community living arrangements. The handicapped persons studied were physically handicapped, blind, deaf, multihandicapped, and moderately, severely, or profoundly mentally retarded.

Prerequisites for Study

Prerequisite to experimenting with generalization methodology are (a) an operational definition of self-sufficient behavior, (b) identification of federal, state, and local regulations for conducting the human delivery system, (c) knowledge of the available instructional and behavioral technology for conducting individualized programs, and (d) identification of subenvironments having sequentially less restrictiveness. We undertook a thorough study of these prerequisite components prior to experimentation and generated procedures and principles from conducting training programs with diverse handicapped populations, environments, and behavioral learning techniques.

Results

Procedures for conducting individualized behavioral programs for self-sufficiency resulted from exploring generalization methodology. The steps involve: (a) definition of minimal motor functioning for self-sufficient behavior of specific individuals for specific environments, (b) determination of the unique needs for self-sufficiency through community-based assessment, (c) identification and development of subenvironments for the purpose of generalizing skills, (d) construction of behavioral programs to help students develop motor skills and to identify cues, contingencies, and correctional procedures that facilitate generalization, and (e) development of strategies for generalization. A brief description of each of the components of the generalization process follows.

Definition of Minimal Motor Functioning in the Community

The first step of generalization methodology is to state an operational definition of self-sufficient functional motor behavior that the handicapped are to demonstrate in specific community environments. Motor skills which are targets of training toward self-sufficiency for specific handicapped persons should match the skill demands of their environments.

Not all handicapped persons can attain motor skills for self-sufficiency in the community. Most, however, may gain motor skill proficiency to achieve goals commensurate with their ability. As a rule, the more severe the handicap, the greater the need for environment-specific training that limits the number of environments in which a handicapped person can function. Specific training also limits choices for types of vocation, domestic living, and recreational opportunities.

Providing Community-Based Assessment

Community-based assessment of what kind of education is needed for self-sufficiency is prerequisite to program development. Thus, for purposeful programming we require a full evaluation of the motor skills which need to be developed. This evaluation process minimized instructional behaviors needed for self-sufficiency in the individual. Brown, Nietupske, Lyon, Branston, Folvey, and Greenwald (1978) and Bellemy, Peterson, and Close (1975) indicate that assessment of the natural environment requires consideration not only of the behavioral responses that need to be generalized but also the types of naturally occurring cues, contingencies, and correctional procedures within the person's environment. From this information, we can construct training environments that increase the person's potential for skill generalization to other environments. We need to develop instruments for providing knowledge of the degree to which specific individuals can generalize responses, cues, consequences, and correctional procedures from training to natural environments.

Identifying Subenvironments

Motor skills acquired by the handicapped in training environments can be expressed in many subenvironments such as extracurricular activities in the public schools, community recreation programs, and play in the neighborhood and at home. The conditions under which the skills will be expressed in each subenvironment differ. If the motor skills attained in training are functional, they can find expression in many subenvironments. Therefore, knowledge of the persons' subenvironments in which learned motor skills will be expressed enables us to plan programs that facilitate generalization in each one. Control of cues, reinforcers, and correctional procedures which link motor behavior with specific subenvironments are thus important considerations.

Training Persons in Subenvironments. The generalization of skills from training to natural environments requires a cooperative effort among personnel of formal training settings and the subenvironments where the handicapped generalize learned skills. In one case applying generalization methodology in a Community Living Arrangement, we contacted more than 30 persons in the community to provide correctional techniques that would enable three handicapped persons to adapt to their natural environment.

Constructing Behavioral Programs

Functional motor skills which lead to self-sufficiency in natural environments develop through individualized behavioral programming. It is desirable for the individuals' abilities to match the demands of their specific environments. To help the handicapped achieve mastery of functional motor skills, we can apply the "relevance of behavioral rule" (Allyon & Azrin, 1968). The rule states: "Teach only those behaviors that will continue to be reinforced after training." Thus, the behaviors that undergo training should be determined through community-based assessment.

Programmed Instruction. The procedure for developing programmed instruction which can be applied to motor skills development is well documented in the literature (Lindval & Bolvin, 1968; Taber, Glasier, & Schaefer, 1965). Once we have developed the behavioral programming, generalization strategies for programmed responses should be undertaken.

What an individual needs in terms of motor skills and other physical/motor prerequisites, determined from community-based assessment, is first task-analyzed into teachable units of instruction. The next step is to match the person's performance with the task-analyzed or programmed sequence of objectives. This behavioral sequence provides a pathway for a person's acquisition of the motor skills required for self-sufficiency in natural environments. The summation of all short-term instructional objectives must equal the goal and the goal must relate directly to the person's performance of the motor skills required for participation in natural community environments.

Environmental Cues and Consequences. Handicapped persons' development of target motor skills is associated with their environmental cues, consequences, and natural correction procedures. Their acquired behavioral skills must be closely studied within the framework of generalization methodology; for instance, environmental cues may be introduced which prompt the desired motor skills. These cues can then be faded into the natural environment until the behaviors are elicited without prompting. Different types of reinforcers (Becker, Englemann, & Thomas, 1971) can be provided that increase the probability of strengthening persons' target behaviors in their natural environments.

Furthermore, correctional procedures in the training environment can be structured to mimic those in the natural environment, which may facilitate generalization of motor skills.

Determining Generalization Strategies

Handicapped persons generalize skills from instructional settings to natural environments most easily when the skills to be acquired are functional. Functional skills are lifetime activities which, when a person participates in them, contribute to self-sufficiency. Fundamental motor patterns, fundamental motor skills, recreational, domestic, and vocational skills can be functional behaviors. If the skills can be performed outside the instructional setting, the chances are good that they will be learned more quickly (*Armstrong vs Kline,* 1979).

Generalization strategies must be planned. Prerequisite information for planning the strategies must include detailed knowledge of the motor skills to be learned and the natural environments in which these skills will be expressed. This knowledge identifies the elements of the training environment and enables us to create strategies for generalization of skills to different natural subenvironments. Generalization does not occur by chance, but must be programmed.

Suggestions for Generalization. Some suggested methods for generalization of trained motor skills to natural environments are listed below.

- Have the handicapped persons practice their newly acquired motor skills in a variety of environments (Popovich, 1980; Sulzer & Mayer, 1977), such as extracurricular activities at school, YMCA/YWCA, community recreation settings, and the home.
- Provide transition time for generalization by the learner when natural cues, correctional procedures, and reinforcers are introduced (Wheman, Abramson, & Norman, 1977).
- Train other individuals in the person's natural environment to carry out generalization programs.
- Emphasize common elements between training and natural settings.
- Teach the learners to administer their own cues and deliver their own consequences through self-instructional training procedures.
- Fade unnatural cues and aids.
- Instruct persons to perform motor skills under a variety of conditions in which cues are different. Teach the skills in different settings with different instructors, and vary the materials.

- Add supplemental stimuli to new situations. In changing from one environment to another, use previous cues to elicit the behavior in the new environment, then fade the added cues to the natural cues.

Natural Correction Procedures and Consequence Generalization. The properties of consequences and correctional procedures in the person's natural environment should be carefully noted. This information enables you to form strategies for structuring reinforcement conditions that facilitate motor skills generalization from one environment to another. Some of these reinforcement principles are listed below.

- Increase the delay of time before presentation of consequences so persons will not expect to be reinforced immediately after the behavior.
- Vary training conditions so the person cannot determine when the consequence will be delivered or by whom and in what setting.
- Vary the time and the persons who deliver the consequence.
- Substitute naturally occurring consequences for artificial, programmed consequences. Artificial consequences may be necessary for the person to learn the skill, but you should fade to natural consequences as soon as possible.
- Use intermittent schedules of consequences in the original training sessions prior to generalization training. This may assist persons in maintaining the new behavior in other environments.

Summary

Functional motor skills which contribute to self-sufficient living among the handicapped are not learned until they have been generalized in natural community environments. Community-based assessment and programming directs training at those behaviors which will continue to be reinforced after training.

Litigation in the US courts has defined the state of the art for applying behavioral and instructional technology to the human delivery system. We can see an imperative need for research to develop procedures for incorporating this technology into human delivery systems in order to enhance self-sufficiency among the handicapped. Motor skill generalization contributes to recreational skills, mobility, vocation, and domestic activity of the handicapped for self-sufficient living in the community.

Critical to the program is teaching the handicapped to generalize skills attained in training environments to their natural environments. Procedures for facilitating generalization of attained skills to natural environments are: (a) determine the motor skills handicapped persons need for self-sufficiency in the community; (b) assess the behavioral needs of handicapped persons for self-sufficiency in the community; (c) determine the subenvironments where skills will be expressed; (d) develop programs that facilitate a person's acquisition of motor skills within the context of cues, correctional procedures and consequences of the subenvironments; and (e) employ strategies of generalization combined with community-based programs.

References

ALLYON, T., & Azrin, N. *The token economy.* New York: Century Crofts Psychology Services, 1968.

BAER, D.M., Wolf, M.M., & Risely, T.R. Some current dimensions of applied behavioral analysis. *Journal of Applied Behavior Analysis,* Spring 1968, 1, 91-97.

BECKER, W., Englemann, S., & Thomas, G. *Teaching: An applied course in psychology.* Chicago: Science Research Associates, 1971.

BELLEMY, T. Testimony in *Fialkowski vs Pittenger* (Civil Action 74-2262) in the United States 3rd District Court for the Eastern District of Pennsylvania, 1976.

BELLEMY, G.T., Peterson, L., & Close, D. Habilitation of the severely and profoundly retarded: Illustration of competency. *Education and Training of the Mentally Retarded,* 1975, 10, 174-186.

BROWN, L., Nietupski, S.H., Lyon, S., Branston, M.B. Folvey, M., & Grenwald, L. *Curricular strategies for developing longitudinal interaction between severely handicapped students and other curricular strategies for teaching severely handicapped to acquire and perform skills in response to naturally occurring cues and correction procedures.* Madison, WI: Educational Services, Madison Metropolitan School District, 1978.

GOLD, M. *Task analysis: A statement and example of using acquisition and production of a complex assembly task by the retarded blind.* University of Illinois at Urbana-Champaign: Institute of Child Behavior and Development, 1975.

HOOVER, T.H. *60F.* 2d 737, 740 2nd Circuit Court, 1932.

LINDVAL, C.M., & Bolvin, J.D. Programmed instruction in the schools: An application of programming principles in individually prescribed instruction. *Sixty-sixth yearbook of the national society of the study of education.* Chicago: University of Chicago Press, 1968.

POPOVICH, D. *Effective behavioral programming for severely and profoundly handicapped students.* Baltimore, MD: Brooks Publishing, 1980.

SULZER, B.S., & Mayer, G.R. *Applying behavior analysis procedures with children and youth.* New York: Holt, Rinehart, Winston, 1977.

TABER, J.I., Glasier, R., & Schaefer, H.H. *Learning and programmed instruction*. Reading, MA: Addison-Wesley Publishing, 1965.

UNITED States Eastern District Court, 3rd District. *Fialkowski vs Pittenger* (Civil Action 74-2262), 1976.

UNITED States Eastern District Court, 3rd District (findings of fact and conclusions of law). *Armstrong vs Kline* (Civil Action 78-132, 133, 172), June 21, 1979.

UNITED States Eastern District Court, 3rd District. *PARC vs Pennsylvania* (Civil Action 72-94), 1972.

UNITED States Eastern District Court, 3rd District. *PARC vs Pennsylvania* (Civil Action 72-94), 1981.

WHEMAN, P., Abramson, M., & Norman, C. Transfer of training in behavior modification programs: An evaluative review. *Journal of Special Education,* 1977, **11**, 217-231.

Bridge over Troubled Waters — Research Review and Recommendations for Relevance

Julian U. Stein
George Mason University

Worldwide differences between researchers and practitioners abound. On the one hand practitioners are charged with not using findings from research, and on the other hand, researchers are accused of not being in contact with reality! Time has long passed for both groups to stop charging and start listening to each other. Provincialisms and petty ego defenses must be cast aside so researchers and practitioners can interact meaningfully. Both are interested in and concerned with furthering the state of the art so that every individual can have more high-quality opportunities and experiences through physical education, recreation, and sport programs. Greater sensitivity and attention to goals and work of each other are basic to shouting causes and whispering specializations.

Need for cooperation among professionals is exemplified in a statement made recently by G. Lawrence Rarick who challenged participants in a statewide leadership workshop on physical education programs for students with handicapping conditions:

> While the findings of research are important, the knowledge thus generated is of value only to the extent that it is effectively used. Thus, the future of

our work with the atypical rests in no small measure on groups such as this, for change must ultimately come from the grassroots. (Rarick, 1981)

Too often results of research and experiences at grassroots levels are *not* consistent.

- Statements are still made about mentally retarded populations functioning 2-6 years below chronological-age peers in measures of physical and motor proficiency despite research and program experiences refuting such statements.
- Emphasis continues to be on the chronological age when individuals attain certain physical and motor milestones while lip service is given to the individual nature of growth and development in which each child reaches these milestones according to his or her personal time schedule.
- Participation in physical activities of a recreational or sport nature continues to be viewed as purely therapeutic and rehabilitative by many segments of both professional and lay communities despite pleas by participants and results of research that indicate individuals with handicapping conditions take part in such activities for all the same reasons as able-bodied persons.
- Focus continues to be on disabilities and deficiencies—perpetuating the medical model—in spite of research evidence and practical experiences emphasizing the importance of focusing on abilities and recognizing potential.
- Emphasis remains on activities that are consistent with mental age, especially for mentally retarded persons, rather than adapting age-appropriate activities so that the fallacy of individuals being relegated to eternal childhood can be dispelled.
- The importance of individualizing instruction to meet each child's needs in terms of special interests, abilities, and ways of learning are stressed, but those who need individualized instruction and are unable to respond effectively to regimented group, class-oriented activities and methods are still labeled as different and/or deficient.
- We still need to identify behavior characteristics, personal traits, and personality differences to make it more likely that individuals will respond effectively to specific activities and techniques that can be used effectively with all youngsters.
- Play, movement, and motor activity are believed to be important prerequisites for sound growth and complete development, yet many early childhood education programs and early intervention projects for children with handicaps continue to place increasing emphasis on academic activities and cognitive development.

- The importance of early informal learning experiences and of even later starting ages for formal schooling for some individuals are receiving greater emphasis for optimal child growth and development, but early childhood education programs continue to emphasize formal learning experiences at earlier and earlier ages.
- Interdisciplinary cooperation and multiagency teamwork are by-words of the day, yet many groups and individuals give little more than lip service to this concept.
- Understanding children, knowing growth and developmental patterns, and having opportunities to observe, teach, lead, and know able-bodied children are felt to be important prerequisites and form a basic foundation for those who work with individuals with handicapping conditions, yet earlier and earlier specialization is advocated by some persons involved in programs for special populations.

Each of us is confronted by many confusing, apparently contradictory and difficult, if not impossible to understand paradoxes. As Rarick has elucidated, researchers have much to learn from grassroots practitioners, and grassroots practitioners have much to gain from researchers. This is a two-way street on which much give and take, cooperation, and coordination are necessary so that both groups can do better jobs of fulfilling their professional responsibilities. Real benefactors in this process will be individuals of all ages in many different settings who will have greater numbers of opportunities in physical activity, recreation, and sport programs to enhance the quality of their lives.

Studies and projects involving subjects with different handicapping conditions provide exciting and important directions which can, should, and *must* be applied to programs. Too often these results have not been widely communicated to practitioners who have been unaware of the results and their implications for programs. Often reports made available focus on research paradigms—design, statistical methodologies, instrumentation, complicated analysis, and recommendations for follow-up research—rather than implications for application to programs. Level of significance is of little relevance to most practitioners whose major interests and concerns are for ways in which results can help the individuals they serve. Many representative examples of studies with implications for immediate application in programs as well as for continued and follow-up research have involved individuals with handicapping conditions.

- Obesity has been shown to result from overeating and lack of physical activity in mentally retarded populations of all types and severity, just as in nonretarded populations (AAHPER, 1975). Carefully controlled studies have shown the combination of overeating and lack of exercise to result in moderately and severely/profoundly mentally retarded subjects being 10 to 110 pounds overweight. Basal metabolism, biochemical factors, medication, and related medical factors were carefully controlled and ruled out as contributing causes for obesity in these populations in all but the smallest number of cases— one individual out of 25. Conversely, reports from residential facilities, public and special schools, camps, recreation programs, and parents indicate that when similar populations have participated regularly in ongoing physical activity programs, the same gains noted in nonretarded populations have been observed—higher levels of fitness, less obesity, and happier, more productive, fun-filled, and healthier individuals—who had less need for medication.

- Reduction in frequency and severity of seizures in individuals with epilepsy has been shown to be a product of improved physical condition. Individuals with epilepsy can participate actively and safely in contact sports such as wrestling, hockey, and American football without fear of increased frequency and severity of seizures (*National Spokesman,* 1973). Longitudinal studies showed that individuals with epilepsy suffered fewer and less severe attacks when they were in good physical condition. Hyperventilation associated with increases in cardiovascular and cardiorespiratory functions did not result in greater numbers and more severe seizures; instead, seizures were less frequent and less severe. However, in activities for which hyperventilation was not associated with such physiological changes, expected frequency and severity of attacks were unaffected. Although researchers did not propose definitive reasons for these findings, they hypothesized that results were influeenced by improved physical condition rather than effects on mechanisms triggering seizures. With appropriate protection— regular headgear—contact sports were no more dangerous for individuals with epilepsy than for those without the condition. Similar positive effects of active participation in vigorous physical activities have been shown consistently with populations of asthmatic and cystic fibrosis children (Stein, in AAHPER).

- Myographic studies have shown the quality of muscular function of Olympiad athletes (paraplegics) to be comparable to that of top-flight Olympic athletes (Royer & Taylor, 1979). Analyses of slow twitch muscle fibers indicated that Olympiad athletes functioned in ranges comparable to average Olympic athletes, whereas analysis of fast twitch muscle fibers showed that Olympiad athletes functioned in ranges comparable to superior Olympic athletes. Results imply that performances of Olympiad athletes, especially in power events such as weight lifting, field events, and sprints, are comparable with highest level Olympic performances in similar events. Results thus have implications for training such individuals for Olympiad competition: training techniques should be no different for athletes in wheelchairs than for their able-bodied counterparts. Equally important and probably more exciting are implications for furthering the potential of others with spinal cord injuries and related conditions resulting in paraplegia, although their possibilities do not include highly competitive sports.

- Cinemographic analyses have shown both quadriplegic and paraplegic swimmers to have some leg movement in water. Although this study was undertaken to compare arm strokes of Olympic and Olympiad level swimmers, the unexpected findings are extremely important. Quadriplegics and paraplegics placed in classes where no functional use of the legs was expected *kicked* while they were competing in swimming events. Review and revision of classification systems for these athletes apparently are needed; a system appropriate for land-based activities may not be applicable to water activities. Some individuals competing in track and field and other land events perhaps should be reclassified for swimming activities. One additional class for paraplegic swimming not found in other competitive Olympiad events already exists.

   Of more importance are questions raised about the potential of using water activities to reeducate neuromuscular functions by developing new pathways to restore muscular functions previously thought impossible. This therapy would have an outcome similar to the different neuromuscular pathways developed by polio victims when synaptic blocks prevented their neural impulses from reaching muscles through the usual routes.

- Comparisons of World War II veterans injured and confined to wheelchairs and those injured but not confined to wheelchairs showed significantly earlier death ages of those in wheelchairs because of cardiovascular/cardiorespiratory degeneration. Autopsies showed that many of these deaths were caused by atherosclerosis. Contrasting results have been noted in studies in which individuals drove bicycle ergometers with hands, used treadmills adapted for wheelchairs, and took part in both aerobic and anaerobic programs in wheelchairs (Byrnes, 1979; Fisher & Patterson, 1981; *IRUC Briefings,* May 1979; Israel & Ordor, 1979; Rendon-Alacaia & Israel, 1979; Note 1). Using a wheelchair as a primary means of locomotion does not guarantee beneficial effects on cardiovascular/cardiorespiratory functions any more than walking from place to place. Specific attention must be given to developing and maintaining necessary levels of cardiovascular/cardiorespiratory fitness by all individuals with handicapping conditions. Training procedures and conditioning approaches used by able-bodied populations are appropriate for individuals with different types of handicapping conditions, not just those confined to wheelchairs. Weight training, circuit approaches, interval techniques, long-slow distance and speed play/fartlek are training methods which are effective with individuals who have handicapping conditions. In need of further investigation are the effects of exercise on individuals classified as severely/profoundly retarded or multihandicapped.

- Factor analytic studies have shown consistently the same physical and motor factor structures in mentally retarded and nonretarded populations (AAHPER, 1975; Rarick, 1968). Studies of this type have been done repeatedly with mildly and moderately mentally retarded persons. Results have indicated that the factor structure of physical and motor characteristics follow the same developmental sequences with retarded and nonretarded populations. Although retarded children attain many of these physical and motor patterns at a later chronological age than nonretarded populations, no differences have been found in the traits themselves. When mentally retarded individuals are provided opportunities in which activities and teaching progressions have been adapted to individual abilities and needs, they show greater progress and achievement.

Review of what has happened three times in the last 20 years shows the folly of seeking special curricula for these populations. When mildly mentally retarded students were brought into programs in the late 1950s and 1960s, traditional and existing physical education curricula and recreation programs did not work! Some individuals attributed lack of success to the inherent characteristics of mentally retarded persons. Others raised a more basic question—why was this happening? This second group recognized the need to modify and adapt existing curricula and programs, not create new ones. They made instructional steps smaller so that participants did not have to progress so far in moving from one step to the next in a total skill sequence. Successes resulted whether activities focused on physical and motor fitness, fundamental motor skills and patterns, or skills in aquatics, dance, and individual/group games and sports. Results of some of these programs and related research showed that mildly mentally retarded participants not only equaled but in many cases surpassed performances of nonretarded populations.

As increasing numbers of moderately mentally retarded students were introduced to programs, progressions adapted for mildly mentally retarded participants did not work. Remembering what had worked several years before, progressions adapted for mildly mentally retarded individuals were taken back to the drawing board. The distance between steps was made even smaller and beginning levels for skills were lowered. These moderately mentally retarded persons then also showed success.

As increasing numbers of severely/profoundly mentally retarded persons came to programs in the mid- to late 1970s, materials developed for and successful with moderately mentally retarded participants did not work. Again, materials were revised in the same two ways—steps were made smaller and entry levels were lowered more for successful participation.

This same process is appropriate for other populations possessing handicaps. Physical, recreational, and sport activities for these populations are not new and different, but rather simple adaptations of tried and true activities enabling these individuals to be successful and enjoy participation. Lip service has long been given to similarities among able-bodied and disabled populations, but programs have focused on differences. Research and practical experiences reinforce the necessity of focusing on similarities, not differences, in planning and implementing physical activities, recreation, and sport programs for persons with handicapping conditions.

- Empirical reports have shown that training principles are no different among disabled and able-bodied athletes. Until recently, disabled individuals training for highly competitive activities did so in their own ways. Often these approaches had little structure and adhered to few, if any, basic principles. Although records continued to be broken, questions had to be raised as to what degrees these accomplishments were consistent with the disabled athlete's abilities, potential, and intensity of training. The same training principles and methods used by able-bodied athletes are being applied by disabled athletes regardless of handicapping conditions. Weight training is commonplace; combinations' of long-slow distance for foundation and interval training are used for speed and pace routines; workouts funnel long-to-short distance in a given session and increase toward race distance throughout the week. Tactics, strategies, and pace splits follow the same patterns as for able-bodied runners.

    Additional study is needed to identify the most effective approaches and procedures for *individuals,* the same as for able-bodied populations. Compared as a group, little if any difference is noted between able-bodied and disabled athletes. In several European countries teams and individuals preparing for Olympiad competition practice with companion Olympic teams and individuals. Opening facilities of the US Olympic Committee at Colorado Springs to individuals and teams of handicapped athletes preparing for international competition is a step in the right direction.

- Sociometric studies have shown that children with handicapping conditions are accepted or rejected for the same reasons as able-bodied peers and classmates (AAHPER, 1975; Lauchmen, 1979). Both research and experimental evidence are important as handicapped students are integrated into regular programs. Able-bodied students need to be aware of handicapping conditions so they understand them as types of human differences. Individuals with handicapping conditions must recognize personal characteristics and traits which appeal to as well as turn off others. This process is no different for developing interpersonal relationships and social graces by any individual. Attitudes of adults—parents, teachers, and various professional providers of services—often influence students negatively before they have chances to meet children with handicapping conditions and make their own judgments regarding likes and dislikes, acceptances and rejections. Social development can be learned and improved; it follows developmental progression in exactly the same way as physical and motor skills—sequentially—and is learned most effectively in planned and systematic ways.

Underlying virtually all negative expectations regarding individuals with handicapping conditions is categorical thinking that dictates decisions based on these same handicaps. We cannot overstress results of studies and empirical evidence in support of emphasizing similarities, not differences, between disabled and able-bodied populations. Application of known techniques and approaches from all fields and specializations contributing to physical education, recreation, and sport is a necessity; recent sports medicine reports reinforce this emphasis.

Just how troubled the waters is uncertain. Whether we are dealing with swift currents and eddies, dangerous rapids, or treacherous undertows varies among places and individuals. However, it can be safely said that the "waters" involving researchers and practitioners are *not* crystal clear and smooth! This is a sad commentary in that each of these specializations has so much to offer to the field.

- When we perform basic research, groups of individuals with handicapping conditions should be considered right along with able-bodied subjects.
- Practitioners need to plan and carry out wildfire research to obtain answers to some of their own questions and concerns about programming.
- Practitioners must communicate problems, needs, concerns, and priorities to the research community.
- Researchers are challenged to come out of their ivory towers and become better acquainted with the realities of practitioners.
- Results of studies, projects, and activities need to be widely distributed as important means of insuring continued program progress and development.

- Both researchers and practitioners have personal and professional responsibilities to seek carefully and thoroughly both research and programming materials that are available from a variety of sources.

Progress must be an important product of all; efforts and use of resources must result in productive findings. Directions must be for moving forward and onward, not simply treading water or being swept downstream, moving backward rather than progressing. In fields for which teamwork and cooperation are basic—physical education, recreation, and sport—researchers and practitioners working *together* can bridge the troubled waters confronting those interested and involved in using fully these activities to enhance the lives of handicapped individuals.

Reference Note

1. Beedle, B. Cross exercise phenomenon and the mentally retarded. Doctoral dissertation. Oxford, MS: University of Mississippi, 1979.

References

ANNOTATED bibliography in physical education, recreation, and psychomotor function of mentally retarded persons. Washington, DC: American Alliance for Health, Physical Education, and Recreation, June 1975.

BYRNES, P. Universal weight training program for paraplegics. *IRUC Briefings,* Nov. 1979, **5**(1), 6.

FISHER, S., & Patterson, R. *Cost of ambulation with assistive devices.* Minneapolis, MN: University of Minnesota Research and Training Center, 1981.

ISRAEL, R., & Ordor, O.E. *Cardiovascular responses to different body positions during maximal arm ergometry in young college males.* Washington, DC: Howard University, March 1979.

LAUCHMEN, D.R. Creative teacher develops innovative P.E. program. *IRUC Briefings,* Jan. 1979, **4**(2), 1 & 3.

PARAPLEGICS, amputees can use unique new bicycle exerciser. *IRUC Briefings,* May 1979, **4**(4), 7.

PHYSICAL stress and epilepsy: An investigation. *National Spokesman,* June 1973, **6**(6), 6.

RARICK, G.L. The factor structure of motor abilities of educable mentally retarded. In (G.A. Jervis, Ed.), *Expanding concepts in mental retardation.* Springfield, IL: Charles C. Thomas, 1968.

RARICK, G.L. *Recent research findings in adapted physical education.* Berkeley, CA: University of California, Sept. 1981.

RENDON-ALACAIA, A.E., & Israel, R.C. *Cardiovascular responses to different cranking rates during arm ergometry.* Washington, DC: Howard University, 1979.

ROYER, D., & Taylor, A.W. *Use of muscle biopsies and enzyme studies in planning a training program for elite wheelchair athletes.* Sherbrooke, Can.: University of Sherbrooke, 1979.

STEIN, J.U. Effects of physical activity and exercise upon asthmatic children: State of the art. *Physical education and recreation for impaired, disabled, and handicapped individuals: Past, present, and future.* Washington, DC: American Alliance for Health, Physical Education, and Recreation, no date.

SECTION 5:
Research Topics in Adapted Physical Activity

The professional literature concerning the movement status of handicapped individuals and special populations is sparse, inconclusive, and often contradictory. In its current state, it is of little value. As program and curriculum theorists, how can we state measurable, predetermined objectives related to recreation, health-related fitness, and movement skills when we have so little data about the learning styles of our clients? We must know how special populations compare to their nonhandicapped peers. We must know common deficient behavioral characteristics and the implication of movement for remediation and normalization. What are the learning styles of the atypical—reinforcers that work, length of attention for learning, and practice environments? Professionals from education and recreation are combining with those in medicine and allied health to provide quality services, but much information is needed. There is hardly a body of knowledge from which to begin!

In this section we are treated to the results of experiments, both applied and laboratory-based. Reid, Collier, and Morin initiate the discussion by providing long-awaited answers concerning the motor performance of autistic individuals. We will discover how they compare to normal, mildly retarded, and moderately retarded populations.

In this age of accountability, we are being asked to individualize our instruction and demonstrate progress toward long-range goals for handicapped students. Ulrich presents research that suggests we should differentiate between quantitative and qualitative assessment tools for decision-making. As we read, we will want to know if quantitative and qualitative assessment instruments correlate concerning differences between mentally deficient and normal children. One of the compounding problems with many special populations is their inability to pay attention during instruction. Stamps, Eason, and Smith examine academically gifted and learning-disabled children to determine if response time scores are different; they help us to understand that some attentional problems may be neurochemically based and as more commonly believed motivationally based. Similarly, Surburg has shown with mildly mentally retarded populations that the uncertainty of time and occurrence of an expected response stimulus can effect the reaction time scores.

The literature recommends fundamentally different programs for the remediation of perceptual motor problems. Two of the most common approaches are balance-oriented programs and vision-oriented programs; Cowden, Eason, and Wright present results comparing the relative effectiveness of each type on motor proficiencies. Finally, Church and Broadhead provide information about how to use an excellent research tool — discriminant analysis.

The Motor Performance of Autistic Individuals

Greg Reid, Doug Collier, and Brian Morin
McGill University

A dearth of information pertains to the motor proficiency of autistic individuals. Furthermore, physical educators have been particularly silent with regard to the role of movement activities for autistic persons (Reid & Morin, 1981). We lack knowledge and direction in program content and objectives, teaching techniques, and effectiveness of motor intervention, despite the fact that physical education is viewed as fundamental by education and government officials for *all* handicapped children.

An initial step in the creation of physical education programs for autistic persons might be a description of their motor skills, the knowledge of which should form a base for curriculum development. Early reports suggested that motor development and motor skills were normal for autistic individuals (Alderton, 1966; Kanner, 1943; Rimland, 1964; J. Wing, 1966). Recently, the notion of adequacy of motor control in autism has been questioned, although much of the evidence is clinical in nature (DeMyer, 1976; Lotter, 1966; Ornitz, Guthrie, & Farley, 1977; L. Wing, 1976; Singleton, Note 1). We need empirical work describing the motor functioning of autistic individuals. Such data should be quantitative and qualitative, as qualitative data are particularly lacking in descriptions of most handicapped persons.

The purpose of the present research was to more clearly describe the motor performance and anthropometric and fitness status of autistic children. The information generated should increase the knowledge base of autism as well as offer some direction for physical activity programmers.

Method

Subjects

Twelve subjects were chosen from a school for the multiply handicapped and from a hospital setting. Those selected were deemed by their physical education teachers to be "testable" on the proposed items and had been diagnosed as autistic by resident psychologists and psychiatrists. The subjects were divided into two groups: a young group, mean age 10.2 years, range 8.3-12.0, and an older group, mean age 16.6 years, range 14.8-19.4. With the exception of two females in the older group, all subjects were male.

Quantitative Tests

A sit-and-reach flexibility test using a modified Wells and Dillon flexometer was selected from the Standardized Test of Fitness (Note 2). Two test items were selected from the Bruininks-Oseretsky Test of Motor Proficiency (1978): catching and balance. The remaining items were taken from a study conducted by Rarick, Dobbins, and Broadhead (1976) and included: anthropometric and fitness measures of height, weight, left and right grip strength (hand dynamometer); abdominal strength (sit-ups); and estimated body fat (tricep subscapular and abdomen; Lange caliper), as well as the following performance measures—vertical and horizontal target throw, standing long-jump, mat crawl, and scramble. Test items were believed to provide a broad assessment of the motor domain. Cardiovascular tasks were excluded because motivating the subjects to sustain performance was not considered possible at this time. The Bruininks-Oseretsky Test and that of Rarick, Dobbins, and Broadhead (1976) also provide comparative norms with nonhandicapped children and in the latter case, norms with mentally retarded youngsters. All items were administered according to procedures outlined in the Standardized Test of Fitness, the Bruininks-Oseretsky Test, and the Rarick, Dobbins, and Broadhead test with any exceptions noted below.

Sit-ups. The number of bent-knee sit-ups in 60 seconds was assessed with the experimenter holding the subject's ankles. Subjects raised the upper body to the vertical plane but were not required to rotate the trunk to touch the contralateral elbow and knee.

Catching. Only the first four items of the Bruininks-Oseretsky upper-limb coordination subtest were employed, all using a tennis ball. The items were (1) bounce and catch the ball with both hands, (2) bounce and catch the ball with preferred hand, (3) catch a tossed ball with both hands from 10 feet, and (4) catch a tossed ball with the preferred hand from 10 feet. Each task included five trials with a maximum score of 5.

Balance. Only the composite balance score was used; it was calculated according to procedures in the Bruininks-Oseretsky *Examiners' Manual*.

Target Throw. A tennis ball was thrown at a 6-foot square target which was divided into 15 divisions of 4.8 inches each. The subjects were required to hit the centermost division which was bright yellow. Subjects threw 20 times at the target with the parallel lines running horizontally and 20 times with the lines running vertically. The target was placed 10 feet from the young autistic children and 15 feet from the older autistic individuals. Scores were the mean of the 20 trials.

Mat Crawl. Remaining on a hands-and-knees position, the subjects were required to crawl as quickly as possible around a pylon 8 feet away and return to the finish-starting line. The score was the mean of three trials to nearest 1/10 sec.

Scramble. Subjects were required to start in the supine position with their feet 10 feet away from a 10-inch wooden baton. The task was to get up as quickly as possible, run to the baton, pick it up and return to the starting position. The score was the mean time of three trials to the nearest 1/10 sec.

Qualitative Assessment

Qualitative components of catching, throwing, and standing long-jump also were assessed. The developmental diagrams and descriptions by McClenaghan and Gallahue (1978) were used to select the following qualitative dimensions for observation: *catching* — eyes tracking ball, arms form basket, hands in opposition, arms give with contact; *throwing* — weight transfer, cross extension pattern, elbow leading wrist, trunk rotation; and *standing long-jump* — initial knee bend with arms retracted in the preparatory crouch, body lean in flight, forward and upward arm swing, knee extension. The qualitative dimensions were measured on a yes/no basis with subjects receiving a "yes" score if the dimension was performed at the mature level (McClenaghan & Gallahue, 1978). The exception was "arms form basket" in the catching pattern which is described at the initial level by McClenaghan and Gallahue.

Procedures

All testing was conducted by two experimenters, one of whom was the student's physical education instructor. One experimenter was responsible for eliciting the performance while the other recorded the quantitative results. Both experimenters assessed the qualitative components of the catching, throwing, and standing long-jump tasks. Each subject was tested individually in a small gymnasium during normal school hours.

Every effort was made to obtain optimal performance. Test items were briefly described and demonstrated with subjects being prompted or manipulated if necessary. Practice trials were not constant as scored performance began only when task comprehension was apparent. If behavior of a subject interfered with testing a particular item, another task was chosen and the subject was returned to the original item later in the session. If a subject did not appear to understand the task or if disruptive behavior persisted, scores were not recorded.

Results

Reliability and Inter-Rater Agreement

Test-retest reliability was determined by a Spearman Coefficient Correlation. The obtained correlations were: balance .73, standing long-jump .93, sit-and-reach .95, and mat crawl .52.

Inter-rater agreement via percentage agreement procedure (ratio of number of congruent recordings to number of recordings) on the qualitative components were: catching, .86; throwing, .78; standing long-jump, .76; and retest of the standing long-jump, .78. Although the mat crawl results must be treated cautiously, the remaining reliability and interrater agreements were viewed as satisfactory.

Anthropometric and Physical Fitness Measures

Height and Weight. The height and weight of each subject was evaluated using the tables in Zaichowsky, Zaichowsky, and Martinek (1980). The percentile rank for each subject compared with nonhandicapped children is described in Table 1.

Estimated Body Fat, Grip Strength and Sit-up. Means and standard deviations for these items as well as normative data with retarded and nonretarded boys from Rarick, Dobbins, and Broadhead (1976) are presented in Table 2. Figures 1-6 graphically show these findings.

Flexibility. The results of the sit-and-reach test and the percentiles with a nonhandicapped sample are listed in Table 3.

Table 1
Percentiles[a] for Height and Weight of Each Subject

Subject	Age	Percentile	
		Height	Weight
Young autistics			
1	9.4	45	15
2	9.2	Below 5	15
3	8.3	10	50
4	11.2	70	70
5	11.0	85	Above 95
6	12.0	25	15
Older autistics			
1	16.5	10	45
2	15.7	25	80
3	16.2	NA[b]	NA[b]
4	16.8	50	65
5	19.4	NA	5
6	14.8	75	55

[a]From Zaichkowsky, Zaichkowsky, and Martinek (1980) based on nonhandicapped boys and girls.
[b]NA, not available.

Motor Performance Measures

Catching and Balance. The catching and balance results are presented in Table 4 with normative data from the Bruininks-Oseretsky Test of Motor Proficiency. The data are shown further in Figures 7 and 8.

With the catching tests, the younger autistic children were particularly weak in placing the hands in opposition while preparing for the ball and tended not to "give" upon contact. The older autistic subjects held their arms in opposition but did not "give" with contact. In general, therefore, a very immature catching pattern was evident for both groups. Although visual tracking was apparent in all subjects, inconsistency in this area was very common, especially with the younger students.

Target Throw. The results of the target throw are presented in Table 5 and are graphed in Figures 9 and 10. An immature throwing pattern was generally observed in the subjects. There were large, interindividual differences regarding weight transfer but the cross-extension pattern and trunk rotation were almost universally absent. Generally the elbow led the wrist during the early throwing action.

Standing Long-Jump. The results of the standing long-jump are presented in Table 2 and are shown in Figure 11. Subjects appeared to

Table 2
Means and Standard Deviations of Motor Performance and Anthropometric Data for Autistic, Educably Mentally Retarded[a], and Nonhandicapped Children[a]

Test	Young autistics			Older autistics			Young EMR boys[b]		Older EMR boys[b]		Nonhandicapped boys[b]	
	n	M	SD	n	M	SD	M	SD	M	SD	M	SD
Left grip strength (kg)	3	10.4	1.1	5	23.9	11.1	14.3	3.0	20.3	6.8	18.7	3.6
Right grip strength (kg)	3	9.9	2.5	5	23.3	11.2	14.9	3.4	20.9	6.3	19.0	3.7
Sit-ups (number/min)	6	10.3	7.9	6	10.8	5.5	16.8	7.8	21.9	8.6	22.6	8.1
Triceps skinfold (mm)	5	20.7	14.5	6	18.4	6.9	10.6	4.9	10.8	5.8	6.0	2.2
Subscapular skinfold (mm)	5	12.5	10.2	5	12.3	3.7	6.7	5.3	9.6	7.1	4.4	1.9
Abdominal skinfold (mm)	5	22.8	22.6	5	23.8	14.0	8.3	6.8	13.5	11.6	4.9	3.3
Standing long-jump (in.)	6	25.0	16.8	6	29.5	41.2	44.4	9.3	50.6	11.0	52.4	7.9
Mat crawl (sec)	6	8.2	1.8	6	9.1	2.2	5.0	.8	4.8	.8	4.2	.6
Scramble (sec)	6	12.1	6.8	6	11.2	2.7	5.8	1.0	5.7	1.1	5.2	.6

[a]From Rarick, Dobbins, & Broadhead (1976).
[b]Young EMR boys = 8.5 years; n = number of subjects; older EMR boys = 11.5 years; M = mean; nonhandicapped boys = 8.4 years; SD = standard deviation.

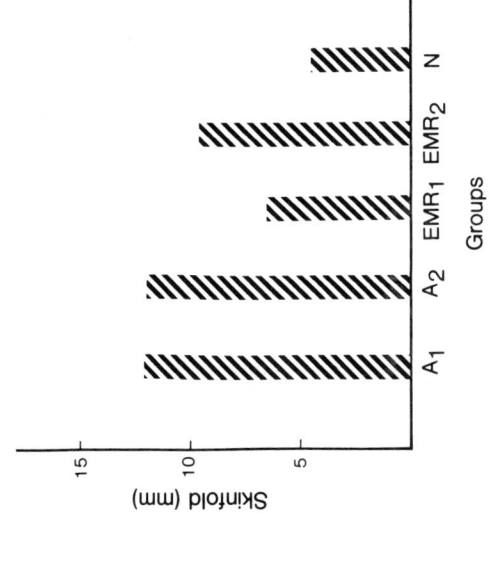

Figure 1 – Triceps skinfold for autistic subjects and for comparison subjects. (A_1 = young autistics, A_2 = older autistics, EMR_1 = young educable mentally retarded boys, EMR_2 = older educable mentally retarded boys, N = nonhandicapped boys.)

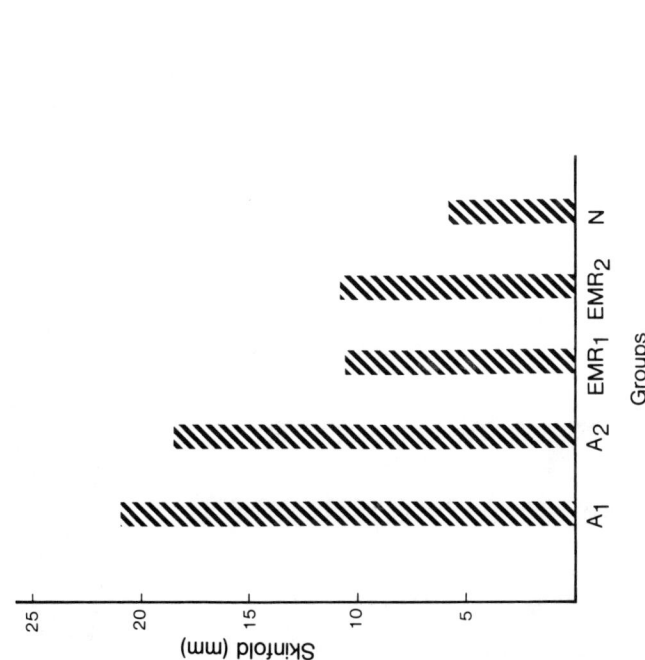

Figure 2 – Subscapular skinfold for autistic subjects and for comparison subjects. (A_1 = young autistics, A_2 = older autistics, EMR_1 = young educable mentally retarded boys, EMR_2 = older educable mentally retarded boys, N = nonhandicapped boys.)

208 / REID, COLLIER, AND MORIN

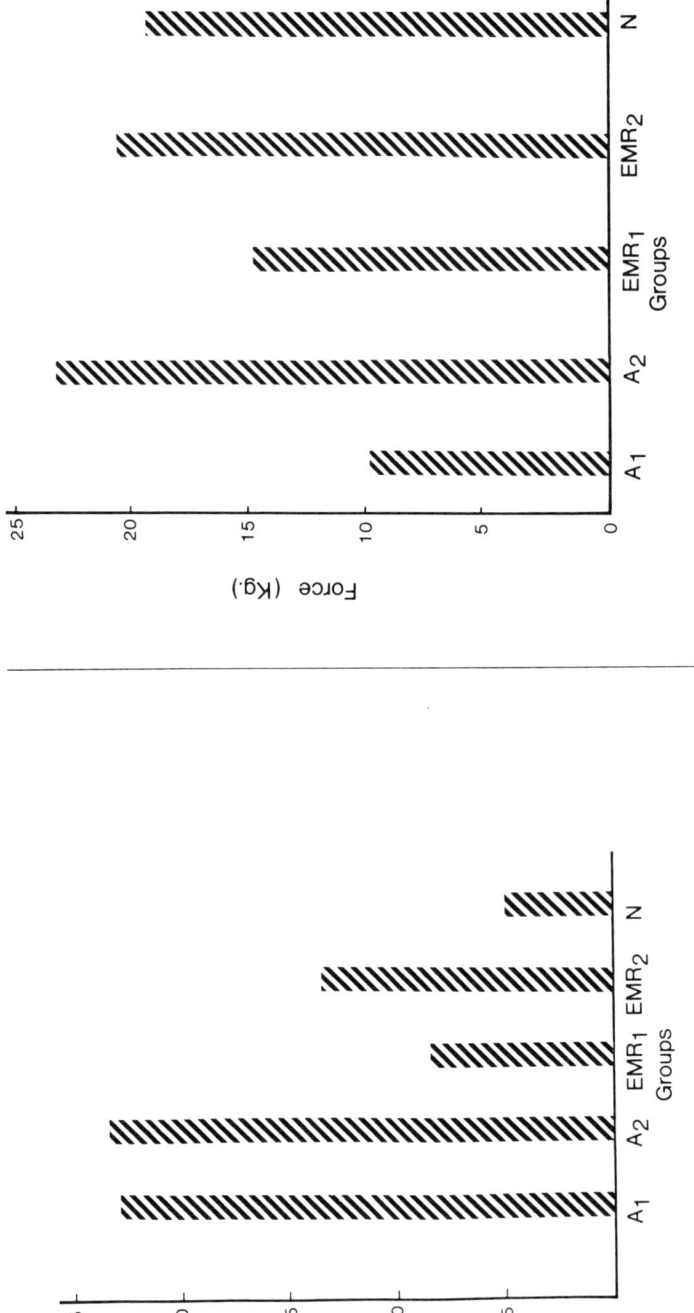

Figure 3 — Abdominal skinfold for autistic subjects and for comparison subjects. (A_1 = young autistics, A_2 = older autistics, EMR_1 = young educable mentally retarded boys, EMR_2 = older educable mentally retarded boys, N = nonhandicapped boys.)

Figure 4 — Left hand grip strength for autistic subjects and for comparison subjects. (A_1 = young autistics, A_2 = older autistics, EMR_1 = young educable mentally retarded boys, EMR_2 = older educable mentally retarded boys, N = nonhandicapped boys.)

MOTOR PERFORMANCE OF AUTISTIC INDIVIDUALS / 209

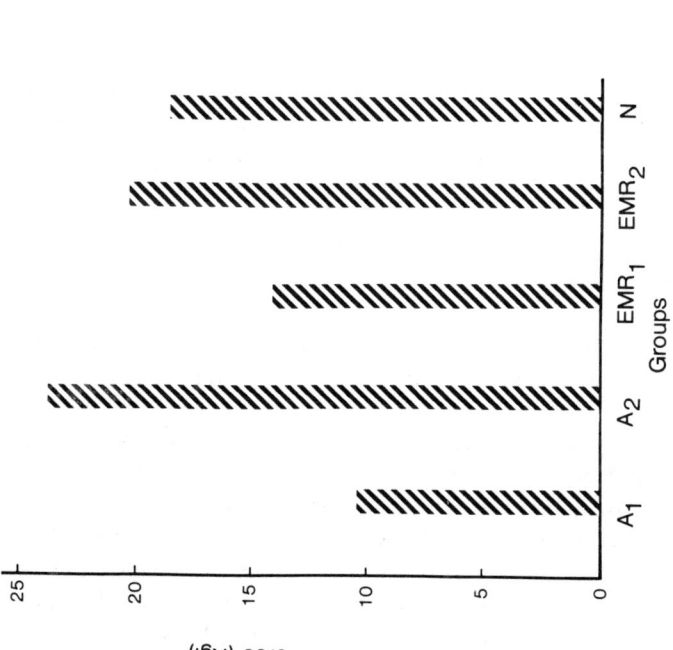

Figure 5—Right hand grip strength for autistic subjects and comparison subjects. (A_1 = young autistics, A_2 = older autistics, EMR_1 = young educable mentally retarded boys, EMR_2 = older educable mentally retarded boys, N = nonhandicapped boys.)

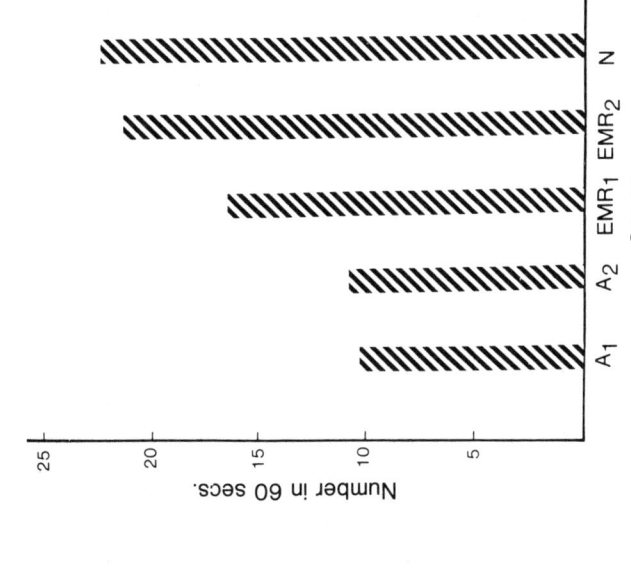

Figure 6—Sit-ups for autistic subjects and for comparison subjects. (A_1 = young autistics, A_2 = older autistics, EMR_1 = young educable mentally retarded boys, EMR_2 = older educable mentally retarded boys, N = nonhandicapped boys.)

Table 3
Means and Standard Deviations for Flexibility: Sit and Reach

Group	n	M	SD	Percentile rank[a]
Young autistics	6	13.3	9.7	
Older autistics	5	12.4	11.7	Below 5

[a]Percentile rank from the Standardized Test of Fitness (1981), males 17-19.

have good imitation and maintenance of the crouch, although difficulty in coordination of leg extension and arm swing was evident. In general, body lean in flight was almost vertical and the arm swing was minimal.

Mat Crawl. The results of the mat crawl test are listed in Table 2 and are graphed in Figure 12. It was noted that verbal encouragement was particularly necessary on the task in order to elicit maximal performance.

Scramble. The results of the scramble test are presented in Table 2 and are shown in Figure 13. As in the mat crawl, it was apparent that verbal encouragement was necessary for subjects to optimally perform the task.

Discussion

Some cautionary notes and restrictions germane to all test items are warranted before discussing the findings. Because of the low numbers in the study, only major trends are described in the ensuing paragraphs. Care must also be exercised in comparing the performance of autistic persons with the various groups presented in the tables and figures. For example, in Table 2, the older autistic group has a mean age of 16.6 years whereas the nonretarded boys are 8.4 years old and the older EMR boys are 11.5 years old. Although these are clearly not ideal groups to compare, it was felt nonetheless that simply reporting averages for autistic persons would be less productive. Indeed, it *is* quite meaningful that autistic adolescents often perform more poorly than much younger retarded or nonretarded children.

Anecdotal comments suggested the subjects were seldom clearly motivated to perform well. It may be that the tasks and their administration were novel; autistic subjects often do not perform well in new environments. Also the students may not have fully comprehended some of the tasks. Although procedures such as familiar experimenters, use of prompts in practice trials, and verbal encouragement were used to elicit optimal performance, it is possible the data are, in part, a reflection of understanding and interest in the tasks rather than purely an indication

Table 4
Means and Standard Deviations for Catching and Balance

Test	Young autistics			Older autistics			Nonhandicapped boys[a] 10 yr		14 yr	
	n	M	SD	n	M	SD	M	SD	M	SD
Catching										
Item 1	6	2.0	1.3	6	1.8	1.2				
Item 2	6	1.8	1.7	6	1.8	1.5				
Item 3	6	1.5	1.4	6	2.7	.5				
Item 4	6	1.2	1.7	6	1.5	1.4				
Balance	6	11.0	4.2	6	13.2	5.9	25.2	4.4	25.7	2.8

[a]From Bruininks-Oseretsky Test of Motor Proficiency (1978).
n = Number of subjects; M = mean; SD = standard deviation.

Table 5
Means and Standard Deviations for Target Throw

Test	Young autistics			Older autistics			Young EMR girls[a]		Young EMR boys[a]	
	n	M	SD	n	M	SD	M	SD	M	SD
Horizontal target throw	3	4.6	1.3	5	3.8	2.9	5.7	1.01	5.9	.75
Vertical target throw	3	5.5	1.4	5	4.1	2.2	6.1	.79	5.99	.69

n = Number of subjects; M = mean; SD = standard deviation.
[a]Young EMR girls = 8.5 years; young EMR boys = 8.5 years. From Rarick, Dobbins, & Broadhead.

of present capabilities. Despite these acknowledged limitations, the data do point to some tentative interpretations and conclusions.

It is apparent from Table 1 that the autistic subjects were, with few exceptions, within the normal bounds of height and weight for their chronological age. However, they appeared to be rather corpulent, judging from the skinfold measures (Figures 1-3). Both younger and older subjects were carrying appreciably more fat than the educable retarded or nonretarded boys.

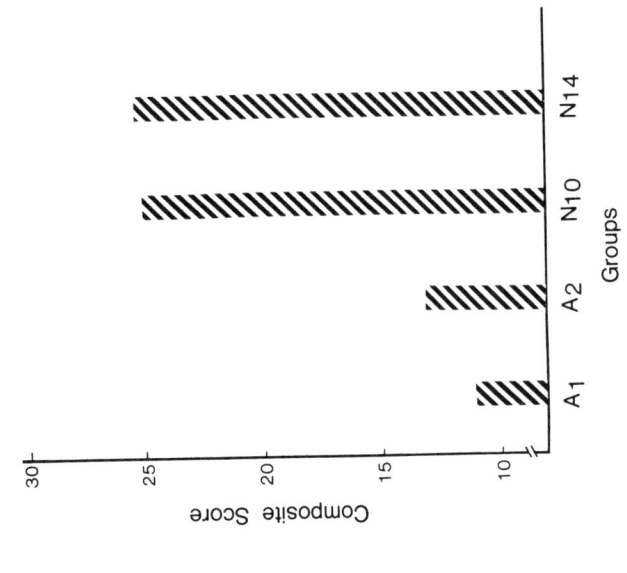

Figure 8 — Composite balance scores for autistic and nonautistic groups. (A_1 = young autistics, A_2 = older autistics, N_{10} = nonhandicapped 10-year-old boys, N_{14} = nonhandicapped 14-year-old boys.)

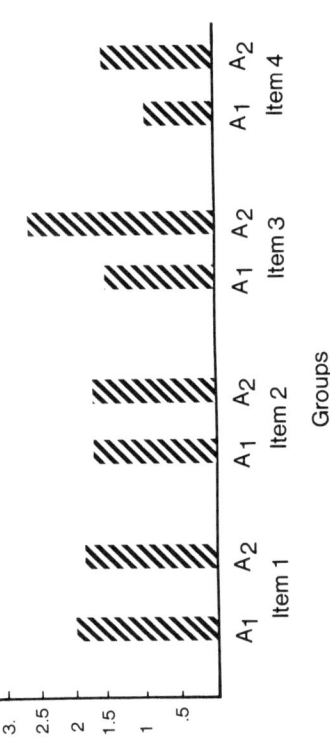

Figure 7 — Performance scores on four catching tasks for autistic subjects. (A_1 = young autistics, A_2 = older autistics.)

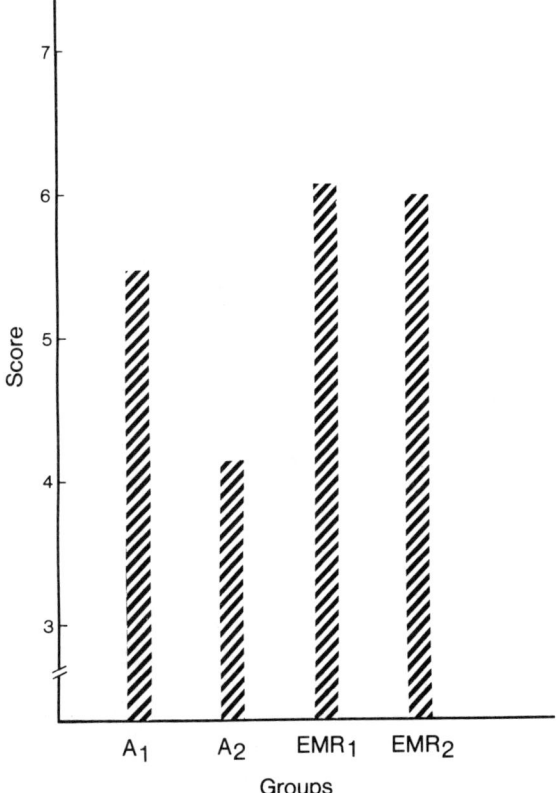

Figure 9 — Horizontal target throw scores for autistic subjects and for comparison subjects. (A_1 = young autistics, A_2 = older autistics, EMR_1 = young educable mentally retarded girls, EMR_2 = young educable mentally retarded boys.)

The young autistic group demonstrated less grip strength than the young mentally retarded children and the nonretarded group although the autistic students averaged 2 years older than either of the comparison groups. The older autistic group did not exert greater force than the nonretarded comparison group despite their being 8 years older (Figures 4 and 5). The notion of strength deficits in the 2 groups of autistic students is also supported by the results of abdominal strength as assessed by sit-ups (Figure 6).

The older autistic pupils did not demonstrate flexibility commensurate with their age, judging from their percentile rank of less than 5 (Table 3). Although data with nonhandicapped children of similar ages to the young autistic pupils were unavailable, flexibility would not be expected to be less in younger subjects. Thus, it can be concluded that both groups of autistic subjects demonstrated a large deficit in trunk flexion. In sum-

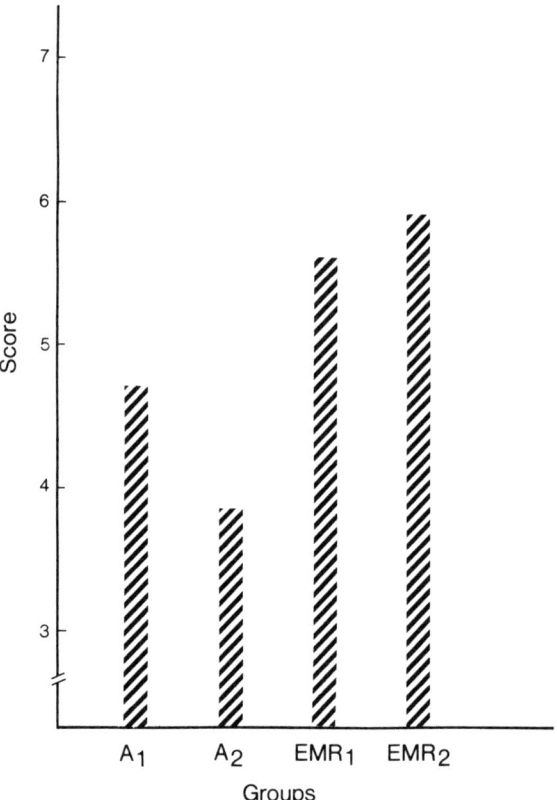

Figure 10 – Vertical target throw scores for autistic subjects and for comparison subjects. (A_1 = young autistics, A_2 = older autistics, EMR_1 = young educable mentally retarded girls, EMR_2 = young educable mentally retarded boys.)

mary, the autistic individuals appear to be within normal ranges of weight and stature but seem to score poorly on physical fitness measures of estimated body fat, grip strength, abdominal strength, and flexibility.

The autistic individuals performed below comparison groups on the balance and target-throwing tasks (Figures 8-10). In addition, target-throwing results indicated immature patterns of throwing. Both groups of autistic students performed quite poorly on the standing long-jump (Figure 11). Furthermore, the autistic groups appeared deficient with regard to qualitative dimensions of the task as immature jumping patterns were evident.

The mat crawl and scramble are complex tasks compared with previously discussed items. They are, for example, dependent on the subject's maintaining enthusiasm for the task over a longer period of time. Also, the tasks have discrete components (e.g., stand up, run). It was noted

MOTOR PERFORMANCE OF AUTISTIC INDIVIDUALS / 215

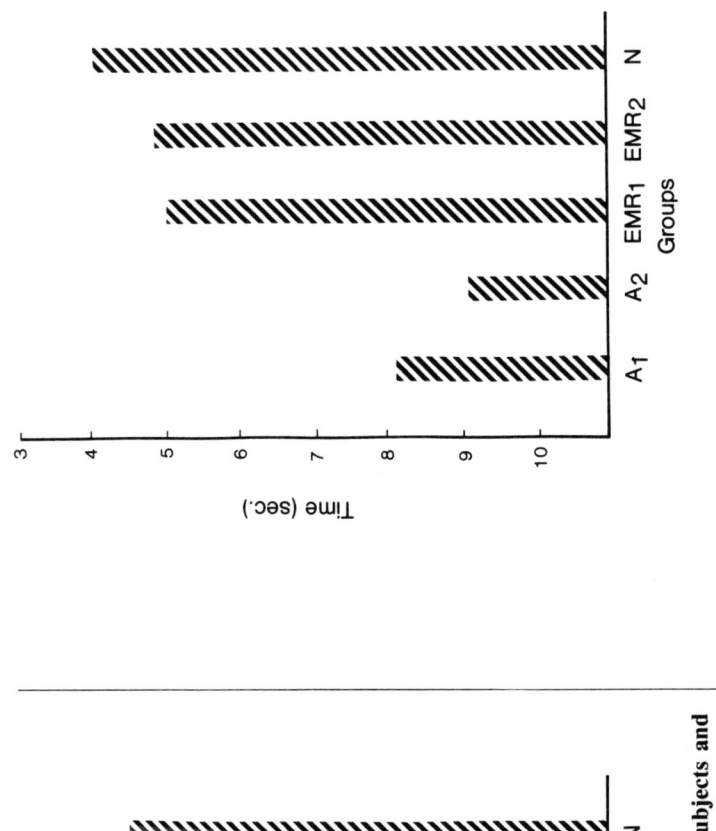

Figure 11 – Standing long-jump scores for autistic subjects and for comparison subjects. (A_1 = young autistics, A_2 = older autistics, EMR_1 = young educable mentally retarded boys, EMR_2 = older educable mentally retarded boys, N = nonhandicapped boys.)

Figure 12 – Mat crawl scores for autistic subjects and for comparison subjects. (A_1 = young autistics, A_2 = older autistics, EMR_1 = young educable mentally retarded boys, EMR_2 = older educable mentally retarded boys, N = nonhandicapped boys.)

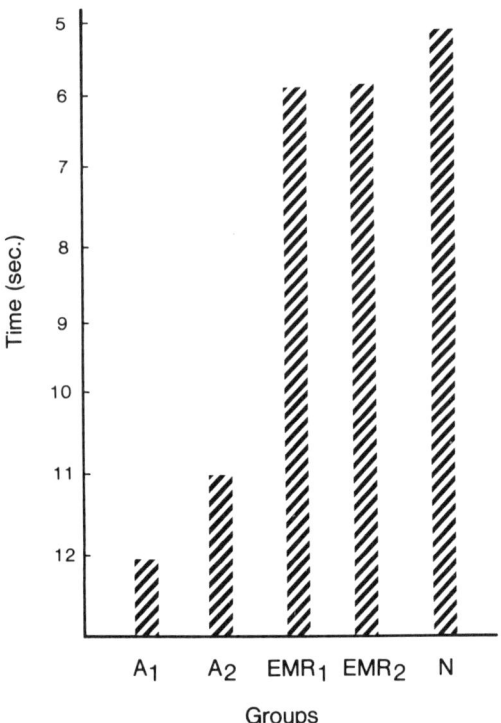

Figure 13 — Scramble scores for autistic subjects and for comparison subjects. (A_1 = young autistics, A_2 = older autistics, EMR_1 = young educable mentally retarded boys, EMR_2 = older educable mentally retarded boys, N = nonhandicapped boys.)

that verbal encouragement was required in order to maintain the subject's interest in the task. On one hand, this is very preliminary evidence that verbal praise is an effective motivator in such "endurance" tasks. On the other hand, it is unclear how effective their performance might have been under another motivational regime. With the mat crawl (Figure 12) and scramble (Figure 13) both groups of autistic pupils were much slower than the mentally retarded or nonretarded groups.

The motor performance data from balance, catching, throwing, standing long-jump, mat crawl, and scramble tests suggest several trends. Minimal differences in performance were evident on most tasks between the younger and older groups. It is possible the older students have not improved for many years, but the explanations for this are unclear. We have no reason to believe that the lack of motor development apparent in this study represents a ceiling effect unique to autism.

Large between-subject variability as demonstrated by standard deviations (see Table 2 in particular) was evident in motor performance tasks.

Such wide variation is common in groups of exceptional children and presents obvious difficulties to the special education teacher.

The present data support previous research and clinical reports which argued that autistic persons do not perform motor skills at a rate consistent with their chronological age (DeMyer, 1976; Geddes, 1977; Ornitz, Guthrie, & Farley, 1977; Singleton, Note 1). Also, the subjects generally scored lower than mentally retarded children, a finding at odds with DeMyer's research. This incongruency might be due to dissimilar autistic students in the two investigations. Because diagnosing autism is still in its infancy, comparing two groups across studies is difficult. Physical activity programmers should be aware that physical fitness and motor performance often are weak in autistic students. Individualized instruction using contemporary educational technology probably is necessary for these youngsters to develop motor skills.

Reference Notes

1. Singleton, D. A physical education program for the autistic child. Paper presented at the Third National Conference on Physical Activity Programs and Practices for the Exceptional Individual, Long Beach, CA, 1974.
2. Standardized Test of Fitness. *Fitness and Amateur Sport.* Government of Canada, 1981.

References

ALDERTON, H.R. A review of schizophrenia in childhood. *Canadian Psychiatric Association Journal*, 1966, **11**, 276-285.

BRUININKS, R.H. *Bruininks-Oseretsky Test of Motor Proficiency.* Circle Pines, MN: American Guidance Service, 1978.

DEMYER, M.K. Motor, perceptual-motor, intellectual disabilities of autistic children. In L. Wing (Ed.), *Early childhood autism* (2nd ed.). New York: Pergamon Press, 1976.

GEDDES, D. Motor development of autistic monozygotic twins: A case study. *Perceptual and Motor Skills*, 1977, **45**, 179-186.

KANNER, L. Autistic disturbances of affective contact. *The Nervous Child.* 1943, **43**(4), 80-81.

LOTTER, V. Services for a group of autistic children in Middlesex. In J.K. Wing (Ed.), *Early childhood autism*. London: Pergamon Press, 1966.

MCCLENAGHAN, B.A., & Gallahue, D.J. *Fundamental movement.* Philadelphia: W.B. Saunders, 1978.

ORNITZ, E.M., Guthrie, D., & Farley, A.J. The early development of autistic children. *Journal of Autism and Childhood Schizophrenia*, 1977, **7**, 208-229.

RARICK, G.L., Dobbins, D.L., & Broadhead, G.D. *The motor domain and its correlates in educationally handicapped children.* Englewood Cliffs, NJ: Prentice-Hall, 1976.

REID, G., & Morin, B. Physical education for autistic children. *CAHPER Journal*, 1981, **48**, 25-29.

RIMLAND, B. *Infantile autism: The syndrome and its implications for a neural theory of behavior.* New York: Appleton-Century-Croft, 1964.

WING, J.K. (Ed.). *Early childhood autism.* London: Pergamon Press, 1966.

WING, L. Diagnosis, clinical description and prognosis. In L. Wing (Ed.), *Early Childhood Autism* (2nd ed.). New York: Pergamon Press, 1976.

ZAICHKOWSKY, L.D., Zaichkowsky, L.B., & Martinek, T.J. *Growth and development: The child and physical activity.* St. Louis: C.V. Mosby, 1980.

A Comparison of the Qualitative Motor Performance of Normal, Educable, and Trainable Mentally Retarded Students

Dale A. Ulrich
Southern Illinois University at Carbondale

Most motor assessment instruments can be classified into two groups: those that measure the quantitative aspects of motor performance and those that assess the qualitative performance. The vast majority of instruments surveyed fall into the first category.

Quantitative measures of fundamental motor skills for primary- and elementary-age children were generated by a number of investigators. Taylor (1941) and Latchaw (1954) collected comparative data for activities found in the context of a physical education curriculum for primary and elementary grades. Carpenter (1942), Glassow and Krause (1957), Johnson (1962), and Kane and Meredith (1953) investigated quantitative performance of what they termed "general motor ability." These studies of fundamental motor skills consisted of measuring distances and times with emphasis on age-appropriate behaviors.

Qualitative analysis of fundamental motor skills was first identified in detail when Wild (1938) studied the overhand throw of 32 children ranging in age from 2 to 12 years. Hellebrandt, Lawrence, Glassow, and Carns (1961) studied the broad jump and were able to document the sequential development of that skill as the 47 subjects demonstrated various stages of the skill. Seefeldt, Henn, and Haubenstricker (Note 1; Notes 3-9), Milne (Note 2), and Wickstrom (1977) have attempted to qualitatively establish common sequences of motor skill development in several fundamental motor skills.

Motor skill acquisition is a sequential and complex process during which attention is focused successfully from simple to more complex competency. The most common levels of motor skill acquisition used to describe the degree of competency in a specific skill are: (1) rudimentary (nonmature) level; (2) mature or qualitative level; and (3) functional (qualitative plus quantitative aspects) level. The rudimentary level represents initial learning of the skill without having all of the required components. The mature or qualitative level represents a degree of competency exemplary of mastery of all the stated qualitative components of a skill. The functional level represents the performance of the mature level plus the quantitative aspects of distance, time, and/or accuracy.

In reviewing the available literature, it is apparent that the majority of studies comparing the motor performance of handicapped and nonhandicapped groups incorporate quantitative test batteries. If they had used qualitative tests, as well, they may have resulted in more complete findings. This unevenness in the literature suggests that more knowledge is needed relative to qualitative comparisons of various student groups.

Procedures

Student assessment data were collected by administering a criterion-referenced test standardized by Ulrich (1981) covering 12 fundamental motor and four physical fitness skills. Each skill test item was subdivided into four performance levels. The mature or qualitative performance level was used as the criterion for each test item. This level was present when a student completed the item according to *all* stated qualitative criteria. The second level or rudimentary performance was present when a student responded to some of the qualitative criteria but not all of them. The third level represented a student who needed some form of physical assistance to perform one qualitative component. The final level of performance for each skill item was represented when a student refused physical assistance or responded inappropriately.

Three testers were employed to collect the data. Prior to any formal data collection, each tester had to meet a 1.0 level of mastery when compared to expert ratings of a videotape demonstrating the 16 skills. Subsequent to reaching the mandatory level of assessment accuracy, the testers evaluated the motor performance of 117 nonhandicapped students, 96 educable mentally retarded students placed in special classes in the regular neighborhood school, and 66 trainable mentally retarded students placed in special classes in intermediate school districts.

The age range of the sample was 36 months to 155 months with sample sizes by age including: 3-year-olds ($n = 18$), 4-year-olds ($n = 21$), 5-year-olds ($n = 29$), 6-year-olds ($n = 29$), 7-year-olds ($n = 33$), 8-year-olds ($n = 39$), 9-year-olds ($n = 46$), 10-year-olds ($n = 26$), 11-year-olds ($n = 21$), and 12-year-olds ($n = 17$). The sample was also stratified by sex: females ($n = 134$) and males ($n = 145$). Each tester administered all test items on an individual basis and was responsible for obtaining the correct data on student classification and age from the student's teacher.

The student performance data were initially analyzed by computing a three-way analysis of variance (ANOVA) to test for a significant interaction effect. If an interaction effect was significant, the means were plotted to determine if it was ordinal or disordinal in nature. Where the interaction was disordinal, or not significant, the main effects of age, student classification, and sex were tested. If main effects were significant, the Tukey Multiple Range Test was conducted to determine the location.

Results

Initial analysis of the data consisted of computing a three-way ANOVA to test for an interaction between sex, age, and student classification (normal, educable, and trainable). The run test item resulted in a significant (.007) disordinal interaction for age by student classification. The horizontal jump test item resulted in a significant (.003) disordinal interaction for sex by age and by student classification. The leap test item also resulted in a significant (.01) disordinal interaction for sex by student classification. The only physical fitness test item to result in an interaction was the sit and reach. This item resulted in a significant (.002) disordinal interaction for sex by age and by student classification.

Subsequent to the initial interaction analysis, the main effects of sex, age, and student classification were evaluated. The mean and standard deviation for each test item (skill) were calculated by converting each performance level into numerical form (criterion level = 4, rudimentary level = 3, physically assisted level = 2, and other level = 1). The only test items to result in significant (.01) differences across sex were the overhand throw ($F = 9.30$) and the two-hand strike ($F = 26.12$). All 12 fundamental motor skill test items resulted in significant (.01) main effects across age (3-12), whereas none of the physical fitness skill items were significant. This may have been due to the fact that the physical fitness items were only administered to students between 8 and 12 years of age. Significant main effects resulted for all 16 skill items across the three student groups.

Where significant main effects were realized, the Tukey Multiple Range Test was conducted. In 10 of the test items, neither of the three student classifications resulted in homogenous student performances. Six of the items (overhand throw, stationary bounce, kick, two-hand strike, sit and reach, and run/walk) had homogeneous student performance in some combination relative to student classification.

Table 1 presents a summary of ages at which the criterion level of performance (mature form) was mastered by 25, 50, and 75% or more of the

Table 1
Age at Which the Criterion Level of Performance Was Mastered by 25%, 50%, and 75% or More of the Students in Each of the Student Classification Samples

Test Item	Classi-fication	Age 25%	Age 50%	Age 75%	Test Item	Classi-fication	Age 25%	Age 50%	Age 75%
Run	N[a]	4	4	9	Catch	N	6	7	9
	E[b]	7	9	12		E	7	10	12
	T[c]	8	—[d]	—		T	11	—	—
Gallop	N	5	5	7	Stationary	N	6	7	9
	E	7	9	12	bounce	E	7	9	9
	T	11	—	—		T	9	—	—
Hop	N	4	5	7	Kick	N	8	10	11
	E	7	9	10		E	8	12	12
	T	8	—	—		T	—	—	—
Skip	N	5	9	9	Two-hand	N	4	9	—
	E	6	—	—	strike	E	7	10	12
	T	12	—	—		T	—	—	—
Horizontal	N	4	5	9	Sit-ups[e]	N	8	9	11
	E	6	9	12		E	11	12	12
	T	8	—	—		T	11	12	—
Slide	N	4	9	11	Sit and	N	8	10	12
	E	7	10	12	reach[e]	E	11	12	—
	T	—	—	—		T	8	—	—
Leap	N	9	10	11	Push-ups[e]	N	9	12	—
	E	—	—	—		E	—	—	—
	T	—	—	—		T	—	—	—
Overhand	N	4	7	—	Run/walk[e]	N	8	8	8
throw	E	7	12	12		E	8	8	8
	T	11	—	—		T	8	9	9

[a]Normal student classification.
[b]Educable mentally impaired student classification.
[c]Trainable mentally impaired student classification.
[d]The criterion level was not mastered by this percentage of the students at any age between 3 and 12.
[e]This test item was administered to students 8 years old and above.

students in each of the student classification samples. Table 2 presents a summary of ages at which the criterion level of performance first appeared for each student classification on each test item.

Reviewing the mean and standard deviation for subtotal scores (locomotor, object control, and physical fitness) for each student classification was the final phase of data analysis. As would be expected, normal students scored the highest, followed by educables and then trainables. These results support the research literature comparing the quantitative performance of the three student classifications.

Table 2
Age at Which the Criterion Level of Performance First Appeared for Each Student Classification

Test Item	Classification	Age	Test Item	Classification	Age
Run	N[a]	3	Catch	N	5
	E[b]	7		E	7
	T[c]	7		T	11
Gallop	N	5	Stationary bounce	N	5
	E	7		E	5
	T	11		T	8
Hop	N	3	Kick	N	5
	E	6		E	7
	T	8		T	8
Skip	N	4	Two-hand strike	N	4
	E	5		E	5
	T	9		T	7
Horizontal jump	N	4	Sit-ups[d]	N	8
	E	4		E	8
	T	6		T	9
Slide	N	4	Sit and reach[d]	N	8
	E	7		E	8
	T	—[e]		T	8
Leap	N	6	Push-ups[d]	N	8
	E	7		E	9
	T	—		T	12
Overhand throw	N	3	Run/walk[d]	N	8
	E	7		E	8
	T	8		T	8

[a]Normal student classification.
[b]Educable mentally impaired student classification.
[c]Trainable mentally impaired student classification.
[d]This test item was administered to students 8 years old and above.
[e]The criterion level of performance did not appear in the age range 3-12.

Discussion

Our findings indicate that student classification differences do exist relative to qualitative motor performance. Using the age at which 50% of the students in each student classification mastered the criterion (mature) level of performance (Table 1), the results indicate that normal students are approximately 3.5 years ahead of educable mentally retarded students on qualitative performance of fundamental motor skills. Normal students are at least 6 years ahead of the trainable mentally retarded group.

In comparing educables and trainables, the data indicate that educables are at least 3 years ahead of trainables. The actual age at which 50% of the trainable group mastered the criterion level is unknown. It was set at 13, but a large measurement error could be present.

The difference in qualitative motor skill performance between the three groups usually is attributed to the lack of adequate opportunities for movement experiences at an early age. Trainable mentally retarded children are not known for their ability to initiate play. If they are left to their own efforts, they will develop very sedentary lives. Another contributing factor is that the majority of motor skill instruction is being delivered by untrained classroom teachers in special education settings. Unless parent or professional pressure is placed on special education administrators, specialists in adapted physical education will not be hired.

The last contributing factor that is evident in a majority of special education centers is the emphasis placed on Special Olympics rather than on a systematically planned program of motor skill development. The Special Olympics, although it is very beneficial, was not designed to take the place of regularly scheduled physical education, but rather to supplement the program. Unless we make efforts to correct the inadequacies for handicapped students, they will remain far below their nonhandicapped peers in motor skill performance.

Reference Notes

1. Haubenstricker, J., Henn, J., & Seefeldt, V. *Developmental stages of hopping*. Unpublished paper, Michigan State University, 1975.
2. Milne, C. *Fundamental motor skill sequences*. Unpublished paper, University of Western Ontario, London, Ontario, 1972.
3. Seefeldt, V. *Developmental sequence of catching*. Unpublished paper, Michigan State University, 1976.
4. Seefeldt, V. *Developmental sequence of running*. Unpublished paper, Michigan State University, 1976.
5. Seefeldt, V. *Developmental sequence of the standing long jump*. Unpublished paper, Michigan State University, 1976.

6. Seefeldt, V., & Haubenstricker, J. *Developmental sequence in skipping.* Unpublished paper, Michigan State University, 1974.
7. Seefeldt, V., & Haubenstricker, J. *Developmental sequence of kicking.* Unpublished paper, Michigan State University, 1975.
8. Seefeldt, V., & Haubenstricker, J. *Developmental sequence of striking.* Unpublished paper, Michigan State University, 1976.
9. Seefeldt, V., (Haubenstricker, J. *Developmental sequence of throwing.* Unpublished paper, Michigan State University, 1976.

References

CARPENTER, A. The measurement of general motor capacity and general motor ability in the first three grades. *Research Quarterly*, 1942, **13**, 444-465.

GLASSOW, R., & Krause, P. Motor performance of girls age 6 to 14 years. *Research Quarterly*, 1957, **28**, 400-406.

HELLEBRANDT, F., Lawrence, G., Glassow, R., & Carns, M. Physiological analysis of basic motor skills. *American Journal of Physical Medicine*, 1961, **40**, 14-25.

JOHNSON, R. Measurements of achievements in fundamental skills of elementary school children. *Research Quarterly*, 1962, **32**, 94-103.

KANE, R., & Meredith, N. Ability in the standing broad jump of elementary school children 7, 9, and 11 years of age. *Research Quarterly*, 1953, **23**, 198-208.

LATCHAW, M. Measuring selected motor skills in fourth, fifth, and sixth grades. *Research Quarterly*, 1954, **25**, 439-449.

TAYLOR, E. Achievement scales in physical education skills for children in grades I, II, III. *The Elementary School Journal.* May 1941, 677-682.

ULRICH, D. *The standardization of a criterion-referenced test in fundamental motor and physical fitness skills.* Unpublished doctoral dissertation, Michigan State University, 1981.

WICKSTROM, R. *Fundamental motor patterns.* Philadelphia: Lea and Febiger, 1977.

WILD, M. The behavior pattern of throwing and some observations concerning its course of development in children. *Research Quarterly*, 1938, **9**, 20-24.

Discriminatory Response Time and Heart Rate Differences Between Gifted and Learning Disabled Children

Leighton E. Stamps, Bobby L. Eason,
and Theresa L. Smith
University of New Orleans

Learning disability has been defined in many ways, often from widely different viewpoints. In examining these definitions, however, we found that they all had at least one point in common. Learning disabled (LD) children are described as having difficulty in paying attention. Most classroom teachers report that learning disabled children are the worst attenders and children who have been identified as gifted tend to be among the best attenders in their classes. The degree of attention that individuals exhibit in a given situation will be based on two factors: (1) their motivation or desire to attend, and (2) their ability to attend, which is related to neurological and other physiological factors.

The simplest form of attention is the orienting response (OR), for which Sokolov (1963) described five response components: (a) increased sensitivity of the sense organs; (b) motor orientation of the sense organs toward the source of stimulation; (c) changes in general skeletal musculature; (d) desynchronization of the EEG pattern with accompanying lowered amplitude and increased frequency; and (e) autonomic responses including decreased skin resistance, decreased respiratory frequency with increased amplitude, and heart rate deceleration. Thus, the

OR facilitates information intake. Lacey and Lacey (1970) have examined the cardiovascular components of the OR in great detail and have reported an inverse relationship between the magnitude of heart rate deceleration and the latency of psychomotor responding in attention-demanding tasks. Thus, the larger the deceleration, the faster the reaction time. These researchers also have found that the performance of simple cognitive tasks, such as mental arithmetic, results in heart rate acceleration. Their findings indicate that when individuals are attempting to take in information from the external environment, their heart rate decelerates. When internal processing takes place and external stimulation is ignored, acceleration occurs.

Much of the research related to heart rate responses has focused on the mechanism of the deceleratory response. According to Lacey's theory, the cardiovascular responses observed during attention-demanding tasks are both stimuli to and responses of the central nervous system. Thus, Lacey and Lacey disagree with the view that the autonomic nervous system is solely an effector system. Based on neurophysiological evidence, they have concluded that the cardiovascular system is a source of a negative feedback pathway to the central nervous system. The negative feedback impulses, coming from baroreceptors in the aortic arch and carotid sinus of the heart, may result in inhibitory effects on several physiological response systems. Increased output from baroreceptors, which would result from increased heart rate, has been shown to produce a number of changes, including decreased muscle tone, increased slow activity in the electroencephalogram, elevation of threshold for a monosynaptic reflex and shortened duration of stimulus produced, increases in neural and muscle activities. Decreased input from the baroreceptors, resulting from heart rate deceleration, would have the opposite effect.

Because heart rate changes seem to play a regulatory role in attentional processes, we have done several previous studies examining relationships between heart rate measures of attention and performance in learning disabled and gifted children. In our first study, the children were given a "Get ready" signal, followed several seconds later by a "Go" signal, at which point they had to run a distance of 11 feet. We were primarily interested in the heart rate changes between the "Get ready" and the "Go" signals, a time when the child had to pay very close attention. We found that the gifted children showed larger heart rate decelerations prior to the "Go" signal than did the LD children. The gifted children also exhibited faster running times than the LDs. In our second study, we compared gifted and LD children on a perceptual search task while we monitored their heart rates. Each child was required to look at a slide and identify certain characteristics as quickly as possible. We found that the gifted children showed larger heart rate decelerations while they were looking at the slides and faster response times than the LDs. Thus, in both of these studies the gifted children showed larger decreases in heart rate and faster response times than the LD children. In the present study, we used a similar paradigm comparing gifted and LD children on a reaction time task while heart rate was recorded.

Method

Sixteen gifted boys and 16 learning-disabled boys were included in the study. Each member of the gifted group had an IQ of 120 or above and was enrolled in a program for gifted and talented children. The LD boys had IQs between 90 and 110, and were at least 2 years below grade level in reading. They also had no diagnosed emotional or perceptual problems.

Each child was tested individually. On each of eight trials, a 2-second warning tone was followed by an interval of 10, 15, or 20 seconds, and, finally, the respond signal. The warning signal was a 70-db, 250-Hz sine wave. The respond signal was the illumination of one of four pilot lights. The child then had to press a button corresponding to the illuminated light. Subjects were told that the tone meant that they were to get ready to push the button. They were then told to push the button as quickly as possible when the light came on. The subjects were also informed that they would receive a prize at the end of the session if their responses were fast enough. All of the boys were given prizes. All stimuli were presented automatically, using electronic timers.

Heart rate was measured during 1 second prior to warning signal onset (baseline) and for a total of 15 seconds, divided into three periods, following warning signal onset. Period I included the first 5 seconds, following warning signal onset; period II consisted of the 5 seconds prior to the respond signal; and period III included the 5 seconds following the respond signal. For analysis, difference scores were calculated for each subject on each trial by subtracting the baseline heart rate for that trial from the heart rate during each of the 15 1-second intervals. Thus, we obtained a total of 15 data points for each trial.

Results and Discussion

An analysis of variance of the reaction times yielded a group difference, $F(1, 30) = 5.83, p < .03$. The mean reaction times were 1.08 seconds for the LD group and .80 seconds for the gifted children. The analysis of the heart rate data indicated a group × period × seconds interaction, $F(8, 240) = 3.17, p < .002$. In period I, which included the first 5 seconds following warning signal onset, both groups exhibited an acceleration, which is typical in a reaction time task for both children and adults. The gifted group showed a heart rate increase of 5.2 beats per minute (bpm), whereas the LD children's heart rate increase averaged only 2.6 bpm. The acceleration to the warning signal may be related to some type of cognitive processing that is occurring as the child thinks about the task. In period II, which consisted of the 5 seconds prior to the respond signal, both groups showed a deceleration in comparison to the heart rate in period I. The decreased heart rate in anticipation of the respond signal should facilitate information intake. The gifted and LD groups showed decelerations of 5.5 and 4.5 bpm, respectively. Period III included the 5 seconds following the respond signal, during which the children pressed the button. Both groups exhibited accelerations which were probably caused by the energy expended in pressing the button. The heart rate response of the gifted group was slightly larger at 7.7 bpm than that of the LD children, which was 7.0 bpm.

The findings of this study are consistent in several ways with other research dealing with heart rate changes during a reaction time task. First, the pattern of responses found in our study was very similar to that found in other studies, with an acceleration to the warning signal, a deceleration in anticipation of the respond signal, and an acceleration following the response. Second, the relationship between the magnitude of the heart rate changes and performance were similar in our research compared to previous work. The gifted group showed larger heart rate decelerations prior to the respond signal and also had faster performance than the LD group. Thus, our findings confirmed those of Lacey and Lacey (1974) who have found an inverse relationship between the magnitude of the anticipatory deceleration and reaction time. As more is learned about the neurophysiological processes that control the cardiovascular system, it may be possible to more precisely determine the brain mechanisms which appear to be related to heart rate changes and attentional processes. As this additional information is acquired, we may be able to understand more fully the attentional deficits seen in learning-disabled children.

References

LACEY, J.I., & Lacey, B.C. Some autonomic-central nervous system interrelationships. In P. Black (Ed.), *Physiological correlates of emotion*. New York: Academic Press, 1970.

LACEY, J.I., & Lacey, B.C. Studies of heart rate and other bodily processes in sensorimotor behavior. In P.A. Obrist, A.H. Black, J. Brenner, & L.V. DiCara (Eds.), *Cardiovascular psychophysiology*. Chicago: Aldine, 1974.

SOKOLOV, E.N. *Perception and the conditioned reflex*. New York: Macmillan, 1963.

Effects of Uncertainty of Time and Occurrence on Reaction Time

Paul R. Surburg
Indiana University

Precision and appropriate measurements are of paramount importance in a motor assessment for an individualized educational program or in experimental research. In an attempt to improve the precision of measurement, researchers such as Baumeister and coworkers (1965, 1966, 1967, 1969) and Brewer and Nettlebeck (1977) have opted reaction time (RT) as a dependent variable. Pachella has stated:

> The most important consideration accounting for the popularity of reaction time measure is the indisputable nature of time as a meaningful quantity. (1974)

Woodworth and Schlosberg (1961) have noted that speed is a readily assessed dependent variable, for speed can evaluate achievement through the dimension of task duration and can be a measure of task demand on an organism. An increase in complexity of a task necessitates a longer time to complete the task.

Measurement of reaction time (RT) has been deemed by investigators as meeting the appropriate criteria for use as a dependent variable. Using uncertainty of time and occurrence in RT studies with special population subjects may help clarify the strategies these people use in learning motor tasks or may confound the results of a study.

Variation of foreperiod as a function of uncertainty of time and use of catch-trials as a function of uncertainty of occurrence have been used as operational protocol or as independent variables in RT studies. Preparatory intervals or variation of foreperiods denote the elapsed time between onset of a warning signal and appearance of a stimulus; intervals of different duration are presented in a randomized or regular order. Baumeister, Dugas, and Erdberg (1967) and Baumeister and Hawkins (1966) reported that with mentally retarded subjects the shortest preparatory interval in a nonrandomized schedule yielded the fastest RTs, whereas the shortest foreperiod in a randomized sequence elicited the slowest RTs.

Although sequencing of foreperiods may influence this dependent variable, duration of foreperiod has been used as an independent variable in studies with mentally handicapped persons. No significant differences in RT following randomized foreperiods of 4, 5, and 6 seconds were found by Baumeister, Hawkins, and Kellas (1965). Two studies found the shortest foreperiods in randomized sequence of 2, 4, 7.5, and 15 seconds elicited the slowest RTs (Baumeister & Hawkins, 1966; Baumeister, Dugas & Erdberg, 1967). More recently, Surburg (1981) found RT following 3 and 4.5 seconds to be faster than latencies following a 1.5-second foreperiod. The significant differences in this study may be a function of foreperiod brevity, an age factor, and/or intellectual capacity. Comparison of intellectual levels and foreperiod brevity was addressed in the present study.

Occurrence uncertainty, a warning signal without a presented stimulus, has been used primarily in RT studies with normal subjects. Näätänen (1970), investigating the effect of diminishing time-uncertainty with varying foreperiods on RT, reported slower RTs when catch-trials were used than when subjects did not have to contend with occurrence uncertainty. A subsequent study by Näätänen (1972) found RT to slow as the number of catch-trials increased; this relationship did not change over a wide range of foreperiods.

Wyrick and Owen (1970) used a 10% catch-trial protocol in determining the effects of practice on RT of trainable mentally handicapped persons. Surburg (1981) used occurrence uncertainty as an independent variable with mildly mentally handicapped (MMH) adolescents. During the first 3 days of testing, 10 and 20% catch-trial groups exhibited significantly slower RTs than a group receiving no catch-trials.

The nuances of time and occurrence uncertainties transcend the protocol role; these variables may address more fundamental questions. Catch-trials are used to eliminate an anticipatory factor. Do MMH adolescents exhibit the same type of strategy? The readiness to act and the inability to complete a task characterizes a catch-trial situation. This inability to complete an act may have an inhibitory effect upon performance and may be viewed as a negative or punishing effect. Will this negative effect differentiate performance between two levels of intelligence? The purpose of this study was to determine the effects of variation of foreperiod and frequency of catch-trials on RTs of normal and MMH adolescents.

Method

Subjects

Subjects were 60 students from Bloomington High School North in Bloomington, Indiana. Thirty subjects were classified as MMH persons with a mean intelligence quotient of 64 and a range of 48 to 80; chronological age ranged from 14 to 18 years, with a mean of 16. Thirty normal subjects were of comparable chronological age; recent intelligence quotients were unavailable for these students but the mean score on the Iowa Test of Basic Skills was 95.

Apparatus

A vertical panel consisting of three lights was located on a table. The top light which served as a fixation point was a 12-volt, white incandescent lamp. The middle lamp, a VE-51 neon lamp located 15.2 centimeters below the fixation light served as the stimulus. The bottom light was illuminated to inform the subjects to begin a trial by depressing a normally open telegraph key. A chronoscope recorded the elapsed time from illumination of the stimulus lamp until key release.

Procedure

Subjects were tested individually in the presence of the researcher using a game format. The game or task was to release the telegraph key as quickly as possible after the illumination of the middle lamp. Foreperiods of 1.5, 3.0, and 4.5 seconds were presented in a random sequence to all subjects; the only constraint was that during a testing session, a foreperiod must be presented seven times. When catch-trials were used, an additional 10 or 20% of total trials was randomly arranged among the trials. A catch-trial consisted of the following sequence: illumination of the bottom light, depression of the key, and the word "stop" being played on a cassette recorder. Subjects had been instructed to slowly take their index finger off the key when the word "stop" was heard. Subjects were randomly assigned by intellectual strata to three treatment groups: no catch-trials, 10% catch-trials, and 20% catch-trials. Twenty-one recorded trials constituted a testing session; subjects were tested on 3 consecutive days.

Results and Discussion

Means and standard deviations for three treatment groups at two intellectual levels are presented in Table 1. Reliability coefficients were calculated by the intraclass correlation method (Safrit, 1976). For the MMH adolescents, no catch-trials, 10% catch-trials, and 20% catch-trials groups exhibited coefficients of .86, .94, and .97, respectively. For the no catch-trials, 10% catch-trials, and 20% catch-trial groups in the normal stratum, coefficients were .95, .94, and .92, respectively.

A four-way analysis of variance (intelligence × treatments × days × foreperiods was conducted to determine the effects of catch-trials and foreperiods on RT. Significant main effects for intelligence ($F = 65.2$, $1/54 \, df, p = .05$), treatments ($F = 3.54, 2/54 \, df, p = .05$) days ($F = 3.12, 2/108 \, df, p = .05$), and foreperiods ($F = 62.8, 2/108 \, df, p = .05$) were found. There were significant interactions for intelligence × treatments ($F = 3.56, 2/54 \, df, p = 0.5$) and intelligence × foreperiods ($F = 15.2, 2/108 \, df, p = .05$).

An analysis of simple main effects for intelligence × treatment interaction indicated a significant difference between the two levels of intelligence with the 20% catch-trial groups ($F = 4.9, 1/54 \, df, p = .05$). Analysis of simple main effects for intelligence × treatments revealed no significant differences between treatments at the two intelligence levels. Helmert comparisons revealed a significant difference between the two

Table 1
Reaction Time Means and Standard Deviations for Two Levels of Intelligence and Two Conditions

Condition	Normal		Mentally Handicapped	
	M	SD	M	SD
Occurrence Uncertainty				
No catch-trials	.22	.03	.28	.04
10% catch-trials	.23	.03	.36	.08
20% catch-trials	.21	.02	.37	.10
Time Uncertainty (sec)				
1.5	.23	.03	.37	.08
3.0	.21	.02	.32	.08
4.5	.22	.03	.32	.09

catch-trial groups and the no catch-trial group, but this difference was found only at the MMH level.

Analysis of simple main effects for the intelligence × foreperiod interaction indicated differences between the two intelligence strata for 1.5 seconds ($F = 96.1$, $1/216\ df$, $p = .05$), 3.0 seconds ($F = 60.0$, $1/216\ df$, $p = .05$), and 4.5 seconds ($F = 56.6\ 1/216\ df$, $p = .05$). An analysis of simple main effects for the foreperiod × intelligence interaction revealed only significant differences among the three foreperiods at MMH level ($F = 7.5$, $2/216\ df$, $p = .05$). One and five-tenths, 3.0, and 4.5 second foreperiods exhibited means of .373, .325, and .326, respectively.

We found significant differences between the two intellectual strata for all three foreperiods. These results replicate the findings of several studies that normal subjects' latencies are faster than RTs of mentally handicapped persons (Baumeister, Hawkins, & Kellas, 1965; Baumeister, Wilcox, & Greeson, 1969; Caffrey, James, & Hinkle, 1971).

Baumeister, Hawkins, and Kellas (1965) have suggested that mentally handicapped persons attend to an RT task with a sensory set whereas normal subjects perform this type of task with a motor set. According to Woodworth and Schlosberg (1961), motor preparation leads to faster RT than another type of preparation; Baumeister, Hawkins, and Kellas (1965) contend a sensory set introduces an adaptive element to an RT task which may account for the slower RTs of mentally retarded persons.

With MMH adolescents a 1.5-second foreperiod resulted in significantly slower RTs than the 3.0- or 4.5-second foreperiods. This difference in part could be attributed to a type of range effect, the shortest foreperiod in a series causing a difference in RT. This range effect was not operant with normal subjects. A more simplistic explanation is that MMH subjects could not attain a suitable level of preparation in a 1.5-second period. Krupski (1977) investigated the role of attention in RT performance and found retarded subjects exhibited greater off-task glancing than normal subjects. This inattention to task may reflect the inability of these subjects to prepare quickly for an RT task.

Although the only significant difference between intelligence strata was with the 20% catch-trial groups, MMH subjects exhibited a significant difference between catch-trial conditions and no occurrence uncertainty. According to Näätänen (1972) catch-trials may lower expectancy when the chance of the stimulus appearing is decreased. A relationship exists between expectancy and motor inhibitory and excitatory processes; these relationships are juxtaposed to the phenomenon of readiness. The reduction in readiness coupled with a sensory-set orientation may explain the influence of catch-trials on MMH subjects. The inhibitory aspect of catch-trials could be considered a punishing effect, for the subjects experience prestimulus tension without the concomitant release as the motor act is executed.

References

BAUMEISTER, A., Dugas, J., & Erdberg, P. Effects of warning signal intensity, reaction signal intensity, preparatory interval, and temporal uncertainty on reaction times of mental defectives. *Psychological Record*, 1967, **17**, 503-507.

BAUMEISTER, A., & Hawkins, W. Variations of the preparatory interval in relation to the reaction time of mental defectives. *American Journal of Mental Deficiency*, 1966, **70**, 689-694.

BAUMEISTER, H., Hawkins, W., & Kellas, G. Reaction speed as a function of stimulus intensity in normals and retardates. *Perceptual and Motor Skills*, 1965, **20**, 649-652.

BAUMEISTER, A., Wilcox, S., & Greeson, J. Reaction time of retardates and normals as a function of relative stimulus frequency. *American Journal of Mental Deficiency*, 1969, **73**, 935-941.

BREWER, N., & Nettlebeck, T. Influence of contextual cues on the choice reaction time of mildly retarded adults. *American Journal of Mental Deficiency*, 1977, **82**, 37-43.

CAFFREY, B., James, J., & Hinkle, B. Variability in reaction times of normal and educable mentally retarded children. *Perceptual and Motor Skills*, 1971, **32**, 255-258.

KRUPSKI, A. Role of attention in the reaction-time performance of mentally retarded adolescents. *American Journal of Mental Deficiency*, 1977, **83**, 79-83.

NÄÄTÄNEN, R. The diminishing time-uncertainty with the lapse time after the warning signal in reaction-time experiments with varying foreperiods. *Acta Psychologica*, 1970, **34**, 399-419.

NÄÄTÄNEN, R. Time uncertainty and occurrence uncertainty of the stimulus in a simple reaction time task. *Acta Psychologica*, 1972, **36**, 492-503.

PACHELLA, R. The interpretation of reaction time in information-processing research. In B. Kantowitz (Ed.), *Human information processing: Tutorials in performance and cognition*. Hillsdale, NJ: Lawrence Erlbaum Associates, 1974.

SAFRIT, R. *Reliability theory*. Washington, DC: American Alliance for Health, Physical Education, Recreation and Dance, 1976.

SURBURG, P. Effects of uncertainties of time and occurrence on reaction time of mentally handicapped students. *Perceptual and Motor Skills*, 1981, **53**, 355-360.

WOODWORTH, R., & Schlosberg, H. *Experimental psychology*. New York: Holt, Rinehart, & Winston, 1961.

WYRICK, W., & Owen, G. Effects of practice on simple reaction time of trainable mental retardates. *American Corrective Therapy Journal*, 1970, **24**, 176-179.

A Comparison of Two Sensory Motor Intervention Programs for Elementary Children Diagnosed as Specific Learning-Disabled

Joey Cowden and Robert Eason
University of New Orleans

Jennifer Wright
Jefferson Parish School Board

Basic knowledge about the importance of sensory stimulation and sensory motor integration have existed in education since the late 1800s when Itard and Seguin developed theories that would later influence Piaget and Montessori (Moran & Kalakian, 1977). These educators developed innovative learning theories encompassing the concepts of individual differences, developmental sequences, sensory stimulation, and the influence of sensory motor learning on cognitive development. Only recently, though, has the significance of planned sensory motor activities and movement experiences been recognized as an important aspect of the total developmental and neurophysiological process.

Children learn about their environments through sensory reception and motor processing. These processes incorporate the interpretation of objects and events through the use of the sensory modalities and thereby assist in the acquisition of learning. Developmental activities which heighten sensory stimulation of the modalities (vestibular, tactile, kinesthetic, olfactory, visual, and auditory) will produce circumstances which require neurological integration and thereby influence the total learning process.

The childhood years are crucial in the growth and development process because they provide a time for sensory stimulus to be linked to movement skills. Thus, complex sensory motor schemas become defined, controlled, and meaningful. The multiple schemas become an integrated sensory motor system which is a sizable and significant part of the foundation for higher human development. Piaget has stated that

> concrete action precedes and makes possible the use of intellect and that sensory motor experiences are the foundation of mental development. Children must experience the environment through afferent pathways, and then interpret, evaluate, and integrate the information before movement occurs. The child's basic movement proficiency is greatly determined by this preceding sensory processing. (Montgomery & Richter, 1978, p. 1)

Early perceptual learning is dependent on a sequential-developmental framework of sensory motor experiences. Numerous children enter school with interferences in their maturation which limit or distort further learning. Grass has found that the interpretation of movement feedback with young children is one of the major interferences:

> A child who experiences incorrect or inconsistent feedback cannot possibly have integrated organization of CNS processing. It has been found that learning disability children have deficits in their nervous systems' organization, preventing them from precisely perceiving and responding to environmental demands. (Grass, 1977, p. 2)

Through appropriate sensory motor activities children can be helped to respond and become more successful at performing psychomotor and cognitive tasks requiring a highly integrated nervous system. Traditional motor programs provided by schools, however, often are geared at too high a level for behaviorally and educationally handicapped children. The programs do not correlate reflex activity and are not based on normal, developmental motor sequences.

Numerous nontraditional programs do exist. Jean Ayres (1973) and many from the field of occupational therapy have developed elaborate motor programs based on sensory motor integration that focus on activities which stimulate vestibular and proprioceptive receptors. Conversely, G.N. Getman (1963) and Marianne Frostig (1964), among others, also are concerned with a movement approach for the remediation of children who have perceptual motor difficulties. They have formulated widely circulated theories expanding the importance of visual training for correcting perceptual problems. They believe that the visual dynamics are so related to motor development that one system cannot adequately develop without the other, and also that most learning is achieved through visual learning.

But the relative importance of one sensory modality over another is controversial. Ayres (1973) has stated that "considerable opportunity exists for the vestibular system to exercise influence over all sensory experiences." Eviatar, Eviatar, and Naray (1974) and deQuiros (1976) have conducted neurophysiological studies that show the vestibular system is intimately connected with the proprioceptive and visual motor systems in the acquisition of muscular and postural control. Other research (Frank & Levinson, 1973; Gregg, Haffner, & Korner, 1976; Weeks, 1979; White & Castle, 1964) also supports the beneficial effects of vestibular input on visual behavior. These authors would suggest that the vestibular system is the coordinating apparatus for all sensory functions.

Although many have listed the effectiveness of the two approaches individually on cognitive and motor proficiencies, few have contrasted the two approaches on their relative effectiveness. The purpose of this study was to determine the effects and intermodality association of two different sensory motor intervention programs on motor proficiencies that comprise the Bruininks-Oseretsky Test of Motor Proficiency (BOTMP) (1978). Two curricula were designed that incorporated sequential developmental skills within the two basic target areas of the psychomotor domain: vestibular/proprioceptive and visual motor. Also, the specific sensory modalities were selected to examine intermodality association.

The sensory intervention programs were designed for use by special education and physical education teachers. One program was restricted to specific visual input and activities which heighten fine motor and eye-hand coordination. Activities included were visual tracking, fixations, visual-motor imitations, eye-hand and eye-foot coordination activities, and visual motor-oriented equipment and games. Activities selected limited use of gross motor involvement. The second sensory curriculum was designed to increase vestibular and proprioceptive sensitivity. Activities were included for neurological organization and reflex inhibition, postural and balance mechanisms, sense differentiation, spatial awareness, and motor planning. In addition, each group received mainstream daily physical education.

Method

Subjects

The 18 children selected had been diagnosed as having specific learning disabilities and had been placed in self-contained learning environments. Children were paired by age, sex, and prescreening motor proficiency scores and then assigned randomly to two experimental sensory intervention groups. The subjects ranged in age from 6 to 11 years with a mean age of 8-2 years for the vestibular/proprioceptive group and a mean age of 8-6 years for the visual group.

Evaluation

A sensory motor screening battery that contained similar items as in the BOTMP was administered to each subject prior to beginning the intervention. Following the 12-week experimental period, the BOTMP was administered. The dependent variables were the eight motor proficiency items and three composite scores of the BOTMP. Cognitive and perceptual variables, except as reflected in the BOTMP tests and reflex screen, were not evaluated.

Scoring procedures of the BOTMP enabled multiple statistical tests for the sensory motor treatment effects. The eight individual motor proficiencies are:

1. Running speed and agility
2. Balance
3. Bilateral coordination
4. Strength
5. Upper limb coordination
6. Response speed
7. Visual motor control
8. Upper limb speed and dexterity

The composite scores include gross motor, fine motor, and total battery. Gross motor incorporates items 1-4; fine motor includes items 6-8; and the fifth item was considered (by Bruininks) as a combination of gross and fine motor and was used with the other seven to comprise the total battery.

Procedure

The vestibular/proprioceptive (VP) group received sequential activities designed to stimulate the VP modality. The second group received specific visual/fine-motor (visual) exercises. Each intervention program was administered by physical education and special education teachers and aides during a 12-week period, three sessions per week for 50 minutes per session.

Results and Discussion

The results of a series of one-way analysis of variance tests are presented in Table 1. The visual group performed significantly ($p < .10$) better than

Table 1
Means, Standard Deviations, and F-Tests Between Two Perceptual Motor Training Programs and Selected Motor Proficiencies from the BOTMP

Tests	n	Visual		Vestibular		F	p
		$\bar{x}$	SD	$\bar{x}$	SD		
Running speed & agility	9	9.56	5.22	5.44	4.96	2.93	< .20
Balance	9	5.11	5.20	3.78	5.07	.30	> .20
Bilateral coordination	9	10.00	3.39	9.78	3.96	.01	> .20
Strength	9	9.33	6.02	5.56	2.46	2.64	< .20
Upper limb coordination	9	14.44	4.13	7.67	5.32	9.13	< .002
Response speed	9	14.89	2.93	10.00	3.24	11.25	< .005
Visual motor control	9	12.33	6.56	16.22	3.70	2.40	< .20
Upper limb speed & dexterity	9	10.33	4.69	8.78	5.67	.40	> .20
Gross motor composite	9	32.22	9.64	25.67	7.33	2.63	< .20
Fine motor composite	9	42.11	7.99	38.78	9.36	.65	> .20
Total battery composite	9	35.67	8.14	29.00	7.57	3.20	< .10

the vestibular group on total battery composite, upper limb coordination ($p < .002$), and response speed ($p < .005$). Also, positive mean differences (p less than .20 but greater than .10) were obtained for running speed and agility, strength, and gross motor composite. No significant differences were found that favored the vestibular group; however, a positive mean difference was obtained for visual motor control.

The results of this study support the use of sensory motor programs that stress visual motor activities for developing motor proficiency as measured by the BOTMP. Means of the visual group were significantly higher or approached significance on four of the eight proficiencies tested. Only the means for the visual motor control favored the vestibular group.

Upon observation, some of the differences found were obvious and predictable. Bruininks item Upper Body Coordination measures hand-eye coordination with gross motor movement. Treatment-influenced performance was expected to be higher for the visual group because they were trained on eye-hand coordination tasks using balloons, bean bags, balls, and other missile-target tasks.

Other findings were less obvious. Response Speed favored the visual motor group even though that group did not receive specific training. One explanation was the possibility that identical elements were present in both the Response Speed test and the tasks used for visual motor training. Response speed was measured by dropping a stick along a wall whereby the students trapped it with their thumbs. The thumb was in juxtaposition to the stick and the subject responded when the stick was released by the experimenter, so it is possible that this task had a heavy eye-hand coordination leading.

Another finding that lacks a clear explanation is the visual group's higher performance for Running Speed and Agility and Strength. We eliminated age as an explanation even though the mean age of the visual group was 4 months older than the vestibular group. The Bruininks scoring system controls for age. One factor that could have been contaminating was motivation. Compared to the visual group, students in the vestibular group exhibited excessive problems with discipline and poor effort. Activities for the visual group appeared to be more intrinsically motivating whereas the vestibular activities required a high degree of concentration and postural management. Also, even though the teachers had received inservice training for the activities, the pedagogical rationale for the vestibular intervention system was more difficult for them to grasp. Thus, it appeared to the investigators that the visual group instructors presented their lessons with more enthusiasm and understanding than those for the vestibular group.

If motivation was a factor, it could have affected the results in at least two ways. First, the group with the highest motivation would have been more efficient during practice. This would have resulted in a higher learning rate for the motivated group. Second, the motivated students would have taken the criterion, the Bruininks Test (perceived by the subjects as still more motor activity), with an attitude of challenge as opposed to passive resistance.

If the vestibular group was undermotivated, it could explain why the group failed to show superiority on proficiencies of balance and bilateral coordination. Using traditional theories of specificity of training, we expected superior scores because the vestibular group received concentrated training on tasks that required balance, body differentiation, postural control, and reflex inhibition.

Another explanation is that the vestibular and visual mechanisms might have been, as postulated by Ayres, highly neurologically interrelated so that intermodality association occurred. The vestibular group did show observable improvement in visual motor control. Perhaps the vestibular group had improved more in sensory motor integration and this improvement transferred to tasks that required both visual and VP control. The tasks used to measure Visual Motor Control on the BOTMP seemed to require a higher loading of internal synchronized organization and rhythmical flow of movement. Teachers commented in support of this fact in that they felt the vestibular group had greatly improved efficient movement patterns and general body control.

Conversely, as the visual group's superiority on balance, agility, and strength has no logical "specificity" explanation, it is feasible that intermodality association arising from the visual mode positively influenced in an unexplainable interaction the VP mode.

Conclusions and Recommendations

Based on the results of this study and within the reported limitations, the investigators conclude that sensory motor intervention programs that emphasize the visual modality result in greater gains on tests of motor proficiency than do programs that emphasize the VP modality. This is especially true for tasks that require upper limb coordination of the hands and eyes with gross motor movements, and for tasks that require visual response speed. To a lesser extent, the study supports the use of VP activities for motor proficiencies that require visual motor control with rhythmical sequence of movement. The investigators recommend that this study be replicated with a larger population and a lower mean age. Psychomotor instuctors should be well trained in the rationale and pedagogy for each treatment condition.

References

AYRES, A.J. *Sensory integration and learning disorders.* Los Angeles: Western Psychological Services, 1973, 28.

BRUININKS, R.H. *Bruininks-Oseretsky test of motor proficiency.* Circle Pines, MN: American Guidance Service, 1978.

DEQUIROS, J. Diagnosis of vestibular disorders in the learning disabled. *Journal of Learning Disabilities*, 1976.

EVIATAR, L., Eviatar, A., & Naray, I. Maturation of neurovestibular responses in infants. *Developmental Medicine and Child Neurology*, 1974, **16**, 435.

FRANK, J., & Levinson, H. Dysmetric dyslexia and dyspraxia. *Journal of American Academic Child Psychiatry*, 1973, **12**, 690-701.

FROSTIG, M. *Administration and scoring manual for the Marianne Frostig developmental test of visual perception.* Palo Alto: Consulting Psychologist Press, 1964.

GETMAN, G.N. *The physiology of readiness.* Minneapolis: Programs to Accelerate School Success, 1963.

GRASS, G. Sensory integration: An overview. Paper presented in partial fulfillment of the Occupational Therapy Field Work Experience, University of Wisconsin (Cincinnati Public Schools, March 1977).

GREGG, C., Haffner, M., & Korner, A. The relative efficacy of vestibular-proprioceptive stimulation and the upright position in enhancing visual pursuit in neonates. *Child Development*, 1976, **47**, 309-314.

MONTGOMERY, P., & Richter, E. *Sensorimotor integration for developmentally disabled children: A handbook*. Los Angeles: Western Psychological Services, 1978.

MORAN, J.M., & Kalakian, L.H. *Movement experiences for the mentally retarded or emotionally disturbed child*. Minneapolis: Burgess, 1977.

WEEKS, Z.R. Effects of the vestibular system on human development, Part 1. Overview of functions and effects of stimulation. *The American Journal of Occupational Therapy*, 1979, **33**(6), 376-381.

WHITE, B., & Castle, P. Visual exploratory behavior following postnatal handling of human infants. *Perceptual Motor Skills*, 1964, **18**, 497-502.

Discriminant Analysis in Adapted Physical Education[1]

Gabie E. Church and Geoffrey D. Broadhead
Louisiana State University

Frequently examined topics in adapted physical education research focus on whether motor performance differences exist between nonhandicapped (NH) and handicapped (H) children or between H children of one category and those of another, and the extent to which motor performance characteristics can be used to help classify H children into more homogeneous groups. The thrust of this paper is to examine appropriate statistical techniques to address such topics.

Some of these issues have traditionally been analyzed through univariate or multivariate analysis of variance (ANOVA or MANOVA) procedures. When the dependent variables consist of a set of interrelated variables MANOVA is the more appropriate procedure. When MANOVA indicates significant differences among groups for the mean vector composed of all the dependent variables, it is important to know which of the

---

[1]Financial support for this study was provided by the State of Louisiana Department of Education, Division of Special Education Services, and the US Department of Education, Office of Special Education and Rehabilitative Services. No endorsement by these agents is implied.

dependent variables actually contribute to the overall significance. Several techniques are available for identifying these variables; one of the most common is examination of univariate F ratios. Of course, if this technique is used multivariate data are once again examined via univariate procedures.

Discriminant Analysis Techniques

Another approach to follow-up of significant MANOVA results is a multivariate procedure, discriminant analysis (DISCRIM), which provides variable identification and classification techniques as well as the examination of group differences. DISCRIM deals with research paradigms where two or more preexisting groups ($g \geq 2$) are measured on several response or discriminating variables ($v \geq 2$). It attempts to answer several questions including: Are there significant differences among g groups based on a set of v interrelated discriminating variables? Which of the v variables contribute most to such differences? What is a good classification rule for assigning each observation to one of the groups and how well does the proposed classification rule perform on existing as well as new sample observations? (Morrison, 1969).

DISCRIM attempts to address such issues by constructing function(s) of the set of the v discriminating variables which maximally discriminate among the groups (Tatsuoka, 1970). A statistical test can be conducted to see if the g group centroids defined by the discriminant function(s) differ significantly. In addition, the standardized coefficients used in the function provide information about the relative contribution of the variables in the function in that larger absolute coefficients indicate greater contribution of a variable to the function. Thus, as a follow-up to MANOVA this multivariate procedure allows determination of which variables in the vector are contributing relatively greater influence to significant overall results.

In order to illustrate DISCRIM the following research paradigm taken from another study (Broadhead, 1982) is considered. Four groups of children: NH first grade (NH-G1), NH kindergarten (NH-K), mildly mentally retarded (MR-MI), and moderately mentally retarded (MR-MOD), were administered the Physical Dexterity (PD) component of the System of Multicultural Pluralistic Assessment (SOMPA) (Mercer & Lewis, 1978) consisting of the items ambulation (AMB), equilibrium (EQ), placement (PLC), fine motor sequencing (FMS), finger-tongue dexterity (FTD), and involuntary movement (IVM). Discriminant analysis produced three functions (Table 1). Hypothesis testing showed that the four groups differ significantly with respect to the first function ($p < .05$) with significant additional discrimination provided by the second function, and, of the variation accounted for by the three functions, ap-

Table 1
Results of Significance Test for DISCRIM among Four NH and MR Groups

Function	df	χ^2	Variation (%)	Cumulative %
1	18	83.18[a]	84.77	84.77
2	10	18.52[a]	12.76	97.53
3	4	3.26	2.47	100.00

[a]$p < .05$.

proximately 98% is due to the first two functions. Thus, considering that the third function does not significantly increase discrimination and accounts for less than 3% of the explained variation, only the first two functions were examined further.

Group centroids describe the location of the center of the four groups in the two-dimensional space defined by the two functions retained. Centroids for the SOMPA data (Table 2) indicate that Function 1 discriminates between H and NH children whereas Function 2 separates within this primary breakdown, that is, NH-G1 vs NH-K in the NH children, and MR-MI vs MR-MOD in the H children. Examination of the absolute values of the standardized coefficients (Table 2) indicates that Function 1 can be described by the variables AMB and EQ, gross motor measures, whereas Function 2 is composed of PLC and IVM, fine motor measures. Signs for the standardized coefficients indicate the direction of the variable's influence with positive coefficients indicating that large values for that variable are characteristic of the group(s) with positive mean (centroid) for that function whereas negative coefficients indicate large values for that variable are characteristic of the group(s) with negative mean (centroid) for that function. Thus, for Function 1, larger scores (larger number of errors) for AMB and EQ identify those groups with positive centroid values for Function 1—MR-MI and MR-MOD, etc.

A major feature of DISCRIM is the production of a rule for the classification of existing and new individuals into the g groups. This classification rule provides information as to which of the g groups an individual is most like and classifies the individual into that group. The classification matrix can then provide information about how well the discriminant function(s) describe the relationship among and within groups by the overall correct classification and by revealing where large numbers of misclassifications occur. The classification matrix for the SOMPA data (Table 3) yields an overall 65.7% correct classification with greater precision for the NH groups (82.6 and 65.4%) than for the H groups (40 and 50%).

Table 2
Group Centroids and Standardized Coefficients of Two DISCRIM Functions

Group	Centroids Function 1	Function 2
NH-G1	−1.30	0.43
NH-K	−0.21	−0.40
MR-MI	1.31	−0.63
MR-MOD	2.78	0.85

Variable	Standardized Coefficients Function 1	Function 2
AMB	0.655	−0.025
EQ	0.566	−0.022
PLC	−0.303	1.082
FMS	−0.190	0.517
FTD	0.208	−0.335
IVM	0.335	−0.725

Table 3
Percentage of Correct Classification from Two DISCRIM Functions

Actual Group	Predicted Group NH-G1	NH-K	MR-MI	MR-MOD
NH-G1	82.6	17.4	0.0	0.0
NH-K	23.1	65.4	11.5	0.0
MR-MI	10.0	40.0	40.0	10.0
MR-MOD	0.0	12.5	37.5	50.0

Research Applications of DISCRIM

The usefulness of DISCRIM and its application to adapted physical education research has been demonstrated in reported research studies. Widdop (1968) examined a group of educable mentally retarded (EMR) children ranging in age from 8 to 18 years old, divided into high and low IQ groups, on 18 variables including the seven-item, modified AAHPER Youth Fitness Test, height, weight, IQ, behavior, and seven family variables. He used discriminant analysis "to determine whether the groups could be distinguished from one another on the basis of the entire profile rather than by the analysis of profile components separately" (Widdop, 1968, p. 118). DISCRIM showed significant differences between high and low IQ groups across all ages for boys and in eight of 11 age groups for the girls. Percentage of correct classifications ranged from 64.8 to 95%, indicating a generally successful discrimination. Because the standardized coefficients for the functions were not reported, though, the primary variables contributing to discrimination could not be identified.

Rarick, Dobbins, and Broadhead (1976) conducted a multifaceted investigation of the motor performance of EMR children in the age range 6 to 13 years. Two of the purposes were classification and variable identification which were appropriately addressed through DISCRIM using four contrast groups: NH boys vs NH girls; NH boys vs EMR boys; NH girls vs EMR girls; and EMR boys vs EMR girls. The classification results were very high, ranging from 84.5 to 96.6% correct classification, indicating that both male/female and NH/EMR discrimination could be achieved through consideration of motor performance criteria. The major separating variables identified through DISCRIM revealed different motor performance criteria involved in male/female discrimination than those involved in NH/EMR discrimination.

This discussion of DISCRIM is not meant to convey an exhaustive review. Examination of the work of Huberty (1975), Lachenbruch (1975), and Tatsuoka (1970) will provide an extension of the basic thrust of this paper.

It is believed that the illustrations used to describe this technique are sufficient to demonstrate the ability of DISCRIM to address some important research issues in adapted physical education. In particular, its multivariate basis and its examination of both among- and within-group relationships are characteristics which make it a research technique to be recommended.

References

BROADHEAD, G.D. A paradigm for physical education for handicapped children in the least restrictive environment. *The Physical Educator*, 1982, **39**, 3-12.

HUBERTY, C.J. Discriminant analysis. *Review of Educational Research*, 1975, **45**, 543-598.

LACHENBRUCH, P.A. *Discriminant analysis.* New York: Hafner Press, 1975.

MERCER, J.R., & Lewis, J.F. *System of multicultural pluralistic assessment: Student assessment manual.* New York: The Psychological Corp., 1978.

MORRISON, D.G. On the interpretation of discriminant analysis. *Journal of Marketing Research*, 1969, **6**, 156-163.

RARICK, G.L., Dobbins, D.A., & Broadhead, G.D. *The motor domain and its correlates in educationally handicapped children.* Englewood Cliffs, NJ: Prentice-Hall, 1976.

TATSUOKA, M.M. *Discriminant analysis: The study of group differences.* Champaign, IL: Institute for Personality and Ability Testing, 1970.

WIDDOP, J.H. The motor performance of educable mentally retarded children with particular reference to the identification of factors associated with individual differences in performance (Doctoral dissertation, University of Wisconsin, Madison, 1967). *Dissertation Abstracts*, 1968, **28**, 3010A. (University Microfilms No. 67-12, 493.)

SECTION 6:
Considérations sur l'Activité Physique pour les Handicapés

Cette partie en francais du présent document contient six textes touchant l'une ou l'autre des populations visées par le symposium.

Le premier texte traite de la plasticité du muscle vieillissant et est suivi d'une réaction d'un deuxième auteur; le second s'adresse aux personnes âgées en ce qui concerne plus particulièrement leurs activités de plein air; le troisième concerne l'évaluation des compétences motrices chez les déficients mentaux; le quatrième présente les résultats d'une étude sur l'enseignement de l'activité physique aux élèves en difficultés d'adaptation et d'apprentissage; le cinquième porte sur l'attitude des éducateurs à l'égard de la personne handicapée; et le sixième texte analyse la relation entre les activités physiques et le stress cardiaque chez les jeunes adultes et les personnes âgées.

This section of the Proceedings contains the papers written in French. The first paper focuses on the modifications of the aging muscle, followed by a reaction from another author on this topic. The third paper suggests a model to follow in preparing an outdoor program for the aged; the fourth studies different methods of evaluating motor competency for mentally deficient individuals. The next paper presents the results of an experimental study on the quality of intervention in physical education with students who have difficulty in adaptation and learning; it is followed by an article concerning attitudes in education and the integration of the handicapped. The seventh and final paper in this section analyzes the energy cost and cardiac stress associated with physical activities in young adults and elderly men. An abstract in English follows the one in French for each article.

La Plasticité du Muscle Vieillissant

Clermont P. Simard
Université Laval

Les muscles vieillissants subissent des modifications à différents niveaux. Doit-on être un observateur passif devant ces phénomènes ou doit-on chercher à comprendre le processus et essayer d'apporter, par un programme d'activité physique approprié, les corrections possibles? Suite à un bref rappel anatomo-physiologique du système musculaire, nous traiterons les changements et les adaptations structuraux, métaboliques et fonctionnels du muscle vieillissant. Nous terminerons par quelques commentaires sur un programme de conditionnement physique.

The aging muscle undergoes different modifications throughout its lifespan at different levels of intensity. Are we supposed to be only observers of this phenomenon? Shouldn't we look for an understanding of these changes and try to offer an appropriate physical activity program? Following a brief anatomo-physiological profile of the muscular system, we will discuss some changes and adaptations at the structural, metabolic and functional levels. Finally, we will present some comments about a physical conditioning program.

L'étude du processus de vieillissement du tissu musculaire squelettique est complexe du fait que les fibres musculaires ne constituent pas un tissu homogène et que son état, à un moment donné de la vie, est tributaire de la nature d'une multitude d'influences trophiques. L'efficacité et la vigueur peuvent subir des influences primaires, intrinsèques aux muscles ou des influences externes, provenant des systèmes nerveux, vasculaire ou endocrinien qui pertuberont les qualités fonctionnelles du tissu. Il est aussi important de savoir si le tissu musculaire, qui subit une invagination avec l'âge, peut, quand certaines conditions sont respectées s'améliorer et maintenir un haut niveau d'efficacité.

Après avoir fait un bref rappel anatomo-physiologique du système musculaire, afin d'informer certains membres de l'auditoire moins sensibilisés à ce processus, nous parlerons des changements et des adaptations structuraux, métaboliques et fonctionnels du muscle squelettique vieillissant. Quelques commentaires sur un programme de conditionnement physique et une brève conclusion complèteront cet exposé.

Rappel Anatomo-Physiologique

Afin de bien comprendre le tissu musculaire, on se doit d'être sensibilisé à sa structure, à la physiologie de la contraction et aux sources énergétiques nécessaires pour effectuer différentes actions.

Le couplage excitation-contraction musculaire permet, suite à la conduction d'une impulsion, la libération du calcium du réticulum sarcoplasmique et son lien avec la troponine qui provoque l'arrêt de l'inhibition de la tropomyosine et l'interaction de l'actomyosine. Ceci est activé par l'ATPasique en dégradant l'ATP et libérant de l'énergie. Les liens actomyosines se font et suite à un changement dans la conformation de la tête de myosine, le muscle se raccourcit.

Les sources énergétiques immédiates sont les réserves en phosphagène de la fibre musculaire et ils peuvent servir pour une courte période. Pour les activités qui durent entre 30 secondes et deux minutes, nous avons du glycogène en réserve. Le métabolisme oxydatif, qui utilise les sucres et les graisses peut fournir de l'énergie pour une très longue période.

Les divers changements anatomo-physiologiques vont entraîner des modifications plus ou moins importantes sur diverses qualités neuro-musculaires: force et endurance isométriques; vitesse maximale d'extension; résistance à la fatigue; flexibilité; coordination; force et endurance dynamiques.

Changement et Adaptation des Éléments Structuraux

Il est accepté depuis longtemps que le volume musculaire décroît avec l'âge (Campbell, McComas, & Petito, 1973; Gutmann & Hanzlikova, 1966). On se doit d'aller voir à l'intérieur de la cellule pour savoir quels sont les éléments les plus touchés afin de mieux comprendre le processus et chercher les solutions pour maintenir le système fonctionnel.

Cette masse musculaire passe d'environ 45% à 25% de la masse totale de l'organisme (Hasselkus, 1974). Ces modifications reliées à l'atrophie musculaire peuvent être dissimulées par une élévation de la masse graisseuse et du tissu conjonctif (Larsson, Sjodin, & Karlsson, 1978).

Nous savons qu'avec l'âge le muscle perd de ses fibres et que cette perte est sélective à certaines fibres (Hooper & Sheil, 1978; Jennekens, Tomlinson, & Walton, 1971; Larsson, 1979). Les causes semblent être myogéniques. Il y a d'une part une diminution du nombre de noyaux et d'autre part, une diminution de l'information génétique qui ralentissent la synthèse des protéines. Toutefois, l'atrophie est aussi associée à l'élévation de la dégradation des protéines. Les travaux de Larsson (1979) à cet effet sont très révélateurs. La distribution des fibres change et nous retrouvons une diminution des fibres 2, à la fois les types 2a et 2b. Toutefois, le rapport entre le % des types 2a, 2b et 2c demeure semblable. Les fibres 1 passent de 40% à 26 ans à 60% à 62 ans. Cette tendance, telle que présentée dans la Figure 1, arrive d'une façon progressive. Ce phénomène n'est pas associé à la transformation des types des fibres dans un autre type mais à une perte sélective de certaines fibres.

La surface des fibres varie aussi d'une façon progressive avec l'âge. Les fibres 2 qui étaient plus volumineuses que les fibres 1, passent de 64% à 43% de l'occupation de la surface par rapport aux fibres 1. La Figure 2 illustre ce rapport.

Certains auteurs vont plus loin (Fujisawa, 1974; Tomlinson, Walton, & Reheiz, 1969) en parlant d'une hypertrophie de compensation des fibres 1. Il est bon de rappeler que les fibres 1 sont davantage des fibres toniques comparativement aux fibres 2 qui sont phasiques. La théorie la plus courante pour expliquer ce phénomène provient du type d'activité physique pratiqué par la personne âgée. Avec l'âge le travail est davantage aérobique et a un seuil d'intensité confortable. L'utilisation préférentielle des fibres 1 protège celles-ci contre une dégénération progressive. Ces données sont aussi concordantes avec une réduction de la force musculaire ainsi que les puissances et capacités aérobiques et anaérobiques.

Au niveau de la longueur des fibres, des sarcomères et de leur nombre, on peut signaler que la longueur des fibres diminue tout en maintenant les sarcomères à une longueur semblable (Hooper, 1981). Toutefois, le nombre de sarcomères décroit avec l'âge. Après la naissance, les augmentations ultérieures de la longueur des fibres semblent être reliées à l'augmentation du nombre de sarcomères (William & Goldspink, 1971). Ce nombre semble être régularisé par la tension active ou passive et cette diminution de tension lors du vieillissement peut être une partie de l'explication (Hooper, 1981). Ces constatations nous permettent de croire

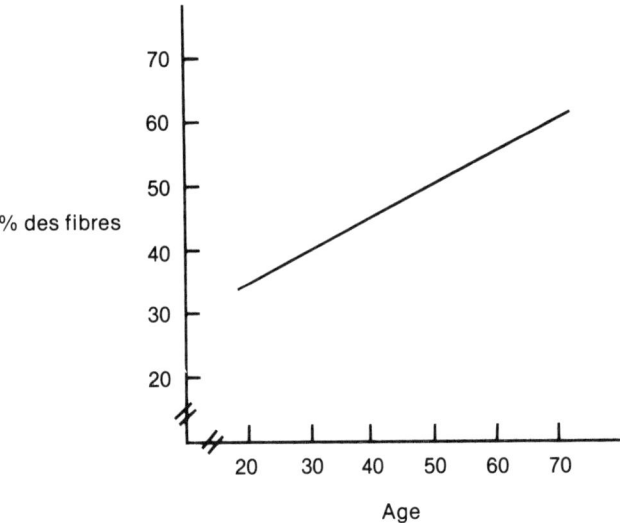

Figure 1 — Pourcentage de distribution des fibres 1 du muscle *vastus lateralis* avec l'âge.

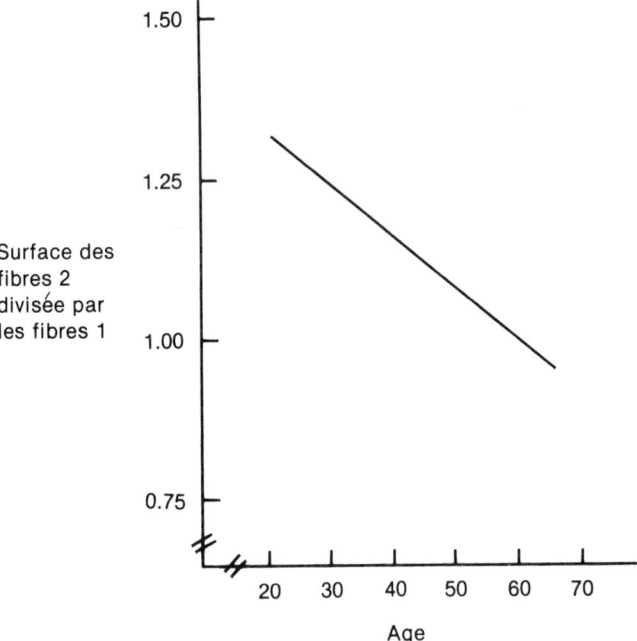

Figure 2 — Le rapport des surfaces des fibres 2 avec les fibres 1 selon l'âge. Le rapport fibre 2/fibre 1 passe de 1.25 à 0.95.

qu'il y a comme une décroissance du muscle. Cette longueur, qui détermine en partie l'amplitude du mouvement, provoque chez les personnes âgées une diminution de la mobilité.

Il est certain que le degré d'atrophie varie d'un individu à un autre du même âge et d'un muscle à l'autre chez un même individu.

Le système neuro-musculaire, au niveau de sa jonction présente certains problèmes et il contribue par la dégénérescence de certaines plaques motrices à la dénervation d'un grand nombre de fibres musculaires (Gutmann & Hanzlikova, 1966; Hooper & Sheil, 1978). La dégénérescence de diverses plaques motrices peut diminuer de presque la moitié les fibres musculaires innervées. On retrouve une réduction du flux axonique et la transmission au niveau des fibres restantes est aussi altérée (Gutmann & Hanzlikova, 1972).

Au niveau des ultra-structures de la cellule, on peut observer une dégénération des myofibrilles ainsi qu'une dilatation et une prolifération du réticulum sarcoplasmique. Le volume et le nombre des mitochondries semblent réduits (Orlander, Kiessling, Larsson, Karlsson, & Aniansson, 1978; Sacktor & Shimada, 1972) ainsi que le nombre de noyaux.

Changements et Adaptations Métaboliques

Selon Gutmann (1972), le montant des enzymes mitochondriales diminuerait. D'autres études vont dans le même sens en indiquant une réduction d'environ 50% de différents enzymes des voies aérobiques comme la succinate dehydrogenase (SDH), la pyrunate dehydrogenase (PDH), la malate dehydrogenase (MDH) et la lactate dehydrogenase (LDH) et peu de changements au niveau de la glycolyse.

Cependant, suite aux études d'Orlander, Kiessling, Larsson, Karlsson, & Aniansson (1978), étant donné une diminution du volume mitochondriale, l'activité des différentes enzymes représentant les principales voies du métabolisme énergétique, s'élèverait par unité de volume mitochondriale. Toutefois, les mitochondries sont des organelles qui peuvent augmenter leur nombre sur demande et synthétiser une partie de leurs protéines par elles mêmes. De fait, la diminution respiratoire du muscle est associée à une perte d'intégrité fonctionnelle des mitochondries en réponse à des altérations de l'environnement.

Nous savons, même avec l'âge que la capacité oxydative mitochondriale s'élève lors d'un entraînement ainsi que la capacité anaérobique. Selon Orlander (1980), la capacité d'oxydation des acides gras demeure inchangée, le potentiel glycolytique s'élève et étant donné la constance au niveau du volume des mitochondries et des gouttelettes de graisse suite à l'entraînement, on doit admettre que l'amélioration des capacités oxydatives se passe à l'intérieur du volume mitochondriale déjà existant.

Changements et Adaptations Fonctionnels

La force, les puissances et les capacités aérobiques et anaérobiques qui avaient diminuées avec l'âge, ont tendance à s'améliorer avec l'activité physique. Cette diminution qui est associée au recrutement des fibres musculaires peut aussi s'expliquer par des changements au niveau des activités endocriniennes, une réduction du sang circulant dans cette zone, par les changements au niveau du système neuro-musculaire (Gutmann & Hanzlikova, 1972), par des modifications des protéines contractiles et des protéines du métabolisme. La force, la puissance et la capacité peut s'améliorer grâce à des facteurs intrinsèques ou extrinsèques au muscle. On voit par les Figures 3, 4, et 5, que l'on peut mesurer l'effet de

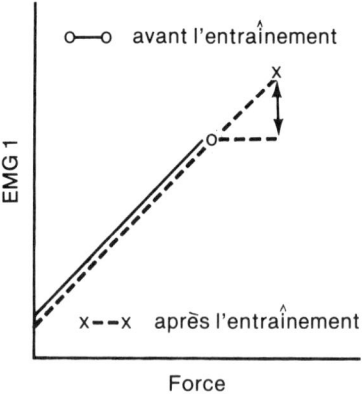

Figure 3 — Amélioration de la force liée aux facteurs nerveux (adapté de Moritani, 1980).

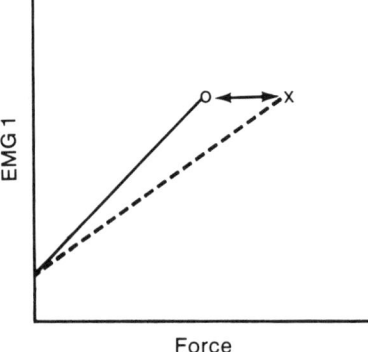

Figure 4 — Amélioration de la force liée à l'hypertrophie (adapté de Moritani, 1980).

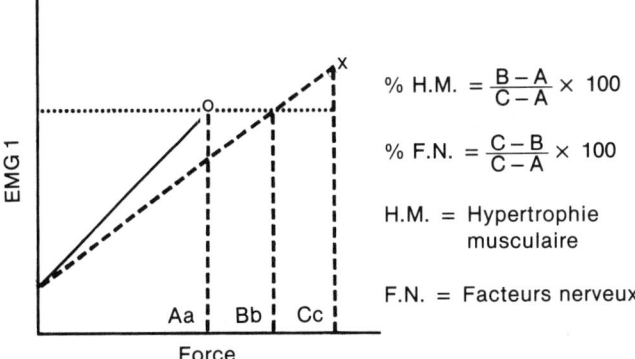

Figure 5 — Evaluation du pourcentage de contribution des facteurs nerveux versus l'hypertrophie (adapté de Moritani, 1980).

différents facteurs dans ce processus. Selon l'étude de Moritani & DeVries (1980), présentée dans les Figures 6 et 7, on retrouve une spécificité dans la réponse à l'entraînement chez les jeunes et les personnes âgées.

Selon certains auteurs (Fujisawa, 1974; Tomlinson, Walton, & Reheiz, 1969), la diminution de la force serait plus grande chez les membres inférieurs que les membres supérieurs. De plus, ce changement serait plus marquant chez la femme et il arriverait plus tôt que chez l'homme (Aniansson, Grimby, & Rundgren, 1980).

Les effets du conditionnement physique peuvent améliorer la force musculaire et la capacité physique au travail. Selon certains auteurs, l'amélioration de la force peut être de 6% à 50% (DeVries, 1970; Moritani & DeVries, 1980; Perkins & Kaiser, 1962). Le Tableau 1 adapté de Shephard (1979) et de Heath (1981), présente les effets du conditionnement physique sur la capacité aérobique des hommes et des femmes en santé de 50 ans et plus.

La Figure 8 illustre les possibilités d'adaptation de l'organisme au travail selon les semaines d'entraînement. On remarque que les premières semaines sont déterminantes dans ce processus.

Programme de Conditionnement Physique

Les objectifs prioritaires qu'on devra se tracer dans le cadre d'un programme de conditionnement physique sont l'amélioration de la flexibilité ou de la souplesse musculaire, le développement de la vigueur musculaire et l'élévation de la capacité physique au travail.

Ces trois objectifs sont reliés aux muscles et on se doit dans le cadre du programme de tenir compte de trois éléments importants: (1) Le niveau de condition physique du bénéficiaire et le pourquoi de son adhésion; on

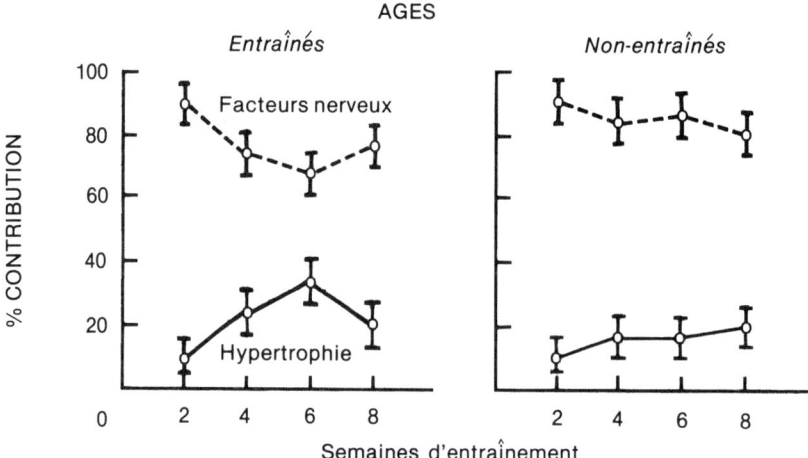

Figure 6 – Moment de l'amélioration de la force associée aux facteurs nerveux ou à l'hypertrophie (adapté de Moritani, 1980).

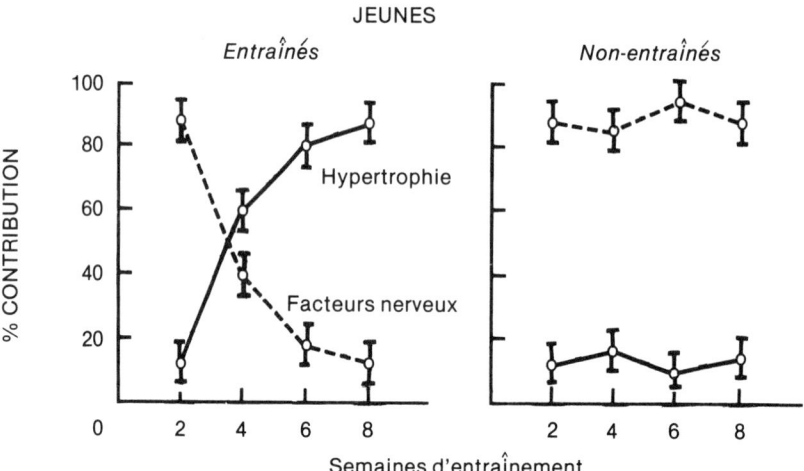

Figure 7 – Moment de l'amélioration de la force associée aux facteurs nerveux ou à l'hypertrophie (adapté de Moritani, 1980).

peut retrouver des gens qui ont besoin d'une normalisation de leurs qualités neuro-musculaires, ou d'un développement neuro-musculaire général, ou encore d'un individu qui désire améliorer sa performance individuelle (Tableau 2). (2) Le niveau de compétence des intervenants qui peuvent offrir des services adaptés et de qualités. (3) La qualité de l'environnement, son accessibilité et un horaire flexible.

Tableau 1
Les Effets du Conditionnement Physique sur la Puissance Aérobique d'Hommes et de Femmes Âgés de 50 Ans et Plus (Adapté de Shephard, 1978)

Investigateur	Sexe	Age	N	Prog. d'entraî. Fréq./	Durée min./	Programme d'entraînement Intensité	Activité	$\dot{V}_{O_2max}$ (ml/kg·min) Pré	Post	Δ	Δ%
Heath et al., 1981	M	59	16	3-5	52 sem.	vigoureuse	C(IT)		58.7		
Wilmore et al., 1970	M	53	7	3	10 sem. (12/24 min)	7.5 mph (600-700 kcal·hr^{-1})	J	40.3	41.8	1.5	4
Kilbom, 1971	F	51-64	12	2-3	7 sem. (18 min)	77% $\dot{V}_{O_2max}$	B(IT)	26.9	29.4	2.5	9
Kiessling et al., 1974	M	54	7	2	13 sem. (24-30 min)	70-90% $\dot{V}_{O_2max}$	B(IT&C)	34.5	37.2	2.7	8
Saltin et al., 1969	M	55	8	2-3	8-10 sem. (45 min)	près maximal	Cal(IT&C)	28.0	33.0	5.0	18
Tzankoff et al., 1972	M	58	8	2-3	25 sem. (55 min)	vigoureux	M,J,G	29.5	35.0	5.5	19
Sidney & Shephard, 1978	M/F	67	8	< 2	14 sem. (45 min)	f_c = 120 min^{-1}	M,J,Cal	19.5[a]	19.2	−0.3	−2(NS)
		63	5	< 2		f_c = 140-150 min^{-1}		24.1[a]	28.1	4.0	17
		64	13	2-4		f_c = 120 min^{-1}		21.7[a]	24.8	3.1	14
		61	8	2-4		f_c = 140-150 min^{-1}		23.4[a]	32.4	9.0	39
	M	65	10	1-4	52 sem. (45 min)	f_c = 120-145 min^{-1}	M,J,Cal	21.7[a]	26.9	5.2	24
	F	65	12	1-4				22.4[a]	27.8	5.4	24

continué

Tableau 1, continué

Buccola & Stone, 1975	M	65	16	3	14 sem. (10-40 min)	$f_c < 144$ min^{-1} (6-7 mets → 8-9 mets)	B	23.7[a]	26.9	3.2	13.5
	M	68	20	3			J	24.2[a]	27.3	3.1	12.8
Suominen et al., 1977	M	69	14	3-5	8 sem. (60 min)	sousmaximal	M,J,N,S,Cal	28.9[a]	32.0	3.1	10.7
	F	69	12	3-5				27.9[a]	31.3	3.4	12.2
De Vries, 1970	M	70	68	3	6 sem. (45-60 min)	$f_c < 120$ min^{-1}	M,J,S(IT)	33.9[a]	35.5	1.6	5
			8		42 sem.		Cal	33.7[a]	36.5	2.8	8(NS)
Barry et al., 1966[a]	M/F	70	8	3	12 sem. (16-25 min)	sousmaximal & maximal	B(IT),Cal	16.1	22.3	6.2	38
Benestad, 1965	M	76	13	3	5-6 sem. (10-34 min)	près maximal	M	27	27	0	0

[a]$\dot{V}_{O_2 max}$ prédit selon le nomogramme d'Astrand.

M = marche   B = bicycle   N = natation
J = jogging   S = sports   Cal = calisthénies
C = continuel   IT = interval training

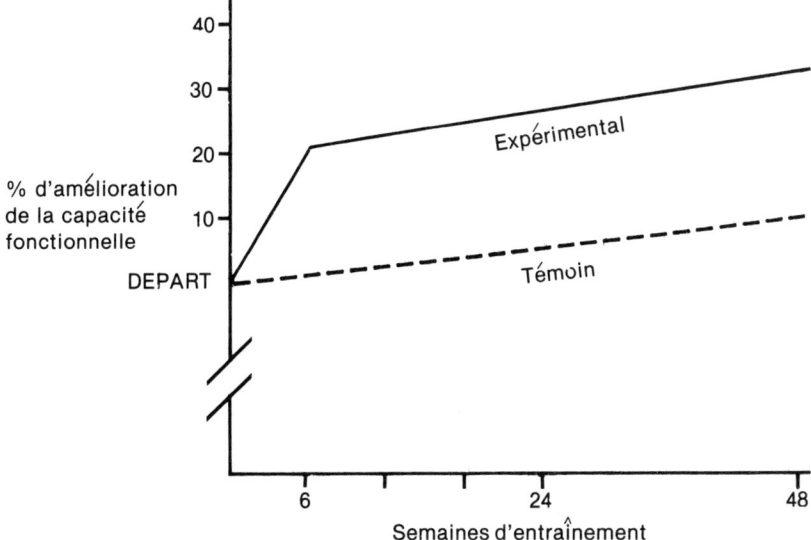

Figure 8 — **Effets importants des 6 premières semaines dans un programme de conditionnement physique adapté à une clientèle âgée (adapté de deVries, 1970).**

Les Figures 9 et 10 présentent une progression dans le programme et dans la séance proprement dite. Il est important d'initier le bénéficiaire à ce nouvel environnement. Les 8 premières semaines du programme permettent de bien s'initier et de poursuivre un processus de maintien et de développement. L'intensité de travail lors de la séance, va varier d'une fois à l'autre et le contenu va dépendre des objectifs recherchés tout au long de l'année.

Tableau 2
Classification des faiblesses musculaires

Nom	Définition
Hémiparésie	Paralysie légère d'une moitié du corps
Paraparésie	Affaiblissement de la contractilité des membres inférieurs
Faiblesse proximale	Faiblesse aux niveaux des ceintures scapulaire et pelvienne et la partie proximale des membres
Faiblesse distale	Faiblesse dans les régions distales des membres
Monoparésie	Faiblesse musculaire spécifique et isolée
Mobilité déficiente	Difficulté de se mouvoir associée à des raisons multiples

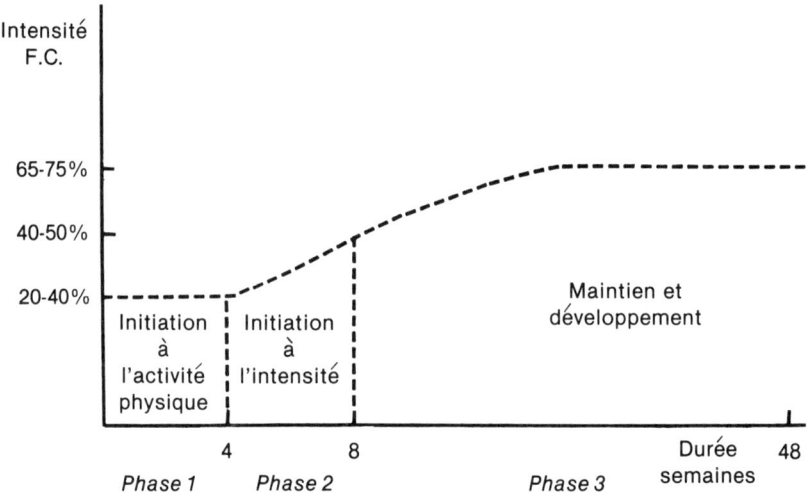

Figure 9 — Phases du programme de conditionnement physique (l'intensité du travail est associée à la fréquence cardiaque).

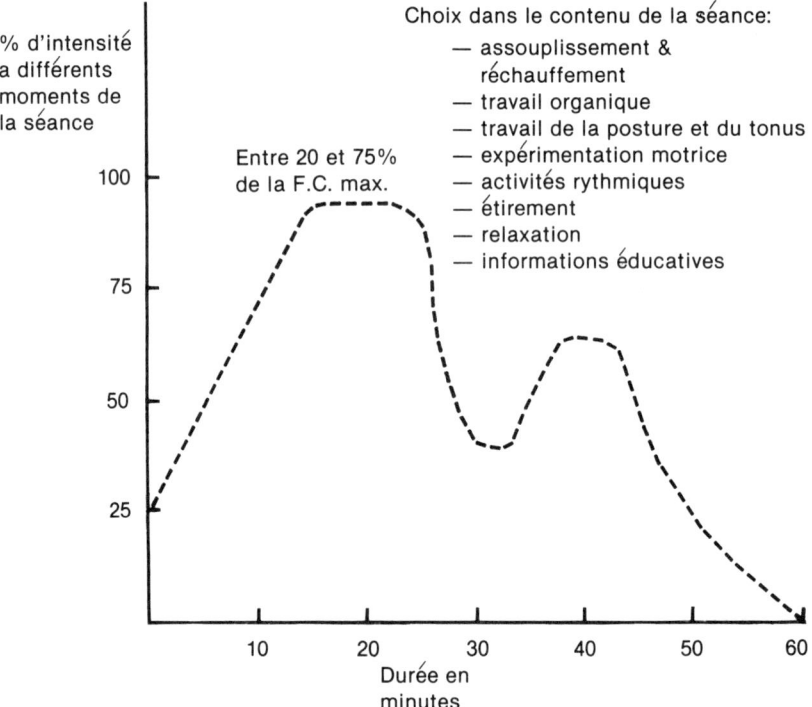

Figure 10 — Courbe de progression selon l'intensité de l'effort à différents moments de la séance.

Conclusion

La plasticité du muscle vieillissant demeure très élevée, aussi bien du côté de sa dégénérescence que du côté de son amélioration. On se doit d'être bien sensibilisé à ces phénomènes de changement afin d'apporter les éléments de solution appropriés dans les programmes offerts.

Les modifications que l'on retrouvent au niveau musculaire sont étroitement associées aux changements que l'on observe dans l'activité physique journalière des personnes âgées. La mobilité diminue en même temps que l'on effectue des gestes moins amples; la puissance et la force s'amenuisent en même temps que la personne effectue un type de travail plutôt léger. Les fibres de travail lentes et oxydatives tendent à se maintenir et à compenser pour l'atrophie des fibres à caractères rapides et principalement glycolitiques.

Nous devons maintenir notre souplesse et notre travail musculaire à un bon niveau en effectuant des mouvements concentriques, à caractère dynamique et en faisant travailler alternativement les fléchisseurs et les extenseurs.

Références

ANIANSSON, A., Grimby, G., & Rundgren, A. Isometric and isokinetic quadriceps muscle strength in 70 year old men and women. *Scandinavian Journal of Rehabilitation Medicine,* 1980, **12**, 161-168.

CAMPBELL, M.J., McComas, A.J., & Petito, F. Physiological changes in aging muscles. *Journal of Neurology, Neurosurgery, and, Psychiatry,* 1973, **36**, 174-182.

DEVRIES, H.A. Physiological effects of an exercise training regimen upon men aged 52-88. *Journal of Gerontology,* 1970, **25**, 325-336.

FUJISAWA, K. Some observations on the skeletal musculature of aged rats. *Journal of Neurological Science,* 1974, **22**, 353-366.

GUTMANN, E., & Hanzlikova, V. Motor unit in old age. *Nature London,* 1966, **209**, 921-922.

GUTMANN, E., & Hanzlikova, V. *Age changes in the neuromuscular system.* Bristol: Scientechnica, 1972.

HASSELKUS, B.R. Aging and the human nervous system. *American Journal of Occupational Therapy,* 1974, **28**, 16-21.

HEATH, G.W., Heyberg, J.M., Ehsani, A.A., & Holloszy, J.O. A physiological comparison of young and older endurance athletes. *Journal of Applied Physiology,* 1981, **51**, 634-640.

HOOPER, A.C.B. Length, diameter and number of aging skeletal muscle fibres. *Journal of Gerontology,* 1981, **27**, 121-126.

HOOPER, A.C.B., & Sheil, E. A study of some muscle and base parameters in mature mice. *Iran Journal of Medical Science,* 1978, **147**, 323-324.

JENNEKENS, F.G.I., Tomlinson, B.E., & Walton, J.N. Histochemical aspects of five limb muscles in old age. *Journal of Neurological Science,* 1971, **14**, 259-276.

LARSSON, L. Muscle strength and speed movement in relation to age and muscle morphology. *Journal of Applied Physiology,* 1979, **3**, 451-456.

LARSSON, L., Sjodin, B., & Karlsson, J. Histochemical and biochemical changes in human muscle with age in sedentary males, age 22-65 years. *Acta Physiologica Scandinavia,* 1978, **103**, 31-39.

MORITANI, T., & DeVries, H.A. Potential for gross muscle hypertrophy in older men. *Journal of Gerontology,* 1980, **35**, 672-682.

ORLANDER, J., & Aniansson, A. Effects of physical training on skeletal muscle metabolism and ultrastructure in 70 to 75 year old men. *Acta Physiologica Scandinavia,* 1980, **109**, 149-154.

ORLANDER, J., Kiessling, K.H., Larsson, L., Karlsson, J., & Aniansson, A. Skeletal muscle metabolism and ultrastructure in relation to age in sedentary men. *Acta Physiologica Scandinavia,* 1978, **104**, 249-261.

PERKINS, L.C., & Kaiser, H.L. Results of short term isotonic and isometric exercise programs in persons over sixty. *Physical Therapy Research,* 1962, **41**, 633-635.

SACKTOR, B., & Shimada, Y. Degenerative changes in the mitochondria of flight muscle from aging blowflies. *Journal of Comparative Biology,* 1972, **52**, 469-477.

SHEPHARD, R.J., & Sidney, K.J. Exercise and aging. In R.S. Hutton (Ed.), *Exercise and Sport Sciences Review,* 1979, **6**, 1-58.

TOMLINSON, B.E., Walton, J.N., & Reheiz, J.J. The effects of aging and of cachexia upon skeletal muscle. *Journal of Neurological Science,* 1969, **9**, 321-346.

WILLIAM, P.E., & Goldspink, G. Longitudinal growth of striated muscle fibres. *Journal of Cell Science,* 1971, **9**, 751-767.

Réaction à la Conférence du Dr. Clermont Simard Portant sur la "Plasticité du Muscle Vieillissant"

André Quirion
Université du Québec à Trois-Rivières

[This author comments on the previous article by Dr. Simard. Abstracts are unavailable.]

Vous venez d'entendre un exposé du Dr. Clermont Simard portant sur la plasticité du muscle vieillissant. Point n'est besoin de vous convaincre de l'importance du sujet traité et de l'importance de la connaissance des divers phénomènes physiologiques et biochimiques associés au processus de vieillissement du muscle. La connaissance de ces divers processus est d'autant plus importante quand nous voyons toute la promotion faite en regard du conditionnement physique chez cette population spéciale. Nous devons, je crois, être très attentifs à cette question quand nous savons que ce type de population spéciale retient de plus en plus l'attention dans notre société occidentale.

J'ai retenu quatre points principaux qui ont été traités dans cet exposé:

1. les changements et adaptations des éléments structuraux;
2. les changements et adaptations métaboliques;

3. les changements et adaptations fonctionnels;

4. les programmes de conditionnement physique.

Point n'est besoin, je crois, de revenir sur la première partie qui traite du rappel anatomo-physiologique. Si on se réfère au premier point concernant les changements et adaptations des éléments structuraux du muscle, vous avez, Dr. Simard, cité quelques travaux (Dr. Larsson, Dr. Hopper, Dr. Jennekens, etc.) portant sur la perte de certaines fibres musculaires et sur la distribution de ces fibres. Cette dégénérescence des fibres de type 2 "glycolitique" serait-elle présente chez l'ensemble de la population observée en tenant compte du passé sportif ou athlétique de la personne? Cette interrogation me vient du fait qu'on a observé une élévation qui est passée de 40% à 60% entre 26 ans et 62 ans au niveau des fibres de type 1 à tendance oxydative, donc aérobique. Nous savons que pour un très haut pourcentage de la population, les types d'activités physiques pratiqués sont à tendance aérobique pendant la vie courante. Ce qui veut dire que ce type de travail ne change pas nécessairement seulement avec l'âge mais semble plutôt constant pendant la vie, et ce, chez un haut pourcentage de la population. Est-ce que, chez un athlète de type résistant, donc, qui a sollicité régulièrement les fibres de type 2a et 2b avec l'entraînement, et ce, pendant une carrière athlétique assez longue, on observe les mêmes rapports que vous avez cités?

Quant aux observations que vous avez faites en regard de la décroissance de la longueur des fibres musculaires sans modification de la longueur des sarcomères, elles sont, je crois, très importantes surtout en associant ce phénomène à la diminution de l'amplitude articulo-musculaire chez la personne âgée. Nous savons tous que la diminution du rendement au niveau de cette qualité physique importante est à la base de l'explication que nous pouvons donner aux problèmes traumatiques tels les lombagos, les lombalgies, les déplacements des disques vertébraux, etc., si fréquents chez les personnes âgées. Toutefois, Dr. Simard, ces observations m'amènent à une deuxième interrogation, à savoir si la diminution du nombre des sarcomères peut être associée à la décroissance du nombre des fibres musculaires, et ce, principalement au niveau des fibres de type 2a et 2b. Le fait que le nombre relatif de fibres de type 1 augmente avec l'âge nous permet-il d'observer aussi une décroissance des sarcomères chez ce type de fibre?

Nous savons, Dr. Simard, que la surface des fibres varie avec l'âge. Ce diamètre augmente durant l'enfance et l'adolescence pour se stabiliser puis diminuer au cours du vieillissement. Cette variation, qui semble aléatoire et qui viserait davantage les fibres du type II pourrait-elle s'expliquer en partie par le fait que le développement nerveux des branches collatérales se fait au niveau des fibres de type I et que ces dernières peuvent être réinversées?

Passons maintenant au deuxième point que vous avez traité, Dr. Simard, à savoir: les changements et adaptations métaboliques. En se référant aux études de Gutmann qui a observé une diminution des enzymes mitochondriales et à celles d'Orlander qui observa quant à lui une diminution du volume mitochondriale, comment peut-on expliquer le fait que la capacité aérobique s'améliore avec l'entraînement chez la personne âgée quand on sait que l'amélioration des capacités oxydatives se passe à l'intérieur du volume mitochondriale déjà existant?

Quand au troisième point traité, les changements et adaptations fonctionnelles, je crois, Dr. Simard, que vos observations sont très importantes car elles reflètent les applications pratiques associées à certaines qualités physiques importantes à développer ou encore à maintenir à un niveau de rentabilité moyenne pour les besoins de la vie courante de la personne âgée. Un point important à retenir concerne la spécificité de la réponse à l'entraînement chez les jeunes et les personnes âgées.

Je me suis toutefois posé une interrogation sur la citation suivante: la diminution de force serait plus importante au niveau des membres inférieurs en rapport avec les membres supérieurs. Est-ce que la diminution de force serait toujours plus marquée au niveau des masses musculaires plus importantes, ou encore, est-ce que ce phénomène prévaut seulement dans la comparaison membres inférieurs-membres supérieurs? En pratique, peut-on tirer la conclusion suivante: l'inactivité des masses musculaires des membres inférieurs est plus courante chez la personne âgée en comparaison de l'inactivité des membres supérieurs?

Votre intervention, Dr. Simard, sur le quatrième point qui concerne le programme de conditionnement est sûrement très importante car vous traduisez en pratique, à partir d'un cadre de connaissances théoriques, les éléments que devait contenir un programme type de conditionnement physique pour personnes âgées.

Les trois objectifs que vous suggérez semblent des plus justifiés. Toutefois, je crois qu'aux trois éléments que vous citez, il y aurait peut être lieu d'en introduire un quatrième qui traiterait des facteurs d'intensité, de durée et de fréquence de travail.

Modèle de Programme d'Education Plein Air Adapté aux Personnes Agées

Georges A. Nadeau et Clermont P. Simard
Université Laval

Suite à notre vécu dans ce domaine, nous suggérons un modèle à suivre dans la préparation d'un programme de plein air. L'approche se veut une démarche individuelle et personnalisée afin de favoriser des activités qui permettront à la personne âgée de maintenir des rapports positifs et harmonieux avec l'environnement naturel. Considérant que la personne âgée doit se rapprocher de la nature en éveillant davantage sa vigilance à l'aide d'un laboratoire dynamique dans lequel elle s'intégrera progressivement, nous devons respecter des préalables tels que les besoins, les intérêts et l'encadrement temporel. Le tout débute par un questionnaire et une interview. La structuration et l'application du contenu sont faites avec l'aide des personnes âgées. La préparation adéquate de notre environnement, la sélection et la préparation d'un personnel compétent sont indispensables. De plus, notre cadre théorique associé au programme se divise en cinq étapes qui passent des caractéristiques de notre clientèle à l'évaluation du processus.

Following our experiences in this area, we suggest a model to follow in the preparation of an outdoor program. The approach is based on an individual, personalized style to favor the activities which permit the aged individual to maintain positive and harmonious relationships with the natural environment. Considering that aged individuals must bring themselves nearer to nature while keeping alert vigilance with the help of a dynamic laboratory in which they've been involved progressively, we must first consider their needs, interests, and time involvement. The process begins with a questionnaire and interview. The structure and application of the content of the program are made with the help of the aged individuals. Adequate preparation of the environment and the selection and preparation of competent personnel are indispensable. Additionally, the theoretical approach associated with the program is divided into five stages which involve the characteristics of the clientele in the evaluation of the process.

Le plein air fait partie de notre culture et de nos moeurs depuis longtemps bien sûr. Depuis fort longtemps, on se référait à la nature comme moyens d'expression utilitaires multiples et variés. Les forces de cette même nature imposaient déjà une symbiose (avec la nature) pour survivre dans des conditions "nordiques" souvent rigoureuses et difficiles.

On peut dire que nos pères et nos grand-pères qui "trimmaient" dur, d'une noirceur à l'autre, vivaient en plein air pour ainsi dire et savaient s'harmoniser à la nature d'une certaine façon. Ils ont connu intimement les grands espaces l'"arpente, l'arrière pays". Ils conciliaient d'une façon remarquable le travail et le loisir (culture, chasse, pêche. . .).

Nous avons tous des leçons à apprendre de ces "riches" pionniers, ceux qui ont façonné le plein air dans ce qu'il a de plus profond. Ces paysans "investis" d'une richesse de vie ont su intégrer admirablement le plein air dans leur vie de tous les jours.

Le "modèle de programme de plein air adapté aux personnes âgées" proposé ici, comprend les 10 étapes suivantes: (1) élément du rationnel; (2) investigation des besoins; (3) identification des objectifs; (4) sélection des expériences d'apprentissage; (5) structuration du contenu; (6) ressources nécessaires; (7) estimé des coûts; (8) limitation temps/espace; (9) implantation du contenu; (10) évaluation.

Eléments du Rationnel

Le concept d'EPA véhiculé ici repose sur une étude auprès des principaux experts dans le domaine répartis à travers le monde afin de dégager, des 97 variables étudiées, les éléments de base de l'EPA au Québec. Plus de vingt-cinq experts américains ont participé à cette recherche (Nadeau, 1976).

Considérant les paramètres étudiés, l'EPA au Québec semble être un mixage des deux concepts suivants: PREMIEREMENT, l'éducation *pour* et au sujet du *plein air* incluant le développement d'attitudes, d'habiletés de plein air et de connaissances et; DEUXIEMEMENT, une éducation plein air incluant l'apprentissage par le plein air comme un processus pour enrichir, revitaliser le curriculum (ensemble des expériences éducatives vécues par l'apprenant) dans lequel le plein air est vu comme un environnement unique pour l'atteinte d'objectifs éducationnels en dehors de la classe. Dimension cognitive fort importante.

Notre approche multi-dimentionnelle du plein air met un accent particulier sur la dimension cognitive (approche globale et pluridisciplinaire) (Nadeau, 1976).

Toute la démarche dynamique d'appréciation, de respect et d'utilisation rationnelle du plein air est supportée inéluctablement par une connaissance éclairée.

Investigation des Besoins des Personnes Agées Plein Air/Caractéristiques Psycho-Sociologiques des Personnes Agées

Tout comme les sciences biologiques en général parlent de l'atrophie par inactivité, il nous est possible d'affirmer que les capacités et fonctions psycho-sociales inutilisées s'atrophient progressivement (Giguère, 1978; Hammerman & Hammerman, 1964; Hassett & Wieseberg, 1972). Ceci dit, nous admettons que le vieillissement est un processus de développement de toute une vie, et plus on avance en âge, plus les variantes intra et inter-individuelles sont élevées. Face à ces "processus," on doit accorder autant d'importance aux facteurs psychosociologiques qu'aux facteurs biologiques.

Sur le plan psychologique, tout en admettant que les différences entre les individus s'accroissent avec l'âge, nous pouvons déterminer certaines tendances comme le repliement sur soi, l'attitude de méfiance et la recherche d'une forme d'auto-défense. De plus, on retrouve progressivement une tendance au *narcissisme* qui devient une forme de refuge face à la diminution de ces ressources (Hassett & Wieseberg, 1972).

Indiquons, suite à une étude de Beckman (1971), que l'index de bien-être sur le plan psychologique, *excellent reflet de la santé mentale*, est associé positivement avec la santé physique des gens. Ajoutons (Karnoven, 1974), que la personne âgée donne autant d'importance à son image corporelle que les personnes des autres tranches d'âge.

Sur le plan sociologique, étant donné qu'on rattache beaucoup la personne à son statut et, qu'à l'âge de 65 ans elle prend sa retraite, ceci provoque un choc et une tendance à l'isolement et au désengagement (Hammerman & Hammerman, 1968). Ajoutons à ceux-ci ses valeurs culturelles et ses allégeances religieuses et politiques. La personne s'identifie à ces rôles et cela favorise son intégration sociale. Toutefois, la personne âgée peut conserver plusieurs rôles sociaux en tant que parent, citoyen, membre d'une association et personne intégrée au monde du loisir.

Besoins Nouveaux de Notre Société

La société moderne en modifiant les standards de vie a créé (Smith, 1972) certains besoins humains fondamentaux qui peuvent en partie, être solutionnés par le plein air: (1) besoin pour une vie créative et enrichissante; (2) besoin pour une bonne forme physique et mentale; (3) besoin pour vivre en rapport plus étroit avec la nature; (4) besoin pour une meilleure compréhension "écologique" de l'environnement: espaces verts et récréatifs utilisés et, (5) besoins pour des satisfactions spirituelles.

Les caractéristiques et les mouvements de notre société "mécanisée" jouent en faveur de l'EPA aujourd'hui.

L'EPA peut rencontrer plusieurs des besoins actuels des gens sur les plans: mental, physique et social aussi bien qu'émotionnel et spirituel.

Si la mécanisation assure la production d'une part, elle permet également plus de temps (libres), de loisirs d'autre part.

Mais il ne faudrait pas que cela conduise à un divorce avec "Dame Nature" et que cette automation vienne trop vite modifier notre sytle de vie.

Les 18 Ans et Plus (Population Estimée à 4,012,000 Personnes)

Le taux de croissance rapide dans la participation des québécois aux activités de plein air a été démontré très clairement dans une étude récente de Parcs Canada, publiée en 1977 et intitulée: "Données longitudinales sur la participation des canadiens aux activités de loisir de plein air, 1967-1976" (Parcs Canada, 1973).

Ce que le Plein-Air Signifie et Implique pour les Personnes Agées

Une communication et une communion avec la nature par le biais d'activités multiples et variées; un contexte de socialisation où il peut partager chaleureusement ses expériences de vie, se préoccuper des autres, se faire des amis; un contexte de valorisation où il pourra se "rendre utile" et faire bénéficier la collectivité de ses expériences de vie.

Le gros bon sens où, dans sa globalité, il choisira des expériences de vie qui lui permettront d'aimer et de vivre pleinement, la vie et ce, dans toute la dignité que cela impose; de se référer au contact du plein air; un "accouchement sans douleur de la connaissance"; "faire l'amour" avec la Nature.

Une occasion de se renouveler, de s'améliorer dans la sécurité et la diversité; un antidote à l'ennui au désoeuvrement, l'inactivité, la tristesse; le goût de vivre.

Contributions du Plein Air vs Personnes Agées

(1) Augmente le pouvoir d'observation par l'utilisation de tous les sens. (2) Stimule l'intérêt et tonifie l'expérience par le développement de nouveaux intérêts ou parfaire ceux qui existent déjà. (3) Fournit en la nature, un laboratoire, tout équipé pour un apprentissage global par des expériences directes. (4) Fournit des occasions pour apprendre des habiletés nouvelles (habiletés pour la vie...) soit en éducation physique, récréation, santé, conservation. (5) Donne de l'extension à l'apprentissage entre quatre murs, en mettant l'accent sur les ressources du milieu. (6) Offre des occasions pour l'exploration et la recherche. (7) Aide à verbaliser les expériences et favorise la communication par une ambiance particulière et unique. (8) Enfin encourage de meilleures relations humaines: par la simplicité, la "globalité" inhérente à la vie en plein air; par les relations personnelles et informelles plus faciles; par la collaboration avec les autres membres du groupe.

Identification des Objectifs

L'implantation d'un programme si court soit-il ne s'est fait sans se poser les quatres questions fondamentales suivantes: (a) Quels sont les fondements philosophiques et le rationnel (nature) du plein air sous-tendant les grandes orientations (objectifs) typiquement québécoises en matière de plein air? (b) Quelles sont les expériences d'apprentissage en plein air qui permettront l'atteinte de ces objectifs? (c) Comment ces expériences d'apprentissage peuvent être organisées d'une façon efficace? (d) Comment vérifier si les objectifs ont été atteints?

En plus de favoriser l'autonomie de fonctionnement des personnes âgées face à différentes activités de plein air, voyons quelques objectifs généraux qui ont sous-tendu le rationnel du programme. (1) Fournir à l'individu des occasions uniques de développer son esprit de créativité et d'initiative dans un contexte significatif. (2) Fournir un milieu très favorable au développement affectif de l'individu. (3) Développer la conscience, l'appréciation et la compréhension de l'environnement naturel et la relation de l'homme avec celui ci. (4) Aider à réaliser, à travers l'éducation plein air, tout le potentiel de l'individu vers un développement complet de l'esprit du corps et de l'âme. (5) Fournir un contexte de socialisation pour l'individu en lui offrant des chances additionnelles de vie sociale intense au sein d'un groupe. (6) Rendre les individus capables de développer de nouvelles habiletés et nouveaux intérêts et fournir une base pour une façon de vivre plus enrichissante. (7) Aider à utiliser judicieusement et protéger l'environnement naturel. (8) Fournir des occasions uniques pour des changements de comportements à cause de l'environnement particulier qu'offre le plein air. (9) Contribuer à l'établissement de meilleures relations entre éduquants et éduqués à travers des expériences directes en plein air. (10) Fournir une occasion pour des expériences d'apprentissage afin de favoriser une approche globale et pluridisciplinaire.

Les objectifs qui ont trouvé un consensus parmi les experts québécois sont listés ici de un (1) à dix (10) par ordre de priorité (Nadeau, 1976).

Sélection des Expériences d'Apprentissage

Le dosage d'intensité des activités apparaît un des points fondamentaux dans la sélection des activités d'apprentissage.

Gordon et al. dans *Handbook for Aging and Social Science* nous laisse entrevoir cinq niveaux d'activités: Niveau 1: *Activités de Relaxation:* sommeil, rêveries éveillées, repos. . . Niveau 2: *Divertissements*: télévision, conversations paisibles, jeux de cartes. . . Niveau 3: *Développement de la personne*: cours, conférences, assistance à des événements socio-culturels, concerts, expositions, activités physiques et sports. . . Niveau 4: *Créativité*: faire des activités artistiques (peinture, musique. . .), jardinage, cuisine. . . Niveau 5: *Activités intenses*: sports, enjeux sportifs, prise de drogues, activités sexuelles.

Les personnes âgées tendent naturellement vers des activités de Niveau 2, plutôt sédentaires (Tableau 1).

Le contenu du programme, en plus de satisfaire aux besoins identifiés au préalable, doit être assez flexible afin de répondre aux intérêts particuliers des participants et de la température lors du déroulement même de l'activité.

Principes

(1) Permettre une intégration sociale (apprivoisement) adéquate et l'atteinte des autres objectifs. (2) Etre progressif: durée/intensité. (3) Intégrer avec équilibre les activités fondamentales: (a) déplacement, (b) abri, (c) nourriture, (d) chaleur (feu. . .). (4) Assurer une bonne acclimatation et le respect de l'environnement; "site": urbain, semi-urbain, naturel. (5) Respect de la personne âgée: type d'animation et leadership adapté. (6) Etre sécuritaire. (7) Permettre des activités libres et des heures suffisantes de sommeil. (8) Impliquer le plus possible les personnes âgées dans l'animation. (9) Promouvoir une compréhension de la nature et de ses interrelations (chaîne alimentaire. . .). (10) Etre évalué adéquatement. (11) Inclure des activités sensorielles: voir, toucher, goûter. (12) Assurer le développement équilibré de: (a) connaissances; (b) habiletés; (c) attitudes sociales.

La programmation doit être orientée vers la détente et l'expérimentation libre des activités de plein-air où on laisse place aux initiatives personnelles.

Tableau 1
Résultats du Sondage Concernant les Intérêts et Expériences en Plein Air Chez les Hommes et les Femmes

Quel serait votre intérêt pour une pratique éventuelle des activités de plein air suivantes et dans un deuxième temps, indiquez votre expérience dans celles-ci.

Hommes et femmes:	A. Experience			B. Intérêt		
	jamais	quelque-fois	souvent	pas du tout	un peu	beaucoup
1. Cuisine de plein air/été	4	8	2	4	9	1
2. Interprétation de nature/arbres	1	11	2	3	7	4
3. Interprétation de nature/pistes/animaux	5	5	4	4	6	4
4. Interprétation de nature/ornithologie	3	8	3	5	7	2
5. Interprétation de nature/MC_____	3	8	3	3	7	4
6. Photographie de plein air	4	6	3	4	7	2
7. Orientation	3	8	3	6	7	1
8. Orientation/cartographie	3	9	2	8	4	2
9. Orientation/secours	2	7	5	7	5	2
10. Trappage/lièvre	4	7	3	10	3	1
11. Trappage/MC_____	10	3	1	11	2	1
12. Premiers soins	1	5	8	6	6	2
13. Autres spécifiez						

Approche Dynamique

Pour une bonne animation: il faut réaliser la transparence de l'action éducative de l'intervenant grandi au rôle de guide, d'inducteur de changement, de générateur d'apprentissage, d'agent socialisant, de catalyseur, de facilitateur, d'unificateur afin de favoriser la congruence et une certaine autonomie chez le "moins jeune."

Ressources Nécessaires

La réalisation d'un programme d'éducation plein air adapté aux personnes âgées peut s'effectuer efficacement et rencontrer les objectifs fixés dans la plupart des centres de plein air reconnus et ayant les services médicaux nécessaires.

Le personnel d'encadrement doit être qualifié et avoir une bonne expérience d'animation avec les personnes âgées. Un animateur qualifié par 5 personnes âgées est recommandable.

Estimé des Coûts

Les coûts devront être réduits au minimum considérant le fait que 70% des personnes âgées vivent en dessous du seuil de la pauvreté.

Il est bon de prévoir 12 à 15$ par jour selon la saison et l'endroit incluant: inscription, hébergement, repas, collation, accès aux salles, ateliers, équipement, animation, premiers soins.

Limitation Espace/Temps

Dans le déroulement des activités de plein air surtout avec les personnes âgées, il importe de prévoir beaucoup de temps et de ne pas sentir le *"poids du temps."* Il faut *savoir prendre le temps.*

C'est là un processus qui demande une progression dans la durée du séjour, il faut débuter avec des expériences de courte durée comme des classes nature d'une journée, pour ensuite pouvoir vivre pleinement des expériences d'une semaine et plus.

Implantation du Contenu

La réalisation du programme en plus de rassembler tout le personnel d'encadrement (directeur du programme, animateur, psychologue, infirmière) regroupe également un groupe de quatre (4) personnes âgées qui font part de leurs besoins spécifiques et participent quotidiennement au bilan quotidien et à l'élaboration du programme/jour du lendemain (Tableau 2).

Evaluation

Sujets à Evaluer

Qualité du programme, satisfaction des attentes, qualités de l'animation.

Tableau 2
Programme de Plein Air Réalisé par les Moins Jeunes

Juin	11-Dimanche	12-Lundi	13-Mardi	14-Mercredi	15-Jeudi	16-Vendredi	17-Samedi	18-Dimanche
Déjeuner 7h45-8h30		Visite du Camp	Int. Nature (centre) (herbier) Plantes comestibles	Premiers soins Sentiers écologiques Etudes des arbres et des plantes	Interprétation de la nature	Orientation et premiers soins Tournoi de pêche	Cimes Brico-Nature cueillette	Evaluation Office religieux
10h00 Collation								
Dîner	Arrivée	Pêche Brico-nature	Erablière Tisane/thé des bois Rond Point Concours de feu Truc-Oscar	Belvédère Jeux extérieurs chaînes	Visite St-Jean-Port-Joli Sculpture Lieux historiques	Concours de feu	Préparation Randonnée en pleinair Tour du Lac	Départ P.A. Départ
Souper	Jeux-présentation Installation Jeux sensoriels: écouter, sentir, toucher	Apprivoisement Jeux de société	"Belvédère" (les grottes) Film	Feu de camp Bivouac Soirée Liquide Contes/ légendes	Bivouac	Jeux sensoriels Films Belvédère	Soirée "vieillotte"	

Modes d'Evaluation

Questionnaire/appréciation, écrit du séjour, rapport final de la direction.

Une évaluation plus systématique peut être faite par les tests suivants: (1) test d'anxiété de IPAT; (2) test de la perception des autres; (3) test de l'estime de soi; (4) test de la satisfaction de vivre. Pour obtenir des différences significatives, la période entre le pré-test et le post-test doit être assez longue.

Conclusion

Le Plein Air Comme un Agent de Changement

Transforme les gens en obtenant de nouvelles perceptions d'eux mêmes et des autres (jeunes/vieux). Pertinent pour prévenir l'érosion humaine aussi bien que l'érosion des sols! Ce qui n'est pas peu dire.

Transforme le processus et les méthodes par lesquelles les gens apprennent par le vécu, la résolution de problèmes, l'expérience directe, concrète indiquant *tout* l'individu *(globalité)*.

Transforme le programme établi en intégrant des sujets nouveaux.

Même si le "aging" ou "vieillissement," caractérisé par la décroissance de la masse métabolique active, appert comme inévitable au point de vue physiologique et fonctionnel cependant les phénomènes pathologiques demeurent "inevitablement."

Bien sûr, l'utilisation intégrée et pertinente du plein air ne viendra pas régler tous les problèmes des personnes âgées.

Références

BECKMAN, P.L. Measurement of mental health in a general population survey. *American Journal of Epidemiology*, **94**, 1971.

GIGUÈRE, L.M. *Le rôle de la personne âgée dans nos sociétés*. Québec: Laboratoire de gérontologie sociale, 1978.

HAMMERMAN, R., & Hammerman, W.M. *Teaching in the outdoors*. Minnesota: Burgess, 1964.

HAMMERMAN, R., & Hammerman, W.M. *Outdoor education: A book of readings* (2nd Ed.). Minnesota: Burgess, 1968.

HASSETT, J.D., & Weiseberg, A. *Open education: Alternatives within our tradition*. Englewood Cliffs, NJ: Prentice-Hall, 1972.

KARNOVEN et al. Longevity of endurance skiers. *Medicine and Science in Sports*, 1974, **6**(1).

NADEAU, G.A. *Outdoor education as seen through a delphi survey of selected groups of experts in the Province of Quebec, Canada, USA and overseas and implications for the outdoor education curriculums at Laval University.* East Lansing: Michigan State University, 1976.

PARCS Canada. Données longitudinales sur la participation des Canadiens aux activités de loisir de Plein-Air, 1967-76, Ottawa, 1973.

SMITH, J.W., et al. *Outdoor education* (2nd Ed.). Englewood Cliffs, NJ: Prentice-Hall, 1972.

Evaluation des Compétences Motrices de Déficients Mentaux

Jean-Claude De Potter
Université Libre de Bruxelles

L'étude porte sur 98 sujets déficients mentaux d'un quotient intellectuel compris entre 50 et 65. Différentes méthodes d'évaluation des compétences motrices ont été appliquées: les mesures des (a) temps de réalisation d'un mouvement limité, (b) coordination dynamique manuelle, (c) rapidité manuelle, (d) coordination dynamique générale, (e) vitesse en course de 25 m. D'importantes corrélations apparaissent entre le *QI* et les différentes épreuves psychomotrices mais aucun lien n'est démontré avec les épreuves plus globales. D'autre part, il apparaît que les coefficients de variation atteignent des pourcentages très élevés dans les trois premières épreuves qui font appel à la vigilance ou à une compétence limitée (de 15,64 à 48,12%). Les coefficients de variation portant sur les résultats obtenus dans des épreuves plus globales et donc plus motivantes comme la course libre (vitesse moyenne de 4,03 m/sec et 4,6 m/sec) n'atteignent que 5,1% et 5,7% respectivement pour les filles et les garçons. Une fiabilité plus grande apparaît donc dans les épreuves globales. Dès lors, il semble que peu de liens existent entre les compétences motrices évaluées par des épreuves très spécifiques et les qualités réelles mesurées par une épreuve globale et motivante. Des méthodes objectives d'évaluation des aptitudes motrices des arriérés mentaux doivent donc reposer sur l'observation et les mesures réalisées dans des conditions les plus ordinaires possibles.

This study used 98 mentally deficient subjects of IQ between 50 and 65. Different methods of evaluating motor competency were applied. The measures were: (a) time required to perform a limited movement, (b) dynamic hand coordination, (c) manual dexterity, (d) dynamic general coordination, (e) speed for a 25-m run. A number of important correlations were obtained between IQ and different psychomotor tasks, but no link was demonstrated with the more global tasks. On the other hand, it appeared that the coefficients of variation reached very high percentage levels for the first three tasks, which dealt with vigilance or limited competency (from 15.64 to 48.12%). The results for the more global and more motivating tasks such as the 25-m run (mean speed of 4.03 m/sec and 4.6 m/sec) reached only 5.1 and 5.75%, respectively, for the girls and boys. Greater reliability was therefore obtained for the global tasks. It appears that few links exist between motor competencies evaluated by specific tasks and real qualities measured by a more global and motivating task. Objective methods of evaluation of motor aptitudes of mentally deficient individuals must therefore rest upon observation and measures obtained during ordinary conditions.

L'évaluation des aptitudes physiques de déficients mentaux relève de différentes méthodologies et notamment des épreuves psychomotrices ou des épreuves sportives globales.

Nous avons présenté cinq épreuves typiques, psychomotrices, techniques et sportives à une population de 98 adolescents arriérés mentaux d'un QI moyen de 56.2 au Wechsler Intelligence Scale for Children et d'un âge chronologique moyen de 16.32 ans (De Potter, 1979).

Expérimentation

La première épreuve porte sur la réalisation d'un mouvement soit limité, soit discriminatif en réponse à un stimulus visuel (Baumeister & Wilcox, 1969; De Potter, 1981). La mesure réalisée porte sur les temps de la réaction et du mouvement soit vers l'extérieur, soit vers l'intérieur, soit vers l'avant. L'appareillage élaboré a fait l'objet d'une communication dans le cadre du 2e Symposium International en Activités Physiques Adaptées (De Potter, 1981). Ces mouvements sont imposés ou répondent à un choix consécutif au stimulus.

Les résultats obtenus démontrent: (a) l'influence de la complexité de la tâche sur le T.R.: selon la direction ou le choix du mouvement à réaliser, le T.R. sera plus ou moins long; (b) que les profils d'évolution des T.R. et T.M. sont semblables entre adolescents normaux et arriérés mentaux à l'exception de tâches trop complexes nécessitant un choix entre les symboles.

La coordination dynamique manuelle (De Potter, 1979), évaluée par l'épreuve II d'Ozoretski-Guilmain démontre un retard très important des adolescents arriérés mentaux, les moyennes étant de 9.72 ans et 9.89 ans respectivement pour les garçons et les filles alors que leur âge est de 16.04 ans et 16.61 ans.

L'épreuve de pointillage de M. Stambak (De Potter, 1979) imposée à la même population d'adolescents arriérés mentaux révèle un retard considérable puisque la rapidité de la main dominante correspond à un âge chronologique de 7.75 ans pour les garçons et 8.26 ans pour les filles.

Evaluation de la coordination dynamique générale (De Potter, 1979) démontre également le retard important dans cette qualité motrice, les résultats étant de 9.63 ans et 10.29 ans.

Dans une cinquième épreuve nous avons soumis les enfants arriérés mentaux à une course de 25 m. La vitesse a été mesurée par cellules photo-électriques placées à 2,5 m, 5, 10, 15, 20 et 25 m. L'ensemble est relié à un enregistreur à grande vitesse stable qui permet de mesurer au centième de seconde. Les mesures traitées sur micro ordinateur portent sur la vitesse moyenne, les vitesses intermédiaires, les variations de vitesse, avec moyenne, variance et écart type.

Les résultats sont les suivants:

- vitesse moyenne pour les garçons: 4,6 m/sec.
- vitesse moyenne pour les filles: 4,03 m/sec.

Si nous comparons ces résultats à la vitesse moyenne qui est de 9,1 m/sec pour un temps total de 12,8 secondes dans une course de 100 m, nous constatons évidemment que la performance est moindre et se situe à 50% environ de la performance normale.

Autre point de comparaison: la vitesse moyenne est inférieure à la vitesse initiale lors d'une course de 100 m réalisée en 12,8 secondes (Murase, Hoshikawa, Yasuda, Ikegami, & Matsui, 1975). Enfin, après le

Tableau 1
Epreuves Motrices

	Garçons 16.04 ans	Filles 16.61 ans
C.D.M.	9.72	9.89
C.D.G.	9.63	10.29
Rapidité	7.75	8.26

départ donné par une poussée dans le dos, un ralentissement apparaît entre 2,5 m et 5 m pour ensuite faire place à un redémarrage.

Résultats

Tous les résultats obtenus, qu'ils le soient sur base du quotient moteur ou d'une course de vitesse, constatent le retard important de cette population d'adolescents arriérés mentaux (Bucher, 1972; Picq & Vayer, 1972; Stambak, 1960; Vayer, 1978; Zazzo, 1958). Mais au-delà de ces lacunes qui n'étaient plus à démontrer, il apparaît que les variations sont les plus grandes lors d'épreuves d'évaluation partielle de la motricité.

Coefficients de Variation

Si nous examinons les coefficients de variation des résultats obtenus à ces différentes épreuves d'évaluation motrice, nous pouvons constater:

Que les épreuves de T.R. et de T.M. présentent un coefficient très élevé de variation, ce qui démontre la motivation des enfants et le lien existant avec les facteurs extérieurs.

Nous pouvons aussi constater que parmi les épreuves psychomotrices — C.D.M., C.D.G. et rapidité — la mesure de cette rapidité manuelle présente le coefficient le plus élevé, car elle fait appel à des notions très strictes de graphisme précis.

Il apparaît ensuite que le coefficient de variation le moins élevé se rapporte à l'épreuve la plus globale à savoir la course.

Ce type d'épreuve apparaît déjà comme plus représentative de l'aptitude motrice des arriérés mentaux.

Enfin, dernière observation basée sur les coefficients de variation: les jeunes filles présentent des niveaux nettement moins élevés que les garçons. Elles semblent donc faire preuve d'une plus grande constance, sauf dans la course.

Tableau 2
Coefficients de Variation

	Garçons	Filles
T.R.	26.4% à 48.8%	20.97% à 29.71%
T.M.	35.55% à 63.98%	30.27% à 46.15%
C.D.M.	19.03%	17.39%
C.D.G.	20.45%	15.64%
Rapidité	36.42%	32.65%
Vitesse	5.1%	5.75%

Corrélations Entre les Epreuves

Si nous recherchons les corrélations existantes, nous pouvons observer la droite de régression entre le QI et les différentes épreuves.

Les corrélations sont très significatives sauf dans le cas de la course de 25 m où seule une probabilité inférieure ou égale à .05 existe.

Par contre, aucune corrélation n'existe entre les épreuves psychomotrices et les résultats obtenus en course. Par conséquent, il semble que peu de liens existent entre les compétences psychomotrices évaluées par des épreuves très fragmentaires et les qualités mesurées par une épreuve globale.

Ces résultats viennent compléter ceux exposés précédemment par le Professeur Levarlet (Levarlet-Joye & Ribauville, 1981). Chaque test psychomoteur est indicatif d'un aspect particulier alors que la course constitue une épreuve motivante qui fait appel à une synthèse des compétences.

Conclusion et Discussion

Après examen de différents types d'épreuves ayant pour but d'évaluer le quotient moteur d'adolescents arriérés mentaux, la question de la méthodologie reste posée. D'une part, sur base de la mesure des T.R. et de T.M. à complexité croissante, nous pouvons cerner les compétences motrices et même établir des normes pour ce type de population.

D'autre part, sur base d'épreuves psychomotrices telles que coordination dynamique manuelle et générale, rapidité manuelle, il est possible de mesurer certains aspects ponctuels de cette motricité pour mieux comprendre le comportement général. Et entre ces deux épreuves, des cor-

Tableau 3
Regression

X	Y	Garçons	Filles
QI	T.R.	S^{++}	S^{++}
	T.M.C.	S^{+}	S^{++}
	C.D.M.	S^{++}	S^{++}
	C.D.G.	S^{++}	S^{++}
	Rapidité	S^{++}	S^{+}
	Course	S	S

$p \leq .050$ S.
$p \leq .010$ S^{+}.
$p \leq .005$ S^{++}.

rélations incontestables existent, mais les coefficients de variation sont très élevés.

Enfin, si nous utilisons une méthode d'observation plus globale telle que la mesure de la course, nous constatons que peu de liens existent avec les résultats précédents. Or, cette course devrait être la traduction de lacunes du développement moteur qui entravent la réalisation des performances. Si l'adolescent arriéré mental doit être considéré comme une intégrité psychomotrice, il y a lieu de l'observer lors d'activités les plus naturelles possibles.

Les méthodes objectives d'évaluation des aptitudes motrices doivent donc reposer sur des mesures réalisées dans des conditions les plus ordinaires possibles.

Il semble donc que les mesures portant sur des épreuves d'activité physique et sportive, si elles peuvent être objectivées, sont complémentaires voire même supérieures aux tests psychomoteurs trop parcellaires et peu attractifs.

Références

BAUMEISTER, A.A., & Wilcox, S.J. Effect of variations in the preparatory interval of the reaction times of retardates and normals, *Journal of Abnormal Psychology*, 1969, **74**, 438-442.

BUCHER, H. *Troubles psycho-moteurs chez l'enfant*, Paris: Masson, 1972, 230.

DE POTTER, J.C. *De la rapidité motrice des adolescents normaux et arriérés mentaux*. Thèse de doctorat en éducation physique, Université Libre de Bruxelles, 1979, nonpublié.

DE POTTER, J.C. Vigilance et rapidité motrice d'adolescents arriérés mentaux. Dans J.C. De Potter (Ed.), *Activités physiques adaptées*, Université de Bruxelles, 1981, 43-50.

LEVARLET-JOYE, H., & Ribauville, A. Les aptitudes sportives et les possibilités motrices des handicapés mentaux de 12 et 13 ans. Dans J.C. De Potter (Ed.), *Activités physiques adaptées*, Université de Bruxelles, 1981, 51-57.

MURASE, Y., Hoshikawa, T., Yasuda, N., Ikegami, Y., & Matsui, H. Analysis of the charges in progressive speed during 100 meter dash. In P.V. Komi (Ed.), *Biomechanics VB*. Baltimore: University Park Press, 1975, 200-207.

PICQ, L., & Vayer, P. *Education psychomotrice et arriération mentale*, Paris: Doin, 1972, 284.

STAMBAK, M. *Manuel pour l'examen psychologique de l'enfant*. Delachaux-Niestlé, 1960, 122-240.

VAYER, P. *L'enfant face au monde*, Paris: Doin, 1978, 272.

ZAZZO, R. *Manuel pour l'examen psychologique de l'enfant*. Tome I: Tests des possibilités motrices de M. Stambak. Delachaux et Niestlé, 1958, 178-217.

Considérations sur l'Enseignement de l'Activité Physique aux Élèves en Difficulté d'Adaptation et d'Apprentissage[1]

Michel Lirette, Claude Paré, Fernand Caron, et Pierre Black
Université du Québec à Trois-Rivières

Cette recherche porte sur la qualité de l'intervention en éducation physique auprès des élèves en difficulté d'adaptation et d'apprentissage. Elle a pour but d'analyser, de secondes en secondes, le comportement du professeur lors de son enseignement afin d'en dégager le "portrait professionnel" dominant. L'instrument d'analyse employé est le "Physical Education Teachers — Professional Functions" qui permet d'identifier différents types d'interventions du professeur. Les sujets retenus pour étude sont des élèves des niveaux primaire ou secondaire faisant partie de l'une ou l'autre des catégories suivantes: déficients mentaux légers, difficultés majeures d'apprentissage, mésadaptés socio-affectifs. Les résultats de l'étude révèlent, premièrement, une plus grande utilisation par le professeur des interventions de type "préparer les activités motrices et observer" lorsque comparées aux interventions de type "guider l'exécution des activités motrices", deuxièmement, un mode d'intervention basée surtout sur l'instruction verbale, troisièmement, une destination des interventions du professeur qui s'adressent davantage à un seul étudiant plutôt qu'à l'ensemble du groupe.

---

[1]Cette étude fait partie d'un programme de recherche qui fut subventionné en 1978-79 par le Ministère de l'Education du Québec, Gouvernement du Québec.

The quality of intervention in physical education with students with difficulty in adaptation and learning was studied. The goal established was to analyze the behavior of the professor during his teaching in an effort to determine a basic "portrait of the professional." The testing instrument used was the "Physical Education Teachers—Professional Functions" test, which permitted the identification of different types of interventions of the professor/teacher. Subjects in the study were students at the primary or secondary school levels in the following categories: mildly retarded, major learning-disabled, or maladapted in the socio-affective domain. The results indicated, first, a much greater use by the professor of interventions to "prepare motor activities and observe" as opposed to "guide the execution of motor activities." Second, the mode of intervention was based primarily on verbal instruction. Third, the interventions of the professor were addressed primarily at one student as opposed to the group in general.

Cette étude veut approfondir certains aspects reliés à l'enseignement de l'activité physique auprès des élèves du secteur adaptation scolaire. Plus précisément, elle s'intéresse au comportement du professeur d'éducation physique lors de son enseignement dans le gymnase. Il s'agit d'une recherche descriptive qui converge vers l'étude du processus d'enseignement plutôt que vers l'analyse de l'efficacité en enseignement.

Le référentiel à la base de la présente étude est le système d'analyse des interventions professionnelles en éducation physique d'Anderson (Note 1) et de Barrette (1977). Il s'agit d'une approche conceptuelle qui se concrétise par un système d'observation descriptif.

Evolution de la Recherche en Enseignement

A cet égard, la préoccupation majeure de la première moitié du XXe siècle fut d'essayer de trouver la réponse à la question suivante: "Quelles sont les caractéristiques d'un professeur efficace?" Un certain nombre de considérations pratiques ont guidé les efforts de recherche sur l'efficacité de l'enseignement. Comme le besoin de fournir des critères pour la sélection des candidats à l'enseignement, le besoin de redéfinir et de modifier les programmes de formation des maîtres. . . Malheureusement, l'obstacle majeur suivant a compromis le succès d'une telle entreprise à savoir: le problème insurmontable d'identification et de sélection de critères valides pour déterminer le succès et l'efficacité de l'enseignement. En conséquence, la valeur relative de ce type de recherche a été sérieusement questionnée et les résultats obtenus ont souvent été vus comme étant fort désappointants.

A la lumière de ces premières expériences, la recherche sur l'enseignement a connu un changement d'orientation important depuis une vingtaine d'années. En effet, l'emphase s'est déplacée de l'étude des qualités et des caractéristiques du professeur vers des recherches descriptives basées sur l'observation, la classification du professeur et de l'étudiant, ainsi que sur les comportements du professeur par rapport à l'étudiant et vice-versa. Comme résultat de cette réorientation, on assiste maintenant à une prolifération d'instruments d'observation systématique.

Situation de la Présente Etude

L'objectif poursuivi par la présente recherche est également orienté vers l'amélioration de l'enseignement. Cependant, son originalité vient du choix qui a été fait de la perspective, du point de départ et de la stratégie choisis pour réaliser ce but; tous trois sont différents des autres études faites jusqu'à maintenant dans ce domaine. L'objectif est plus modeste en ce que la description et l'analyse du comportement observable sont orientées de façon à ce qu'elles puissent aider à mieux comprendre ce qui se passe réellement lors d'une leçon d'éducation physique à des élèves en difficulté d'adaptation et d'apprentissage.

Objectif de l'Etude

L'objectif majeur de cette étude était de répondre à la question fondamentale suivante: en référence au système d'analyse des interventions professionnelles en éducation physique d'Anderson (Note 7) et de Barrette (1977), quels sont les types d'interventions à caractère professionnel employés par le professeur dans ses interactions lors d'un cours d'éducation physique s'adressant aux élèves du secteur adaptation scolaire?

Méthodologie

Echantillon

Les trois groupes retenus pour étude étaient formés d'élèves des deux sexes fréquentant le secteur adaptation scolaire. Ce sont, au niveau primaire: (a) des perturbés ou mésadaptés socio-affectifs légers, moyens et graves (MSA); (b) des déficients mentaux légers (DML); et (c) au niveau secondaire: des élèves en difficultés majeures d'apprentissage (DMA).

Les sujets de l'étude ont été choisis parmi les groupes suivants: (a) MSA, 9 classes au primaire, 73 élèves, (b) DML, 6 classes au primaire, 70 élèves, (c) DMA, 6 classes au secondaire, 82 élèves.

Les 21 classes ainsi retenues pour l'étude étaient réparties entre sept professeurs à raison de trois classes pour chacun.

L'âge moyen des sujets était le suivant: (a) MSA, 10 ans et 3 mois, (b) DML, 10 ans et 5 mois, (c) DMA, 14 ans et 1 mois.

Système d'Analyse des Interventions Professionnelles

L'observation et le codage systématique du comportement du professeur comprennent un ensemble de catégories définies d'une façon opérationnelle. Il s'agit d'un instrument de mesure multidimensionnel qui fait appel à une unité naturelle qui est l'intervention du professeur. Le système vise ainsi à procurer un instrument de mesure qui peut notamment être utilisé pour décrire le comportement du professeur d'éducation physique et, subséquemment, pour communiquer cette description aux autres membres de la profession.

Les interventions professionnelles du professeur ont été codées selon les cinq dimensions suivantes:

1. Intervention : but du comportement
2. Mode d'intervention : façon selon laquelle les messages sont transmis ou reçus
3. Destination de l'intervention : personne(s) vers qui le comportement est dirigé
4. Contenu : sujet de la matière enseignée (ex., basketball, volleyball, etc.)
5. Durée : temps (en secondes) qui s'écoule entre le début et la fin de l'unité de comportement observé

Chacune de ces dimensions est divisée et subdivisée en catégories et les 18 catégories d'interventions identifiées sont regroupées en 6 domaines interactifs. Ces domaines sont les suivants: (1) préparer les activités motrices, (2) guider l'exécution des activités motrices, (3) observer l'exécution des activités motrices, (4) participer aux activités motrices, (5) autres interventions interactives reliées aux activités motrices, (6) autres comportements interactifs. De plus, deux autres catégories noninteractives sont identifiées de manière à pouvoir comptabiliser d'autres comportements ou événements. Il s'agit: (7) d'intervalles non-interactifs et (8) d'intervalles nonidentifiables.

Fidélité des Mesures Prises

Pour calculer la fidélité de vérité du système d'analyse des interventions professionnelles, trois bandes magnétoscopiques témoins ont minitieusement été codées par trois expérimentateurs. Ces bandes témoins étaient d'une durée de 5, 9 et 13 minutes chacune et représentaient des segments de leçon de 3 professeurs différents. Parla suite, ces bandes ont été codées par 4 codeurs et le pourcentage moyen d'acord de .88 fut obtenu.

Pour calculer la fidélité de consensus inter-codeurs, trois autres segments de leçons de 5, 9 et 13 minutes assumées par des professeurs différents ont été codés par chacun des 4 codeurs. Un coefficient correspondant à .91 fut obtenu entre les différents codeurs. Le pourcentage moyen d'accord intercodeurs de .91 fut obtenu.

Cueillette des Données

Tenant compte de la procédure suggérée par Anderson (Note 1) et Barrette (1977) et des ressources (humaines et matérielles) mises à notre disposition, un système assez complexe de prise de vue et d'enregistrement de la voix du professeur a pu être conçu.

Le système de prise de vue, comprenant deux caméras placées l'une près de l'autre dans un coin du gymnase, a permis d'enregistrer les 42 leçons sur bandes magnétoscopiques d'un demi-pouce EIAJ. Une caméra équipée d'un objectif Zoom télé-photo isolait continuellement les déplacements du professeur, tandis que l'autre caméra équipée d'un objectif Zoom avec des effets grands angulaires permettait d'avoir une vue d'ensemble de l'action principale de la classe. Un microphone émetteur sur bande FM fixé à l'aide d'une ceinture à la taille du professeur transmettait au récepteur les données relatives au comportement verbal de celui-ci. De cette façon, les professeurs pouvaient se déplacer et interagir sans être gênés par le matériel requis pour la transmission audio.

De plus, le système de prise de vue était doté d'un générateur d'effets spéciaux qui permettait de diviser l'image en deux sections égales dans le plan horizontal. La moitié supérieure de l'écran diffusait l'image du professeur et la moitié inférieure celle de l'ensemble de la classe.

Enfin, un compteur de temps où l'on retrouvait les heures, les minutes et les secondes était incorporé à l'image. La cueillette des données fut effectuée en différé à l'aide des bandes magnétoscopiques préalablement enregistrées. Quatre codeurs ont été assignés à la transcription des données relatives aux 42 cours pré-sélectionnés.

Présentation des Résultats

Identification des Données

Les données de l'étude furent dégagées des 42 bandes magnétoscopiques correspondant chacune à une leçon particulière. Les 42 bandes magnétoscopiques se répartissaient comme suit: 18 leçons pour la population des MSA, 12 leçons pour la population des DML et 12 leçons pour la population des DMA.

La durée totale de temps d'enseignement retenu pour l'étude fut, pour l'ensemble des populations, de 2082 min (124,906 sec); ce qui équivaut à

905.5 (54,330 sec) pour les MSA, 601.6 min (36,097 sec) pour les DML et 574.6 min (34,478 sec) pour les DMA. La durée moyenne des 42 leçons fut de 49.87 min; elle fut de 50.46 min chez les MSA, de 50.13 chez les DML et de 47.88 min chez les DMA.

Rappelons que l'objectif opérationnel de l'étude était de déterminer la fréquence, la durée et la distribution des comportements de l'enseignant dans le gymnase.

Répartition du Temps de Classe en Fonction d'un Regroupement de Catégories d'Interventions Interactives

La Figure 1 informe sur la façon dont les enseignants en éducation physique emploient leur temps de classe. Cette information est basée sur les catégories du système d'analyse des interventions professionnelles en éducation physique retenues dans la présente étude. Le regroupement correspond aux 6 domaines interactifs déjà identifiés à savoir.

1. Préparer les activités motrices (catégories 1, organiser; 2, consignes préliminaires à l'enseignement; 3, préparer l'équipement ou l'environnement).
2. Guider l'exécution des activités motrices (catégories 4, enseignement simultanée; 5, arbitrage; 6, parade; 7, direction des exercices; 8, rappel du contenu).
3. Observer (catégorie 9, observer l'exécution des activités motrices).
4. Participer (catégorie 10, participer aux activités motrices).
5. Autres interventions (catégorie 11, autres interventions interactives reliées aux activités motrices).
6. Autres comportements interactifs (catégories 12, administrer; 13, établir et mettre en vigueur des codes de comportement; 14, autres interactions).

En analysant la Figure 1 nous constatons que des différences marquées apparaissent entre les populations. Tout d'abord à l'item "préparer les activités motrices," il existe chez les DML un net détachement de la catégorie "organiser" (22.0%). Les pourcentages associés aux autres catégories de ce même groupement sont approximativement de même valeur entre les populations. Pour les catégories "guider l'exécution des activités motrices" on remarque chez les DMA que les professeurs utilisent un bon pourcentage de leur temps de classe pour l'enseignement simultané (18.1%) et pour l'arbitrage (12.7%). Tandis que pour l'ensemble des populations les professeurs accordent peu de temps de classe aux catégories "parade" (.3%), "direction des exercices" (.1%) et "rappel du contenu" de la matière (2.7%).

La catégorie "observer" forme à elle seule un groupement. Le pourcentage est élevé chez les MSA (24.5%) tandis qu'il est semblable chez les deux autres populations.

La catégorie "participer aux activités motrices" forme également à elle seule un groupement dont la principale remarque se situe au niveau de la population DML. Son pourcentage est peu élevé (3.5%) comparativement à ceux des deux autres populations (MSA, 12.1% et DMA, 8.5%). Le plus fort pourcentage se situe chez les MSA.

Le groupement suivant est constitué de la catégorie unique "autres interventions interactives reliées aux activités motrices." Il n'y a pas de temps de classe alloué à cette catégorie chez les MSA et les DML alors qu'un très faible pourcentage apparaît chez les DMA (1.0%).

Le dernier groupement présente les différences qui suivent: à la catégorie "administrer," le plus haut pourcentage concerne les DMA (3.9%) alors qu'il est inexistant chez les DML; par contre à la catégorie "établi et mettre en vigueur des codes de comportement," le plus haut pourcentage se trouve chez les DML (10%); la dernière catégorie "autres interactions" révèle un pourcentage de 14.1% chez les MSA alors qu'il est semblable chez les DML et les DMA (7.9 et 8.0%).

Mode d'Intervention

Le Tableau 1 présente la fréquence et le pourcentage de la fréquence totale associés à chaque mode, pour chacune et pour l'ensemble des populations. Nous remarquons que le mode "parle" a une fréquence élevée comptant pour plus de la moitié de la fréquence totale, soit 55.6%. Ensuite, suivent dans un ordre décroissant les modes "écoute," "observe" et "participe" dont les pourcentages respectifs de la fréquence totale sont de 15.9%, 13.5% et de 7.9%. D'une façon générale, plus de 92.9% de la fréquence totale est composée des quatre modes précédemment identifiés. En ce qui a trait aux autres modes leur pourcentage est à toutes fins pratiques, négligeable.

Les différences entre les populations révèlent chez les DML que le pourcentage de la fréquence totale associé au mode "parle" est le plus élevé, soit 64.5%; chez les MSA que les modes "écoute" (20.3%) et "observe en silence" (16.0%) sont différents des DML et des DMA; et chez les DMA que les modes "utilise des instruments signalitiques" (7.1%) et "participe" (11.3%) les différencient des deux autres populations.

Destination de l'Intervention

Les fréquences et les pourcentages de la fréquence totale en fonction des éléments de la destination de l'intervention apparaissent au Tableau 2. D'une façon générale pour l'ensemble des populations, le Tableau 2 in-

Tableau 1
Fréquences et Pourcentages de la Fréquence Totale des Modes pour Chacune et pour l'Ensemble des Populations

Nom des modes	MSA (%)	DML (%)	DMA (%)	Tous
1. Parle	2970.0 (48.3)	3483.0 (64.5)	2809.0 (55.0)	9262.0 (55.6)
2. Ecoute	1250.0 (20.3)	656.0 (12.1)	744.0 (14.6)	2650.0 (15.9)
3. Observe (en silence)	982.0 (16.0)	741.0 (13.7)	532.0 (10.4)	2255.0 (13.5)
4. Démontre	10.0 (0.2)	88.0 (1.6)	23.0 (0.5)	121.0 (0.7)
5. Utilise un étudiant comme démonstrateur	5.0 (0.1)	9.0 (0.2)	4.0 (0.0)	18.0 (0.1)
6. Utilise des aides audio-visuelles ou visuelles	3.0 (0.0)	2.0 (0.0)	0.0 (0.0)	5.0 (0.0)
7. Utilise des instruments signalitiques	93.0 (1.5)	40.0 (0.7)	362.0 (7.1)	495.0 (3.0)
8. Ecrit au tableau ou fournit un texte imprimé	0.0 (0.0)	0.0 (0.0)	3.0 (0.1)	3.0 (0.0)
9. Aide manuellement	9.0 (0.1)	49.0 (0.9)	0.0 (0.0)	58.0 (0.3)
10. Participe	485.0 (7.9)	250.0 (4.6)	580.0 (11.3)	1315.0 (7.9)
11. Exécute une tâche "physique"	348.0 (5.7)	82.0 (1.5)	54.0 (1.1)	484.0 (2.9)

dique que les interventions sont majoritairement orientées vers un seul étudiant (43.8%), que 31.9% de la fréquence totale est dirigée vers le groupe et que 24.1% de la fréquence totale est constituée d'une combinaison "étudiant et groupe." Quant aux deux catégories restantes, elles peuvent être écartées de la présente analyse en raison de leur faible fréquence d'apparition.

Au niveau des différences entre les populations, le Tableau 2 révèle aussi que la répartition des pourcentages est semblable chez les MSA et les DML, alors qu'une différence majeure apparaît chez les DMA. En effet, chez cette dernière population la catégorie "un étudiant" constitue seulement 27.5% de la fréquence totale, alors que la catégorie "groupe" occupe 48.4% de cette même fréquence. Cette proportion est inversée chez les deux autres populations.

Analyse et Discussion des Résultats

Cette section a comme but d'expliquer les résultats présentés précédem-

Tableau 2
Fréquences et Pourcentages de la Fréquence Totale en Fonction des Eléments de la Destination de l'Intervention pour Chacune et pour l'Ensemble des Populations

Destination	MSA (%)	DML (%)	DMA (%)	Tous (%)
Un étudiant	2186.0	2243.0	1038.0	5467.0
	(50.6)	(51.2)	(27.5)	(43.8)
Groupe	970.0	1176.0	1829.0	3975.0
	(22.5)	(26.9)	(48.4)	(31.9)
Combinaison 1 et 2	1154.0	951.0	899.0	3004.0
	(26.7)	(21.7)	(23.8)	(24.1)
Autres personnes	7.0	6.0	8.0	21.0
	(0.2)	(0.1)	(0.2)	(0.2)
Combinaison 1, 2 et 4	2.0	3.0	4.0	9.0
	(0.0)	(0.1)	(0.1)	(0.1)
Total	4319.0	4379.0	3778.0	12476.0

ment en répondant à la question de base initialement soulevée. "Quels sont les types d'intervention à caractère professionnel employés par le professeur dans ses interventions auprès des élèves?"

Interventions Professionnelles

Pour l'ensemble des populations MSA, DML et DMA, les trois grands types d'intervention "préparer les activités motrices," "guider l'exécution des activités motrices" et "observation de l'activité motrice" schématisés à la Figure 1 attirent notre attention d'une manière particulière. En ce qui touche l'aspect "préparer les activités motrices," près du quart des fréquences totales observées se retrouvent dans cette catégorie. Cette grande concentration d'interventions laisse entendre que les enseignants ont souvent dû intervenir pour structurer la démarche de leur classe. Ce pourcentage (23.8%) de planification pédagogique de la part de l'enseignant semble raisonnable à l'exception des 22% de la catégorie "organiser" chez les DML. Il faudrait possiblement viser une réduction de fréquences de ce type d'intervention au profit de celles portant sur l'enseignement plus actif. De plus, une planification plus ordonnée permettrait vraisemblablement de prévoir les problèmes de fonctionnement et ainsi de pallier aux lacunes provenant de l'organisation pédagogique de la classe.

En ce qui a trait aux catégories regroupées sous la rubrique "guider l'exécution des activités motrices" un pourcentage de 20.7% pour l'ensemble des populations semble nettement insuffisant. Ceci peut

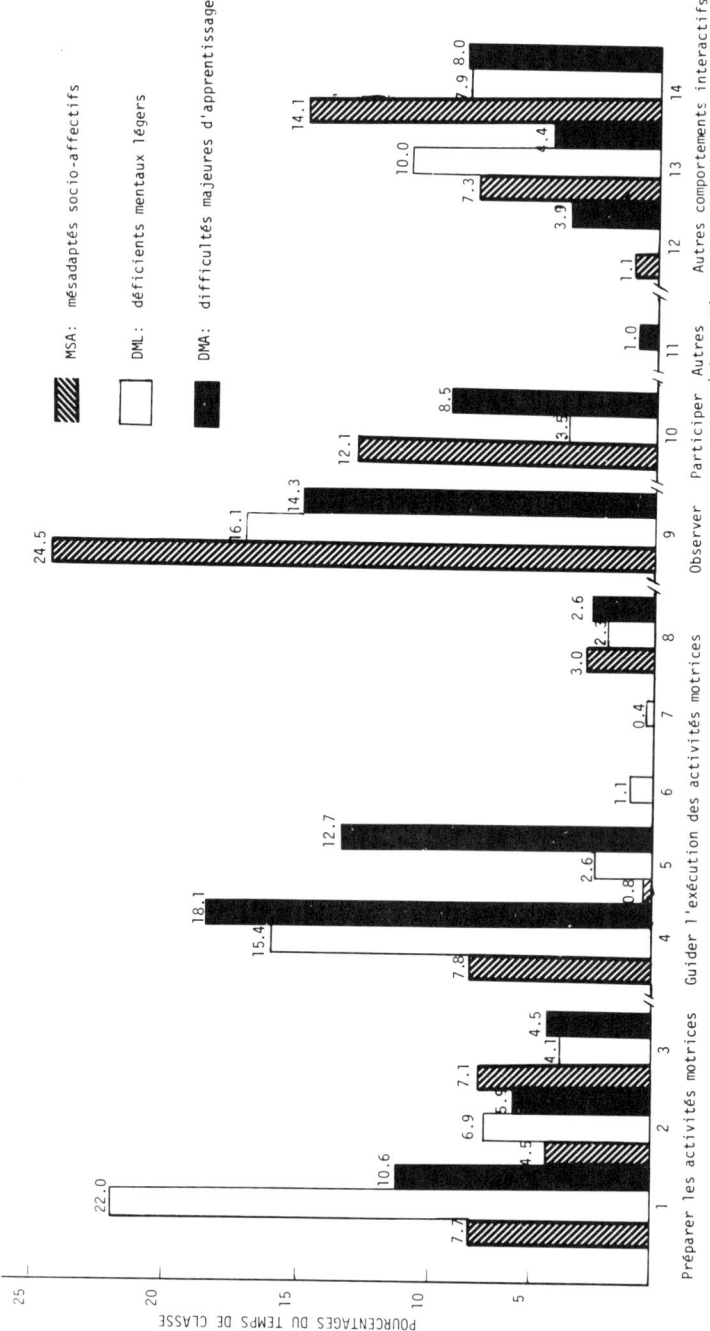

Figure 1 — Pourcentage du temps de classe en fonction des groupements de catégories pour chacune des populations.

révéler, de la part des enseignants, un manque de suivi des activités d'apprentissage des étudiants ou une absence significative d'objectifs d'apprentissage.

La catégorie "observer l'exécution des activités motrices" apparaît assez importante pour s'y attarder quelque peu. Bien que les fréquences de ce type d'intervention ne représentent que 13.3% de l'ensemble des fréquences, ce pourcentage dévoile quand même l'importance accordée à l'exécution de l'activité motrice demandée sous la surveillance du professeur. Cependant, une trop grand fréquence d'apparition de ce type d'intervention incite à penser que le professeur n'utiliserait pas suffisamment son rôle de motivateur, correcteur et enseignant. Le temps de classe occupé par cette catégorie viendra appuyer ces propos.

Le relevé des différences entre les diverses populations en ce qui concerne le temps de classe permet de constater que les professeurs du groupe DML ont émis plus d'interventions par leçon que ceux du groupe DMA et surtout que ceux du groupe MSA. La faible fréquence des interventions pour les groupes MSA provient, semble-t-il, du type d'enseignement donné à ces groupes. L'approche pédagogique de ces professeurs pourrait être décrite en soulignant l'existence d'une programmation très souple tirant sur le "laisser-faire." De ceci découle une attitude pédagogique très permissive. Par contre en ce qui concerne les deux autres populations, les interventions du professeur s'inspiraient un peu plus de la façon traditionnelle d'enseigner.

Ces observations se confirment à la Figure 1 dans la comparaison des catégories (2, 4, 8) touchant l'enseignement actif. Il apparait alors une moyenne de fréquence par classe qui est très inférieure pour les MSA, lorsque comparés aux deux autres populations (MSA, $\bar{X}$ = 53; DML, $\bar{X}$ = 89; DMA, $\bar{X}$ = 81). Concernant la catégorie "observer l'activité motrice," elle n'indique pas de différence entre les populations (MSA, $\bar{X}$ = 42; DML, $\bar{X}$ = 43; DMA, $\bar{X}$ = 37).

Après avoir analysé les résultats obtenus par rapport aux interventions professionnelles, il sera maintenant intéressant d'analyser succinctement quelques résultats reliés aux modes d'interventions observés et à la destination de l'intervention. Les données qui suivent sont tirées directement du rapport général qui sert de base au présent texte (Lirette, Paré, & Caron, 1981).

Modes d'Interventions

Nous avons vu précédemment que le mode "parle" totalise une fréquence de 9262 apparitions pour 55.6% d'utilisation. Les données relatives à ce mode permettent de constater que c'est au niveau des catégories "organiser," "enseignement simultané" et "établir et mettre en vigueur des codes de comportement" que ce mode est le plus utilisé.

Un deuxième exemple à donner de l'utilisation des modes est celui de la catégorie "consignes préliminaires à l'enseignement." Il est composé majoritairement d'instructions verbales (578), d'écoute de l'enseignant (170), de démonstrations occasionnelles par l'enseignant (57) et de rares démonstrations par un étudiant (17). Il semble qu'on pourrait ainsi déduire de ce qui précède que le professeur d'éducation physique parle passablement et que les élèves ne semblent pas encouragés à discuter, interroger, s'informer au sujet de la matière ou autres domaines.

Destination de l'Intervention

En ce qui a trait à la destination de l'intervention, certaines tendances générales peuvent être déduites des résultats obtenus à ce chapitre. En effet, il apparaît clairement, lorsque les enseignants font de l'organisation qu'ils s'adressent davantage à un étudiant plutôt qu'au groupe. Cette tendance se confirme aux catégories "préparer l'équipement," "enseignement simultané," "rappel du contenu d'enseignement" et "établir et mettre en vigueur des codes de comportement." Par contre, elle est dans le sens opposé en ce qui concerne les catégories "consignes préliminaires à l'enseignement," "arbitrage," "direction des exercices," "participer aux activités motrices," et "autres interventions interactives reliées aux activités motrices."

Finalement, il faut souligner qu'à la catégorie "observer l'exécution des activités motrices," un fort pourcentage apparaît sous le code "combinaison 1 et 2." Ce haut pourcentage peut se justifier par le fait qu'il était difficile aux codeurs de toujours discriminer la situation où l'enseignant observait un seul étudiant de celle où il observait le groupe. La plupart du temps, le code 3 était préféré aux deux premiers en raison du manque d'évidence de la priorité d'une situation par rapport à une autre.

Conclusion

Cette étude a permis, entre autres, de mettre en relief la concentration des interventions professionnelles des professeurs aux trois groupements de catégories suivants: (a) préparer les activité motrices, (b) guider l'exécution des activités motrices, (c) observer l'activité motrice. Les résultats obtenus dénotent également que dans l'ensemble les professeurs du secteur adaptation scolaire auraient avantage à augmenter le temps qu'ils consacrent aux fonctions de guide de l'exécution des activités motrices et à diversifier leurs moyens pédagogiques afin d'en arriver à une meilleure répartition des interventions professionnelles.

Note de Référence

1. Anderson, W.G. *Teacher behavior in physical education classes. Part I: Development of a descriptive system*. Unpublished paper, Department of Physical Education, Teachers College, Columbia University, 1974.

Références

BARRETTE, G.T. *A descriptive analysis of teacher behavior in physical education classes*. Unpublished doctoral dissertation, Teachers College, Columbia University, 1977.

LIRETTE, M., Paré, C., & Caron, F. *Analyse de la qualité de l'intervention en éducation physique auprès des élèves en difficulté d'adaptation et d'apprentissage*. Rapport présenté au Ministère de l'Education du Québec, Gouvernement du Québec, octobre 1981.

Attitude des Educateurs à l'Egard de la Personne Handicapée

Pierre Potvin
Université de Montréal

Depuis quelques années, le Québec s'oriente vers l'intégration des personnes handicapées. Nombre d'auteurs (Anthony, 1972; Donaldson, 1980; Wong & Perkins, 1978) soulignent que l'intégration ne sera pas réalisable tant que la population en général ne changera pas d'attitude à l'égard de la personne handicapée. D'autre part, il est reconnu que l'information et le contact sont deux moyens fréquemment utilisés pour modifier les attitudes à l'égard des personnes handicapées. Le but de la présente communication est de présenter quelques principes directeurs favorisant une utilisation efficace de l'information et du contact pour modifier dans une direction positive les attitudes. Ces principes s'inspirent des résultats des recherches en psychologie sociale et tout particuliérement d'une théorie récemment utilisée dans certaines universités québécoises, soit le béhaviorisme social de A.W. Staats.

L'auteur tient à remercier les organismes qui ont subventionné cette communication: le Ministère des affaires intergouvernementales du Québec, le service de recherche de l'Université de Montréal, l'Ecole de Psycho-éducation de l'Université de Montréal.

In recent years, Quebec has directed its efforts toward integration of the handicapped. Many authors (Anthony, 1972; Donaldson, 1980; Wong & Perkins, 1978) emphasize the fact that the success of such integration depends on a change in attitude of the average population. This article introduces some key principles for an efficient use of "information" and "contact" as a contribution to more positive attitude. These principles are drawn from research in social psychology and particularly from Staats' social behaviorism, a theory which is now favored in some Quebec universities.

Depuis quelques années au Québec suite aux documents du Ministère de l'éducation intitulés l'Ecole Québécoise (1979) et le Rapport COPEX (1976) nous assistons à une orientation vers l'intégration scolaire maximale des élèves en difficulté. D'autre part, durant cette même période le Québec s'est doté d'une charte des droits et libertés de la personne qui complète cette politique sociale.

Dans cette même orientation, afin de mieux préparer les éducateurs physiques à faire face aux conséquences de l'intégration des personnes handicapées, un comité de travail sur la formation et le perfectionnement en activité physique adaptée, propose deux cours obligatoires, soit six crédits d'éducation physique adaptée, à intégrer au programme universitaire de formation initiale en éducation physique. L'un des objectifs de ces cours vise à développer chez les éducateurs physiques une attitude positive à l'endroit de la personne handicapée.

Le but principal de la présente communication, est de réaliser une synthèse des écrits concernant les principes directeurs pouvant favoriser l'apprentissage d'attitudes positives à l'égard de la personne handicapée.

Attitudes Envers les Personnes Handicapées

Avant d'entrer dans le vif du sujet de cette communication, il est important de définir les principaux concepts utilisés soit, celui d'attitude, de personne handicapée et d'éducateur.

Staats (1975) définit les attitudes comme étant des réponses affectives apprises, qui peuvent être positives ou négatives et reliées soit à des personnes, soit à des objets ou soit à des événements.

Notre définition de personne handicapée se réfère à celle de la Commission des Droits de la Personne du Québec (1980) soit, toute personne souffrant d'une anormalité pathologique ou congénitale de son corps ou de son développement émotif ou cognitif ou qu'on croit telle. Cette définition englobe l'ensemble des handicaps que ce soit l'handicap physique ou l'handicap mental.

Le terme éducateur quant à lui, désigne les intervenants en éducation ou en éducation spécialisée, comme les enseignants, les orthopédagogues, les éducateurs physiques, les éducateurs spécialisés, les psycho-éducateurs, etc.

Attitudes de la Population Envers les Personnes Handicapées

Depuis les dernières décennies (Donaldson, 1980; Yuker, Block, & Younng, 1970) le sujet des attitudes a reçu une grande attention de la part des psychologues, des médecins et du personnel s'occupant de réhabilitation.

Selon Wright (1973) l'attitude envers les personnes handicapées n'est pas un phénomène isolé, elle a suivi le développement social en général. Depuis la deuxième guerre mondiale, l'emphase a été mise au niveau des droits humains et civils.

L'un des problèmes reliés à la promotion des droits et libertés de la personne, de même qu'à l'intégration des personnes handicapées, réside dans les attitudes négatives de la population envers ces personnes (Donaldson, 1980; Spreen, 1977).

Nombre d'auteurs (Anthony, 1972; Donaldson, 1980; Wong & Perkins, 1978) soulignent que le mandat d'intégration ne sera pas réalisable tant que la population en général ne changera pas d'attitude à l'égard de la personne handicapée. Pour leur part Johnson et Johnson (1980) soulignent que l'intégration ne peut être un succès que si elle permet des interrelations constructives entre les sujets handicapés et leurs pairs nonhandicapés.

Concernant ces différentes réactions négatives, il semble que la plupart des personnes se sentent inconfortables lorsque misent en contact avec une personne handicapée. Elles ont peur, sont curieuses, se sentent coupables et souvent ne savent pas quoi faire. A ce sujet Wong et Perkins (1978) citant Guskin (1977) indiquent que les groupes qui apparaissent étranges ou différents semblent déclencher de l'anxiété, qui elle, mêne à des attitudes défavorables.

Attitudes des Educateurs Envers les Personnes Handicapées

Hughes (1978) citant Mitchell (1976), souligne que l'aspect qui a recu le moins d'attention au niveau de l'intégration c'est l'attitude des enseignants envers les handicapés. Pourtant, c'est l'une des variables importantes dans le succès de l'intégration. En effet, l'attitude de l'enseignant affectera sa relation avec les étudiants handicapés de même qu'avec les étudiants nonhandicapés.

Hughes (1978) précise à ce sujet, que l'attitude de l'enseignant envers les étudiants handicapés modèle un style d'interaction qui peut influencer énormément l'attitude des étudiants nonhandicapés vis-à-vis de leurs pairs handicapés. D'autre part, les attentes de l'éducateur modèlent graduellement le comportement des étudiants handicapés. Ceci rejoint la célèbre étude de Rosenthal et Jacobson (1968) qui fait ressortir que lorsque les enseignants reçoivent l'information qui leur dit qu'ils peuvent attendre un grand rendement d'étudiants sélectionnés au hasard, ces étudiants effectivement démontrent du progrès.

Enfin, Ensher (1973) indique que les attitudes négatives existent chez les enseignants et qu'elles maintiennent la continuité du comportement mésadapté chez les sujets déficients mentaux.

L'apprentissage et le Changement des Attitudes Selon la Théorie du Béhaviorisme Social de Staats

L'apprentissage des Attitudes

Le béhaviorisme social développé par A.W. Staats conçoit la personnalité comme étant composée de trois systèmes interreliés et interdépendants, à savoir: le système instrumental, le système cognitif-linguistique et enfin celui qui nous intéresse présentement le système affectivo-motivationnel, que Staats qualifie aussi de système A-R-D. Ce système A-R-D s'appuie principalement sur le conditionnement classique ainsi que sur l'interrelation entre le conditionnement classique et instrumental.

Le système A-R-D se caractérise donc pour un individu, par l'ensemble des stimuli ayant acquis pour lui les trois fonctions suivantes: Affective, c'est-à-dire qui déclenche une émotion; Renforçante, dans le sens de maintenir et de renforcer un comportement; Directive, en déclenchant la classe de comportements soit d'approche ou d'évitement. Pour Staats (1968, 1970, 1975) c'est le système de personnalité responsable des émotions, des motivations des attitudes d'un individu. A titre d'exemple, un éducateur ou un adolescent qui ont appris des attitudes positives à l'égard des personnes handicapées, lorsque mis en leur présence, celles-ci (jouant le rôle de stimuli A-R-D positifs) déclencheront chez l'éducateur ou chez l'adolescent, la grande classe de comportements d'approche. Ces réponses d'approche pourront être variées, comme par exemple: encourager, aider, coopérer, promouvoir, etc.

D'un autre côté, s'ils ont appris des attitudes négatives et il semble que c'est dans la majorité des cas, la grande classe de comportements d'évitement sera déclenchée. Selon leur répertoire de comportements, ils pourront avoir tendance à éviter les personnes handicapées, les rédiculiser, les ignorer, les surprotéger, les prendre en pitié, etc. Ces attitudes positives ou négatives peuvent être apprises de nombreuses façons, entre autres, par la communication verbale, par l'imitation, par les mass média ou par l'intermédiaire de la personne handicapée.

L'apprentissage d'Attitude par la Communication Verbale. La théorie de Staats fait clairement ressortir que les mots peuvent être des stimuli A-R-D positifs ou négatifs. Par exemple, les mots comme handicapé, infirme, inadapté, malade mental, qui au début pouvaient être neutres, deviennent négatifs, étant donné qu'ils sont continuellement jumelés avec des aspects négatifs comme, incapacité, difficulté, incompétence, déficience, maladie, etc.

L'apprentissage d'Attitude par L'imitation. L'enfant et l'adolescent observent et sont influencés par les attitudes et les comportements des personnes qui leur servent de modèle (parent, éducateur, idole). Si ceux-ci en présence des personnes handicapées, ont tendance à s'éloigner, à être mal à l'aise, à témoigner de la pitié; les enfants ou les adolescents pourront graduellement apprendre ces mêmes attitudes et les comportements qui en découlent.

L'apprentissage d'Attitude par les Mass Média. La télévision, les journaux, les livres, lorsqu'ils mettent l'accent sur le handicap de la personne, sur ses manques, sur ses difficultés plutôt que sur ses compérences, ses qualités, amènent les récepteurs du message à concevoir la personne handicapée comme étant inférieure, incapable, incompétente, etc. Cette orientation du message peut favoriser la formation d'attitudes négatives.

L'apprentissage d'Attitude par L'intermédiaire de la Personne Handicapée Elle-même. Les caractéristiques physiques de la personne handicapée peuvent servir de stimuli A-R-D positifs ou négatifs, que ce soit au niveau visuel, sonore ou tactile. Par exemple, les paralytique cérébral par sa démarche incoordonnée, son langage désarticulé, peut déclencher des émotions négatives et provoquer des comportements d'évitement. Contrairement l'enfant sourd ou aveugle, physiquement très beau, peut déclencher des comportements d'approche. De plus, les comportements de la personne handicapée peuvent exercer une influence positive ou négative au niveau de l'interaction sociale. Ainsi, un adolescent qui a un comportement d'aide envers autrui, manifeste de l'honnêteté au jeu et est non violent, pourra être attirant. Contrairement, le délinquant qui a des comportements compétitifs, violents, qui triche au jeu, pourra déclencher des émotions négatives et par ce fait être rejeté.

Le Changement des Attitudes

Plusieurs auteurs (Gellis, 1976; Goldberg, 1977; Harth, 1974) mentionnent l'importance de changer les attitudes négatives à l'égard des personnes handicapées. Ainsi Gellis (1976) souligne que les attitudes déterminent un standard de vie et établissent un modèle de conduites sociales et de comportements, tant pour les handicapés que pour les nonhandicapés. Cet auteur mentionne de plus que les attitudes négatives à l'égard d'un sous-groupe peuvent avoir des effets négatifs sur le concept de soi, sur l'apprentissage et les comportements sociaux des membres du sous-groupe.

L'une des modalités efficaces pour changer les attitudes selon le béhaviorisme social, consiste à utiliser le contreconditionnement classique. Celui-ci peut être utilisé pour qu'un stimulus, qui déclenche une réaction affective négative, en vienne à déclencher une réaction affective positive ou vice versa. C'est un processus au cours duquel un stimulus qui déclenche la réponse affective appropriée est jumelé un certain nombre de fois avec le stimulus qui déclenche la réponse affective inadéquate. Par exemple, la personne handicapée jumelée de nombreuses fois avec des stimuli A-R-D positifs (sa compétence, son originalité, ses habilités, etc.) peut en arriver graduellement à modifier dans une direction positive les attitudes des sujets.

L'utilisation de L'information et du Contact Pour Modifier Positivement les Attitudes

Plusieurs auteurs (Anthony, 1972; Donaldson, 1980; Harth, 1974; Wong & Perkins, 1978; Yuker, Block, & Younng, 1970) mentionnent que l'information et le contact sont deux moyens frequemment utilisés pour modifer les attitudes à l'égard des personnes handicapées. D'autres moyens comme la simulation et le jeu de rôle sont aussi utilisés, mais moins fréquemment.

L'information

Le concept sous-jacent à l'information selon Wong et Perkins (1978) est que la connaissance de la personne handicapée va promouvoir une attitude plus positive envers celle ci. Ajoutons que certaines conditions essentielles sont nécessaires pour que l'information soit efficace. En effet, il ressort des recherches, que l'information doit accentuer les aspects nontraditionnels et non stéréotypés de la personne handicapée et présenter les situations et les personnages le plus positivement possible.

Voici quelques exemples d'information: cours en enfance inadaptée, conférence par un spécialiste de la question, lecture spécialisée portant sur des personnages célèbres qui ont vécu avec un handicap, discussion sur le vécu des personnes handicapées, etc.

Le Contact

Selon Allport (1954) on a soutenu qu'en assemblant les personnes, peu importe la race, la couleur, la religion, l'origine nationale, on pourrait détruire les stéréotypes et développer des attitudes amicales. Cela ne s'est pas avéré aussi simple.

Suite au nombreuses recherches utilisant le contact, que ce soit en ce qui a trait aux ethnies, au racisme, ou à l'intégration des personnes handicapées, ce moyen d'intervention s'est avec les années raffiné. Ainsi, il s'est avéré que certaines conditions sont nécessaires pour que le contact produise des effets positifs. Comme le mentionnent nombre d'auteurs (Allport, 1954; Harth, 1974; Ségal, 1978) le contact peut être une arme à deux trachants, favorisant aussi bien des attitudes négatives, dépendamment du genre d'expériences vécues.

Certains auteurs (Allport, 1954; Donaldson, 1980; Harth, 1974; Yuker, Block, & Younng, 1970) indiquent des conditions pour que le contact soit efficace. Les critères qui reviennent sont les suivants: que les statuts entre les personnes soient relativement égaux; que le climat soit gratifiant; qu'il y ait réduction de la tension ou de l'inconfort; que les activités soient de type coopératif où les personnes objets de discrimination et non objet de discrimination travaillent ensemble sur une tâche particulière; que le contact soit structuré.

Voici quelques exemples de contact: faire une visite guidée d'un centre pour handicapés; assister à des sports pour handicapés; participer à une table ronde dont les conférenciers sont des personnes handicapées; réaliser des activités physiques avec des personnes handicapées; visionner un film ou un vidéo sur le vécu des personnes handicapées.

Principes Directeurs pour Modifier dans une Direction Positive les Attitudes a l'Égard des Personnes Handicapées

Il est reconnu par nombre d'auteurs (Donaldson, 1980; Harth, 1974; Richardson, 1975) que changer positivement et significativement les attitudes à l'égard des personnes handicapées, n'est pas chose facile. L'analyse des recherches indique à ce sujet que des procédures directes et bien organisées sont nécessaires.

Concernant les enseignants Harth (1974) citant Polonsky (1961) conclu qu'il faut dès la formation des éducateurs incorporer des moyens pour modifier positivement les attitudes à l'égard des personnes handicapées. Les programmes d'entraînement des enseignants qui sont trop centrés sur les aspects cognitifs, ne touchent pas les attitudes de ces intervenants.

Quant à la recherche de Stephens et Braun (1980) elle fait ressortir clairement que les enseignants qui ont reçu des cours en éducation spécialisée étaient plus enclins à accepter des étudiants handicapés dans leur classe. Cette acceptation augmente avec le nombre de cours suivis en éducation spécialisée.

D'autre part, les écrits en psychologie sociale en ce qui a trait à l'intégration des personnes handicapées, démontrent qu'un accent mis uniquement sur l'adaptation des programmes, reste insuffisant. L'une des raisons importantes, réside au niveau des attitudes de rejet de la part des groupes qui reçoivent les personnes intégrées. Il faut donc modifier dans une direction positive les attitudes à l'égard des personnes handicapées.

En guise de synthèse des analyses des écrits concernant la modification des attitudes à l'égard des personnes handicapées, nous proposons différents principes directeurs favorisant une utilisation efficace de l'information et du contact. Certains de ces principes resteront à être vérifiés dans le cadre de recherches expérimentales.

Principes Directeurs pour une Utilisation Efficace de L'information

- Centrer le message sur les aspects positifs des personnes handicapées.
- Centrer l'attention du récepteur du message sur la personne, plutôt que sur le handicap.
- Eviter l'utilisation de mots "étiquette" comme: délinquant, déficient, infirme, etc.
- Présenter des personnages qui peuvent servir de modèle par exemple, des personnes qui avec un handicap physique ont bien réussi, soit dans le domaine des arts, de la musique, de la science, des sports, etc.
- Utiliser des mots qui ont une valeur A-R-D positive.
- Utilser les média (film, livre, journal) dont le contenu fait la promotion des personnes handicapées.

Principes Directeurs pour une Utilisation Efficace du Contact

- Structurer le contact avec une personne handicapée, ne pas le laisser au hasard.
- Utiliser un contact in vivo ou par l'intermédiaire de l'audio-visuel, les deux formes sont efficaces.
- Favoriser des interactions positives entre les personnes handicapées et nonhandicapées.
- Voir à ce que les statuts soient égaux, par exemple, la personne handicapée ne doit pas être toujours celle qui reçoit de l'aide.
- Utiliser des activités d'intégration qui permettent aux personnes handicapées d'être compétentes.
- Voir à ce que la personne handicapée soit elle-même active à réduire l'anxiété, la peur que provoque le contact. L'un des moyens est de parler ouvertement de son handicap.
- Organiser des visites de milieux pour personnes handicapées. Choisir des milieux reconnus pour leur compétence. Débuter par les cas les plus lourds et s'attarder aux cas moyens et légers. Centrer la visite sur les compétences des personnes handicapées.

- Offrir aux personnes nonhandicapées la possibilité d'observer des modèles d'interactions positives entre personnes handicapées et nonhandicapées.

Conclusion

Le changement dans une direction positive des attitudes à l'égard des personnes handicapées, peut se réaliser grâce à l'information et au contact. Pour ce faire, le contenu de ces deux modes d'intervention doit être positif.

D'autre part, la personne handicapée doit être perçue par elle-même, par l'éducateur et par les étudiants, comme une personnes ayant un statut égal.

De plus, lorsque l'on veut modifier positivement les attitudes, à cause des apprentissages négatifs antérieurs, il faut alors mettre l'accent surtout sur les compétences afin de contre balancer les effets négatifs des attitudes stéréotypées.

Efin, les principes directeurs proposés dans le cadre de cette communication, sont tirés des écrits concernant le changement des attitudes à l'égard des personnes handicapées. Certains de ces principes directeurs, nécessiteront d'être vérifiés par des recherches expérimentales.

Références

ANTHONY, W.A. Societal rehabilitation: changing society's attitudes toward the physically and mentally disabled. *Rehabilitation Psychology,* 1972, **19**, 117-126.

ALLPORT, G.A. *The nature of prejudice.* Addison Wesley, 1954.

COMMISSION des Droits de la Personne du Québec. Le droit à l'égalité pour les personnes handicapées. Document inédit, 1980.

DONALDSON, J. Changing attitudes toward handicapped persons: A review and analysis of research. *Exceptional Children,* 1980, **46**, 504-514.

ENSHER, G.L. The hidden handicap: Attitudes toward children and their implication. *Mental Retardation,* 1973, **11**, 40-41.

GELLIS, H.M. A model for affecting attitudinal and behavioral changes in primary age normal children toward severely mentally handicapped trainable children based on contact frequency in favorable school. Dissertation submitted to the graduate school faculty of applied and professional psychology of Rutgers, The State University of New Jersey, 1976.

GOLDBERG, R.T. Rehabilitation research on disability. *Journal of Rehabilitation,* 1977, **42**, 14-18.

GUSKIN, S.L. Paradigms for research on attitudes toward the mentally retarded. In P. Mittler (Ed.), *Research to practice in mental retardation* (Vol. I). University Park, 1977.

HARTH, R. Attitude and mental retardation: Review of the literature. *Training School Bulletin,* 1974, **69**, 150-164.

HUGHES, J.H. Attitude is keystone to success. *School Shop, 1978,* **37**, 76-80.

JOHNSON, D.W., & Johnson, R.T. Integrating handicapped students into the mainstream. *Exceptional Children,* 1980, **47**, 90-98.

MINISTÈRE de l'éducation: Gouvernement du Québec. *L'Ecole Québécoise.* Edité par le Service général des communications du ministère de l'éducation, 1979.

MINISTÈRE de l'éducation: Gouvernement du Québec. L'Education de l'enfance en difficulté d'adaptation et d'apprentissage au Québec. *Rapport COPEX.* Edité par le Service général des communications du ministère de l'éducation, 1976.

MITCHELL, M.M. Teacher attitudes. *The High School Journal,* 1976, **59**, 302-311.

POLONSKY, D. Belief and opinions concerning mental deficiency. *American Journal of Mental Deficiency,* 1961, **66**, 12-17.

RICHARDSON, S.A. *Reactions to the handicapped: A review of theory and research.* Proceedings of the special study institute: Fostering positive attitude toward the handicapped in school setting. Erick Reports, 115068-I, May 1975.

ROSENTHAL, R., & Jacobson, L. *Pygmalion in the classroom: Teacher expectation and pupils' intellectual development.* New York: Holt, Rinehart, and Winston, 1968.

SEGAL, S.P. Attitudes toward the mentally ill: A review. *Social Work,* May 1978.

SPREEN, O. Attitudes toward mental retardation and attitude change: An experimental study. *Zeitschrift fur Experimentelle.* und angewandte Psychologi Band xxiv. Heft: 1977, **2**, 303-323.

STAATS, A.W. Social behaviorism and human motivation: Principles of the attitude-reinforcer-discrimination system. In A.G. Greenwald, T.C. Brock, & T.M. Ostom (Eds.), *Psychological foundations of attitudes.* New York: Academic Press, 1968.

STAATS, A.W. Social behaviorism, human motivation and the conditioning therapies. In B.A. Maher (Ed.), *Progress in experimental personality research.* New York: Academic Press, 1970.

STAATS, A.W. *Social behaviorism.* Homewood, IL: Dorsey Press, 1975.

STEPHENS, T.M., & Braun, B.L. Measures of regular classroom teachers: Attitudes toward handicapped children. *Exceptional Children,* 1980, **46**, 292-294.

WONG, N., & Perkins, S.A. *Attitude toward the mentally retarded: A review of the selected literature.* Conférence présentée au: Wórld Congress on Future Special Education, Scotland, 1978.

WRIGHT, B.A. Changes in attitudes toward people with handicaps. *Rehabilitation Literature*, 1973, **34**, 354-357.

YUKER, H.E., Block, J.R., & Younng, J.R. *The measurement of attitudes toward disabled persons.* Alberton, NY: Human Resources Center, Erick Reports EC030615 et ED044853, 1970.

Stress Cardiaque Produit par Deux Activités Physiques Chez des Personnes Agées

Clermont P. Simard, Jean Jobin, Julien Vallières
Henri Bessette, Renée Caron, et Martine Dupuis
Université Laval

Le coût énergétique et le stress cardiaque associés au patinage libre et comparé à la marche ont été mesurés afin de voir si les réponses à ces activités étaient semblables chez les adultes et les personnes âgées. Dix-huit sujets masculins, 10 de 22.8 ± 2.3 ans et 8 de 62.4 ± 4.7 ans furent choisis. Les personnes âgées devaient, avec une fréquence cardiaque à 60-65% de leur maximale, effectuer deux kilomètres en 10 minutes. Sur la glace, les sujets patinèrent 8.6 tours à 35 secondes au tour, avant de commencer à prendre les mesures. En laboratoire, les sujets marchaient sur un tapis roulant à 3 milles à l'heure avec une pente de 6% pendant 5 minutes. Les prélèvements duraient 5 minutes. En utilisant le même $\dot{V}O_2$ sur la glace et sur le tapis roulant, 1.61 L/min, l'index de tension cardiaque chez les personnes âgées est semblable dans les deux cas. Toutefois, on remarque que dans leur travail les personnes âgées sont moins économiques que les adultes. Cette différence est de 11% sur la glace et de 21% sur le tapis roulant.

Energy cost and cardiac stress associated with ice skating and walking were measured in young adults and elderly men. For this study, 18 subjects, 10 young (22.8 ± 2.3 years) and 8 old (62.4 ± 4.7 years) volunteered. The elderly individuals had to be able to cover 2 km in 10 min at 60-65% of their age-predicted maximal heart rate. On the ice, subjects skated 8.6 times around the rink at 35 seconds per circuit before any physiological measurement was taken. In the laboratory, subjects walked on a treadmill at 3 mph at a 6% incline for 5 min. Measurements were taken over the following 5 minutes in both situations. Working at the same $\dot{V}O_2$, 1.61 L/min, on ice as well as on the treadmill, the elderly men had the same TTI. Elderly subjects, however, appeared to be less efficient than the younger ones. This difference was 11% on the ice and 21% on the treadmill.

Les diverses activités physiques pratiquées, même quand elles présentent un niveau de dépense énergétique similaire, ne provoquent pas nécessairement le même stress pour le myocarde. Certains auteurs (Adams & DeVries, 1973; Astrand, 1960; DeVries & Adams, 1977; Limb & McNicol, 1967) démontrèrent que le stress cardiaque était plus élevé lors d'un travail avec les bras par rapport à un travail avec les jambes de même que lorsque les bras étaient au dessus des épaules par rapport à devant soi (Freyschuss & Strandell, 1968); de plus, le travail du myocarde est plus grand lors d'un exercice sur bicyclette ergométrique comparativement à un exercice sur tapis roulant. La marche, qui implique un mouvement rythmé des membres inférieurs et peu de travail musculaire statique, semble être l'activité qui minimise le plus l'effort cardiaque pour une même dépense énergétique (DeVries & Adams, 1977; Freyschuss & Standell, 1968; Kemp & Ellestad, 1969).

Les réactions cardio-vasculaires sont aussi affectées par l'âge et un même niveau de dépense énergétique entraîne un plus grand stress cardiaque au fur et à mesure que la personne avance en âge (Amsterdam, Price, Beman, Hughes, Riggs, DeMaria, Miller, & Mason, 1977; DeVries, 1970; Niinimaa & Shephard, 1978[b]).

Cette dernière caractéristique de l'adaptation cardio-vasculaire à l'effort est importante à considérer dans le choix des activités physiques pour les citoyens âgés (Sidney & Shephard, 1978; Schneidman, 1972). Dans cette étude, nous avons voulu évaluer le stress cardiaque imposé par le patinage sur glace pour les personnes âgées par rapport à celui créé par la marche à une même dépense énergétique. De plus, nous avons voulu comparer la pratique de ces activités pour des individus d'âges différents. L'indice de tension cardiaque (ITC: TASXFC) étant hautement corrélé avec la consommation d'oxygène du myocarde (Feinberg, Katz, & Boyd, 1962; Katz & Feinberg, 1958; Niinimaa & Shephard, 1978(a); Sarnoff, Brunwald, Welch, Case, Stainsby, & Macruz, 1958), nous avons choisi cette variable pour estimer le stress imposé au coeur.

Méthodologie

Chacun des sujets signa une lettre de consentement et par la suite, ils furent soumis à un examen médical, à un ECG 12 dérivations et à un test d'effort progressif sur bicyclette, ECG en CM5, avant de prendre part à l'étude.

Les 18 sujets masculins, 10 dont l'âge moyen était de 22.8 ans et 8 dont l'âge moyen était de 62.4, furent choisis parmi des étudiants en éducation physique et des personnes âgées. Ces derniers furent sélectionnés pour leur habileté à patiner à l'intensité désirée parmi un groupe de 25 personnes âgées impliquées dans un programme de conditionnement physique par le patinage sur glace.

Tous les 18 sujets avaient été soumis aux procédures expérimentales une fois avant le prélèvement de données. La première activité physique consistait à patiner pendant 5 minutes, 8.6 tours de patinoire à 35 secondes au tour avec l'équipement de mesure sur le dos, mais sans que les mesures soient prises. Pendant les 5 minutes suivantes, toujours à la même vitesse, on mesurait la ventilation, le $\dot{V}O_2$ et la fréquence cardiaque.

En laboratoire, les sujets furent soumis à une marche de 3 mph à une pente de 6% sur un tapis roulant. Comme sur la glace, les sujets marchaient pendant 5 minutes avant que les mesures soient prises pendant les 5 minutes suivantes. Cette vitesse et cette pente ont été choisies parce qu'elles entraînaient une dépense énergétique similaire à celle du patinage sur glace à une vitesse moyenne de 5 minutes au kilomètre (12 km/hre) chez les personnes âgées de l'étude. Cette vitesse de patinage correspondait à environ 60 à 65% de la fréquence cardiaque de réserve maximale des personnes âgées (Sheffield, Ratman, & Reeves, 1968).

La fréquence cardiaque était mesurée à partir d'un ECG en dérivation CM5 transmis par télémétrie tout au long de l'exercice. L'ECG était enregistré pendant 6 secondes à chacun des tours de la patinoire et à la fin de chaque minute sur le tapis roulant.

La tension artérielle était mesurée immédiatement après l'arrêt de l'exercice par auscultation à l'aide d'une colonne de mercure. Elle était prise en position debout. Le délai entre l'arrêt de l'exercice et l'audition du premier bruit de Korotkov ne dépassait pas 13 secondes. Le stéthoscope était fixé au bras du sujet sous le brassard tout au long de l'exercice. Toutes les tensions artérielles furent mesurées par la même personne.

La ventilation et un échantillon de l'air expiré était prélevé à l'aide du respiromètre de Kofranyi-Michaelis. La ventilation était mesurée sur 5 minutes. 5% de l'air expiré était collecté à chaque expiration dans un sac à anesthésie de 5 litres. Un échantillon de celui-ci était placé dans une colonne d'échantillonnage jusqu'à l'analyse des F_eO_2 et F_eCO_2 par la méthode de Scholander (Shephard, 1977).

L'indice de tension cardiaque (ITC) était calculé par le produit de la tension artérielle systolique et la fréquence cardiaque à l'arrêt de l'exercice. Chez tous les sujets, les 5 minutes de travail avant les mesures étaient amplement suffisantes pour atteindre un état physiologique stable tel qu'il fut évalué par la fréquence cardiaque.

Les différences entre groupes et entre les activités furent vérifiées à l'aide du test T de Student.

Résultat

Le Tableau 1 présente les caractéristiques des deux groupes. Le groupe jeune a une moyenne d'âge de 22.8 années comparativement à 62.4 années pour le groupe âgé.

Le $\dot{V}O_2$ en litre par minute, la fréquence cardiaque, la tension artérielle systolique et l'indice de tension cardiaque pour les deux activités physiques chez les hommes âgés et les hommes jeunes sont présentés dans les Tableaux 2 et 3.

Les paramètres mesurés sur la glace pour les deux groupes ne montrent pas de différence significative. L'index de tension cardiaque est de 18.24 chez les hommes jeunes comparativement à 17.88 pour les hommes âgés.

Le travail sur le tapis roulant entraîne cependant pour les personnes âgées, une dépense énergétique plus élevée, 1.61 L/min. comparativement à 1.33 L/min. chez les personnes jeunes ($p < 0.01$). De plus, la tension artérielle systolique est aussi plus élevée chez les personnes âgées lors du travail sur le tapis roulant, 156 mm/Hg comparativement à 135 mm/Hg chez les personnes jeunes ($p < 0.05$).

L'indice de tension cardiaque est de 17.88 sur la patinoire comparativement à 18.61 sur le tapis roulant pour les personnes âgées. Chez les jeunes, l'indice de tension cardiaque passe de 15.87 sur le tapis roulant à 18.24 sur la patinoire ($p < 0.05$).

La marche sur tapis roulant provoque un stress cardiaque plus élevé chez les personnes âgées comparativement au groupe jeune ($p < 0.05$).

Discussion

L'indice de tension cardiaque pour le myocarde révèle que le stress, lors de la marche, est de 18.61 comparativement à 17.88 lors du patinage. Ces

Tableau 1
Caractéristiques Physiques des 18 Sujets

	n	Age (ans)	Poids (kg)
Hommes âgés	8	52.4 ($\pm$ 1.9)[a]	75.0 ($\pm$ 2.3)
Hommes jeunes	10	22.8 ($\pm$ 0.8)	70.5 ($\pm$ 2.1)

[a]Écart-type.

Tableau 2
Stress Cardiaque Lors d'une Marche sur Tapis Roulant et en Patinage sur Glace Chez les Hommes Âgés

Activités	$\dot{V}O_2$[a] L/min	$\dot{V}O_2$ mL/kg/min	FC batt/min	TAS mm/Hg	$\frac{ITC}{TAS \times FC}$ 1000
Patinage $\bar{X}$	1.61 (± 0.2)	21.5 (± 2.8)	110 (± 7.0)	161 (± 9.7)	17.88 (± 1.6)
Marche $\bar{X}$	1.61[b] (± 0.06)	21.5 (± 0.6)	119 (± 3.8)	156[b] (± 6.62)	18.61[c] (± 1.1)

[a] STPD.
[b] ($p < 0.05$) entre groupes.
[c] ($p < 0.01$) entre groupes.
± = Erreur standard.

Tableau 3
Stress Cardiaque Lors d'une Marche sur Tapis Roulant et en Patinage sur Glace Chez les Hommes Jeunes

Activités	$\dot{V}O_2$* L/min	$\dot{V}O_2$ mL/kg/min	FC batt/min	TAS mm/Hg	ITC $\frac{TAS \times FC}{1000}$
Patinage $\bar{X}$	1.45 (± 0.05)	20.6 (± 0.6)	120 (± 3.4)	152[a] (± 4.2)	18.24[b] (± 0.6)
Marche $\bar{X}$	1.33[c] (± 0.06)	18.5 (± 0.6)	117 (± 3.7)	135[a,c] (± 3.0)	15.87[b,d] (± 0.4)

*STPD.
[a]($p < 0.01$) entre activités.
[b]($p < 0.05$) entre activités.
[c]($p < 0.01$) entre groupes.
[d]($p < 0.05$) entre groupes.
± = Erreur standard.

données indiquent que pour une même dépense énergétique, le stress cardiaque est identique dans les deux activités. Les études de DeVries (1977) dans ce domaine, montrent des courbes de régression différentes entre les indices de tension cardiaque et la consommation d'oxygène pour les activités comme la marche, la bicyclette ergométrique et l'action de ramper. A une intensité très faible de travail, autour de 0.5 L/min. d'oxygène, la bicyclette ergométrique est moins stressante pour le coeur que la marche. Si l'intensité est à 1.6 L/min. d'oxygène, la marche et la bicyclette ergométrique exigent le même stress cardiaque alors que l'action de ramper produit un indice de tension plus élevé.

Lors de notre étude, nous avons utilisé cette même intensité de travail et nous pouvons voir que le patinage provoque un même indice de tension cardiaque que la marche sur tapis roulant pour les personnes âgées. Les données de divers auteurs (Adams & DeVries, 1973; Barry, Doly, Pruett, Steinmetz, Page, Birkhead, & Rodahl, 1956; Astrand, 1960) vont dans le même sens que nous, à savoir qu'il est avantageux d'utiliser les gros groupes musculaires et d'effectuer un travail dynamique et rythmique.

Toutefois, le stress cardiaque imposé par le patinage sur glace fut plus grand que celui de la marche sur tapis roulant à une même consommation d'oxygène sur tapis roulant pour les jeunes adultes. De plus, cette consommation d'oxygène sur tapis roulant pour jeunes adultes était inférieure à celle des personnes âgées. L'indice de tension cardiaque pour la marche sur le tapis roulant entre les jeunes adultes et les personnes âgées allait aussi dans ce sens. Cela peut s'expliquer par le fait que le premier groupe travaille d'une façon plus économique que le second groupe. DeVries (1977) a rapporté des données semblables entre les jeunes adultes et les personnes âgées lors d'un travail sur bicyclette ergométrique. Cette différence au niveau de l'indice de tension cardiaque s'accroît lors de l'augmentation de l'intensité de l'exercice.

Il est cependant intéressant de noter que si l'indice de tension cardiaque est exprimé par unité d'oxygène consommé (L/min.), il est de 10.26 et 10.31 pour la marche et le patinage respectivement. Une meilleure efficacité mécanique à la marche serait donc aussi une autre cause du plus bas stress comparé au patinage sur glace pour les jeunes adultes. De même, la différence dans l'indice du stress cardiaque disparaît entre les jeunes adultes et les gens âgés lorsqu'il est exprimé par unité de consommation d'oxygène, 10.30 et 10.15 respectivement. Ces chiffres sont sensiblement proches des données rapportées antérieurement.

La différence de l'indice de tension cardiaque entre les deux groupes de sujets lors de la marche est sans doute dans une bonne mesure due à un $\dot{V}O_2$ plus bas chez les jeunes. Le stress total étant plus bas, le stress cardiaque a aussi été diminué. L'indice de tension cardiaque des jeunes adultes à un $\dot{V}O_2$ de 1.3 L/min. sur bicyclette fut d'environ 17 dans l'étude de DeVries (1977), une valeur identique à celle obtenue dans la présente étude pour la marche sur tapis roulant.

La différence de l'indice de tension cardiaque chez les jeunes adultes peut être attribuée surtout à une différence au niveau de la résistance périphérique, les tensions artérielles systoliques étant respectivement de 152 et 135 pour des fréquences cardiaques semblables.

L'estimation du travail cardiaque durant différentes activités physiques est très importante pour les personnes âgées parce que nous voulons travailler à un seuil minimal d'intensité pour obtenir des effets bénéfiques lors de notre travail et protéger le myocarde contre une défaillance possible (Kramer, Paulin, & Werkö, 1966; Schwade, Blomqvist, & Shapiro, 1977). Nous savons que la consommation d'oxygène est associée au travail cardiaque (Feinberg, Katz, & Boyd, 1962; Niinimaa & Shephard, 1978[a]; Shephard, 1977) et qu'il peut y avoir une relation entre les attaques d'angine et le travail cardiaque. Il est certain qu'aujourd'hui, plusieurs chercheurs travaillent sur l'influence de l'exercice en fonction de la prévention et du traitement des ischémies du myocarde (Benestad, 1965; Hellerstein, 1968; Robinson, 1967; Stamford, 1972, 1973; Wehren & Rygdeman, 1971).

Nos données permettent de dire que le patinage libre ne représente pas un stress cardiaque plus élevé que la marche pour les personnes âgées qui savent patiner et que nous pouvons recommander cette activité.

Ces résultats obtenus sont très intéressants pour nous où les activités d'hiver peuvent être pratiquées douze mois par année et où les personnes ont une tendance à diminuer leurs activités de plein air, suite à un climat souvent humide et froid. De plus, notre clientèle âgée a acquis, lors de son jeune âge, les apprentissages nécessaires pour contrôler convenablement cette activité. Elle peut alors patiner à une intensité assez élevée pour en obtenir les effets bénéfiques et en même temps, elle possède les techniques nécessaires pour se protéger contre les chutes. Toutefois, les écarts existants entre les individus sont très grands et on se doit de pratiquer cette activité avec un niveau d'intensité tolérable pour la personne. Il est aussi nécessaire de respecter certaines mesures de sécurité qui peuvent s'énumérer comme suit:

1. Utiliser un casque protecteur, des coudes et des genouillères pour ceux qui craignent une chute.
2. Assister les personnes qui veulent recommencer cette activité et leur fournir les conseils appropriés.
3. S'habiller en fonction d'un milieu plus froid et plus humide qui peut provoquer des problèmes de thermo-régulation.
4. Ajouter d'autres éléments au patinage comme de la musique, des jeux et des activités rythmées, seul ou avec un partenaire, tout en

faisant attention aux chutes ou au contact avec la bande ou une autre personne.

Une autre étape à franchir au niveau de ces études sera de savoir si nous pouvons pratiquer ces activités en augmentant la qualité de notre travail et en s'exerçant d'une façon plus économique à différentes intensités. Différents auteurs (Barry et al., 1956; Benestad, 1965; Shneidman, 1972; Sidney & Shephard, 1978; Stamford, 1972) observèrent avec l'entraînement, une fréquence cardiaque plus basse à un certain niveau de travail et d'autres personnes observèrent en parallèle un pouls d'oxygène plus élevé (Adams & DeVries, 1973; DeVries, 1970). Toutefois, DeVries (1977), Niinimaa (1978) n'observèrent pas d'amélioration de l'indice de tension cardiaque. D'autres études avec Stamford (1973), DeVries (1977) trouvèrent que l'entraînement provoque une diminution de la pression systolique et aucun changement de la pression diastolique.

Il est possible de croire que les prochaines études sur le patinage libre nous permettront, suite à un programme d'entraînement, de diminuer la tension artérielle systolique à une même intensité de travail.

Nous terminons en signalant qu'une approche plus scientifique pour offrir des programmes d'activité physique à une clientèle âgée permettra à la fois d'améliorer les effets positifs et de diminuer les possibilités d'une complication.

Références

ADAMS, G.M., & DeVries, H.A. Physiological effects of an exercise training regimen upon women aged 52-79. *Journal of Gerontology,* 1978, **28**, 50-55.

AMSTERDAM, E.A., Price, J.E., Beman, D., Hughes, J.L., Riggs, K., DeMaria, A.N., Miller, R.R., & Mason, D.T. Exercise testing in the indirect assessment of myocardial oxygen consumption. In E.A. Amsterdam, J.H. Wilmore, & A.N. DeMaria (Eds.), *Exercise in cardiovascular health and disease.* New York: York Medical Books, 1977.

ASTRAND, I. Aerobic work capacity in men and women with special reference to age. *Acta Physiologica Scandinavia,* 1960, **49**, suppl. 169.

BARRY, A.J., Doly, J.W., Pruett, E.D.R., Steinmetz, J.R., Page, H.F., Birkhead, N.C., & Rodahl, K. The effects of physical conditioning on older individuals. *Journal of Gerontology,* 1956, **21**, 182-191.

BENESTAD, A.M. Trainability of old men. *Acta Medica Scandinavia,* 1965, **178**, 321-327.

DEVRIES, H.A. Physiological effects of an exercise training regimen upon men aged 52 to 88. *Journal of Gerontology,* 1970, **25**, 325-336.

DEVRIES, H.A., & Adams, G.M. Effects of the type of exercise upon the work of the heart in older men. *Journal of Sports Medicine and Physical Fitness,* 1977, **17**, 41-47.

FEINBERG, H., Katz, L.N., & Boyd, E. Determinants of coronary flow and myocardial oxygen consumption. *American Journal of Physiology,* 1962, **202**, 45-52.

FREYSCHUSS, U., & Strandell, T. Circulatory adaptation to one and two legs exercise in supine position. *Journal of Applied Physiology,* 1968, **25**, 511-515.

HELLERSTEIN, H.K. Exercise therapy in coronary disease. *Bulletin of the New York Academy of Medicine,* 1968, **44**, 1028-1047.

KATZ, L.N., & Feinberg, H. The relation of cardiac effort to myocardial oxygen consumption and coronary flow. *Clinical Research,* 1958, **6**, 656-669.

KEMP, G.L., & Ellestad, M.H. The maximal treadmill stress test for the evaluation of medical and surgical treatment of coronary insufficiency. *Journal of Thoracic and Cardiovascular Surgery,* 1969, **57**, 708-713.

KRAMER, J., Paulin, S., & Werkö, L. Coronary angiographic findings in correlation with age, body weight, blood pressure, serum lipids and smoking habits. *Circulation,* 1966, **33**, 888-900.

LIMB, A.R., & McNicol, G.W. Circulatory responses to sustained handgrip contractions performed during other exercise, both rhythmic and static. *Journal of Physiology,* 1967, **192**, 595-607.

NIINIMAA, V., & Shephard, R.J. Training and oxygen conductance in the elderly. I. The respiratory system. *Journal of Gerontology,* 1978(a), **33**, 354-361.

NIINIMAA, V., & Shephard, R.J. Training and oxygen conductance in the elderly. II. The cardiovascular system. *Journal of Gerontology,* 1978(b), **33**, 362-367.

ROBINSON, B.F. Relation of heart rate and systolic blood pressure to the onset of pain in angina pectoris. *Circulation,* 1967, **35**, 1073-1083.

SARNOFF, S.J., Brunwald, E., Welch, G.H., Case, R.B., Stainsby, W.N., & Macruz, R. Hemodynamic determinants of oxygen consumption of the heart with special reference to tension-time index. *American Journal of Physiology,* 1958, **192**, 148-156.

SCHWADE, J., Blomqvist, C.G., & Shapiro, W. A comparison of the response to arm and leg work in patients with ischemic heart disease. *American Heart Journal,* 1977, **94**, 203.

SHEFFIELD, L.T., Ratman, D., & Reeves, F.J. Hemodynamic consequences of physical training after myocardial infarction. *Circulation,* 1968, **37**, 192-202.

SHERPHARD, R.J. *Endurance fitness.* Toronto: University of Toronto Press, 1977.

SHNEIDMAN, N.N. Soviet studies in the fitness of the aged. *Canadian Journal of Female Physical Activity,* 1972.

SIDNEY, K.H., & Shephard, R.J. Frequency and intensity of exercise training for elderly subjects. *Medicine and Science in Sports,* 1978, **10,** 125-131.

STAMFORD, B.A. Physiological effects of training upon institutionalized geriatric men. *Journal of Gerontology,* 1972, **27,** 451-455.

STAMFORD, B.A. Effects of chronic institutionalization of the physical working capacity and trainability of geriatric men. *Journal of Gerontology,* 1973, **28,** 441-446.

WEHREN, J., & Bygdeman, S. Onset of angina pectoris in relation to circulatory adaptation during arm and leg exercise. *Circulation,* 1971, **44,** 432-441.

SECTION 7:
Summary Papers

The IIIrd International Symposium on Adapted Physical Activities was a catalyst for the dissemination of over 100 pedagogical and research papers. It was reported that the New Orleans Symposium produced the most comprehensive set of papers ever presented at a single conference on adapted physical activity. As adapted physical activity leaders, however, we must ask ourselves some penetrating questions: As an emerging subdiscipline, do we now have a comprehensive body of knowledge? Does our literature give direction and focus for meeting the physical activity needs of special populations? Are learning and performance theories relating to the handicapped being generated so that scholars can begin scientific inquiry? Are we sharing our information with leaders from other countries and from related disciplines? Are we synthesizing this information into a vital format for rapid and efficient dissemination?

With these and other questions in mind, we asked Lawrence Rarick and Geoffrey Broadhead, two proven theorists and scholars, to summarize the papers presented at the Symposium. Did they come to praise or to bury?

Summary of Pedagogy Sessions

G. Lawrence Rarick
University of California, Berkeley

The papers in the pedagogy sessions covered a variety of topics which, for convenience, can be sorted into those dealing with adapted physical education and those concerned with recreation and leisure for the handicapped. Some of the papers in both areas described model programs, others dealt with program developments including procedures for facilitating integration, whereas some described procedures for improving delivery services. The sections that follow provide highlights of the papers, providing a summary of the thoughts presented without reference to specific papers.

Adapted Physical Education

Curricular Adaptations

The need to adapt the program of activities for meeting the developmental, psychological, emotional, and motor capabilities of the handicapped individual was stressed universally. This can be accomplished only if those responsible for the conduct of adapted physical education programs are fully knowledgeable about the characteristics and needs of the handicapped and are equipped to put this knowledge to use in designing and conducting physical activity programs of an appropriate nature. This means that continued emphasis must be placed on preparing teachers with the competence needed to achieve this end.

Several of the papers described the unique features of the programs that were currently underway. Although authors differed in particulars, there was general agreement in the sense that all stressed the need for (1) early identification of the disabled child, (2) assessment of each child's capabilities, (3) individualization of instruction, (4) regular and frequent evaluation of progress, (5) integration where appropriate, and (6) support of the school administration, teachers, community, and parents.

The following were some of the more specific ideas expressed in the various papers that have implications in curriculum planning:

- Importance of considering the developmental level of each participant, sequential progression of activities, maximal participation, and a safe and secure learning environment.

- Need for establishing both long- and short-term goals and the maintenance of cumulative records on each child, including neurological, motor, and psychological test scores, and the dynamics of personal and group relationships.

- Making certain that the program is an integral part of the total education program.

- Recognition that many internal factors and environmental forces may be operating to elicit motor development delays.

- Understanding of the value and limitations of norm-based and criterion-referenced tests.

- Appreciation of the significance of the affective domain in program planning and implementation.

- Recognition that although integration (mainstreaming) may be beneficial for some, this procedure is inappropriate for many handicapped children.

- Appreciation of the wide range of motor experience that should be made available to the handicapped and that the development of a range of motor skills is as important for them as for their normal peers.

- Recognition of the worth of the humanistic approach in physical education, particularly for the socially sensitive handicapped child who is placed in a mainstreamed instructional setting.

- Understanding that complex motor patterns represent "an unfolding of a sequence of body postures" which can be incorporated into instructional units in a program of "developmental gymnastics."
- Recognition of the failure syndrome in many handicapped children; countering this by avoiding student selection of teams, elimination games, and posting of best scores.

Teacher Preparation and Development of Effective Delivery Services

Many papers stressed the need for improved delivery services in adapted physical education. It is apparent that most teacher training institutions give only limited attention to preparing adapted physical education teachers. Likewise, in-service training programs in terms of the numbers of physical education teachers served and the quality of such programs as reflected by improved services to the handicapped have met with only limited success. To improve the situation the papers emphasized the following:

- Initiation of competency-based requirements.
- Clear definition of what competencies are needed for the specialist in adapted physical education and for the generalist who will be working with the handicapped in an integrated setting.
- The need for state certification requirements for the adapted physical education teacher.
- Recognition that an appropriate delivery system should include the capability of providing prescriptive and/or developmental instruction, counseling, coordination of related services, assessment, and individualized educational programming.
- Development and use of instructional modules to influence favorably the attitudes, knowledge, and teaching competencies of the specialist and the generalist responsible for adapted and integrated physical education programs.
- Where appropriate, offer occupational therapy services to children with sensory limitations, those who exhibit gravitational insecurity, motor planning problems, tactile defensiveness, and a poor body precept.

Recreation and Leisure

The recent past has witnessed many changes in recreation programs and leisure time activities for handicapped individuals. Many forces have been operating in expanding recreational opportunities for this segment of the population, such as the growth of the welfare state, the interest of the medical profession and educational agencies in recreation, and the federal mandate as specified in PL 94-142. The directions that recreation programs for the handicapped are now taking is indicated by the following summarized examples taken from the papers presented here:

- Reasonable skill proficiency is important for satisfying recreation pursuits. Whereas a wide range of skills many be beneficial to the normal individual, skill mastery for the handicapped should be restricted to a small number of skills — those that are within the limitations of the individual and those that can be used in the immediate environment.

- Recreational services for certain special populations may effectively employ an intervention strategy. Such an approach with autistic children, for example, would focus on skill development using the task analysis method coupled with the use of equipment which would provide self-correcting feedback, thus providing the basis for self-stimulating behaviors under socially acceptable conditions.

- Use of neuro-linguistic programming in leisure counseling is a promising development for studying the structure of human experience, particularly useful in organizing recreation and leisure behaviors with handicapped populations of all ages and cultures, because it is content-free and relies on universal internalized responses.

- The need for the development of recreational centers for those with severe disabilities who are not currently served by community recreation centers was stressed. The Recreation Center for the Handicapped in San Francisco, operating over the past 29 years, has served over 10,000 severely handicapped persons of all ages. It currently enrolls 1,600 individuals in six programs: (1) children's, (2) day care, (3) adult's, (4) aquatics, (5) physical education, and (6) outreach. As the director says, the program has dispelled many myths about the disabled and "has demonstrated that programming for them is limited only by the imagination and conviction of the recreation providers."

Research Directions in Adapted Physical Activity

Geoffrey D. Broadhead
Louisiana State University

Beginning this presentation with an apology is not how I first anticipated the occasion. But I believe I need to change the title which appears on the Program as "Summary of Research Presentations," because that is an impossible task. We have had more than 100 formal presentations at this Symposium, more than half of which have dealt with research; indeed, this has been a feast we've all enjoyed. But you can imagine the predicament of someone faced with the task of listening to and evaluating almost 60 papers, many of which were scheduled simultaneously. Hence, I need to change the orientation of this paper somewhat.

    I am quite sure that no one here has managed yet to grasp the full significance of all the research which has been described, but I do not doubt that in the future some fruitful developments will have been sparked by what was presented this week. Therefore, I will entitle my talk "Research Directions in Adapted Physical Activity," and I promise to include a discussion of the papers themselves. Upon realizing I could

---

    Requests for reprints should be sent to Geoffrey D. Broadhead, School of Health, Physical Education, Recreation and Dance, Louisiana State University, Baton Rouge, LA 70803.

not listen to all the presentations, I opted to read the abstracts, which is not a very satisfactory research procedure, but what an experience that turned out to be! There were two kinds of abstracts: those which described the research concept, purposes, sample, procedures, analysis, results, and implications; and those which gave a more generalized commentary but promised that the study would eventually be completed and the results discussed! This left a lot for me to imagine, but I cannot fault the program committee for allowing such flexibility, for it has encouraged the completion of research which might not otherwise have been shared with us. We all need to be encouraged in our research endeavors; we need to be pressed not only to begin but also to continue to research so that we do not rely too much on our intuition.

At this time I should define what I mean by "research," especially because views differ and the research papers presented at this Symposium have been wide-ranging. I can sidestep the issue quite neatly, by quoting something the late Louis Armstrong used to say about jazz, which I feel can apply just as well to research: "If you have to ask what jazz is, you'll never know."

But it is critical for me to discuss just what we mean by the phrase "adapted physical activity" (APA), for I assume it means far more than mere activities which can be adjusted to suit the needs of individuals and heterogeneous groups. One way of finding out what APA means is to ask the rhetorical question of whether there has been something of real value for all of you here. In other words, it seems important to judge whether the Program actually reflected the involvement of those in APA. I shall return to this topic. I am not sure that I know what APA is meant to mean, but I can readily accept that it encompasses more than what I perceive to be the interests of the majority of conference participants, namely adapted physical education and therapeutic recreation. It includes education, therapy, and more, such as activities, settings, and interests which call to mind concepts like care, correction, development, learning, rehabilitation, and remediation. And perhaps it is a useful simulation exercise for each of us to try and recall individual presentations we attended to see if these words or concepts have any specific meaning in that research context.

Let me spend a few moments suggesting another way of looking at APA. It is useful, for example, to consider a small part of the factor analytic work of Rarick and his colleagues (1972, 1976, 1977). Working mostly with children in educational settings, and therefore being aware of any curriculum implications, he (Rarick) hypothesized that at least 12 components exist in sufficiently distinctive form that they can be measured with our currently available instrumentation. Table 1 shows the hypothesized structure, listing for each component a good example of items which indicate the type of motor ability that leads to the labeling of the component. Using the Harris and Harris (1971) factor analysis interpretation strategy, more than half the components were robust across different solutions, for boys and girls over a wide chronological age (CA) range, and for children of normal intelligence as well as those with mild and moderate intellectual and other impairments. A development of that work is the continuing project of Winnick (1979) which extends the range of persons for whom adaptations in motor activities can be conceived. That study involves persons who are less mobile, having orthopedic, sensory, and multihandicapping conditions.

Also of particular significance is the work of Harrow (1972) with her elaborate descriptive taxonomy of the psychomotor domain. This work could be called a companion volume to those by Bloom (1956) and by Krathwohl, Bloom, and Masia (1964) on the cognitive and affective domains, respectively. Table 2 provides a capsulated picture of the six-level classification of movement experiences. Time prevents a discussion of this work, but I would draw your attention to the last and first levels of the paradigm, for they appear to provide somewhat novel directions for many persons involved in APA. Involving our clients in research settings which emphasize expressive and interpretive movement using body postures, gestures, and facial expressions for symbolic or social dance choreographies seems important to me. Likewise, our interest in involuntary movements that are functional at birth and develop through maturation, becoming controlled early in life for most infants, but not at all in our most profoundly multihandicapped individuals, seems of obvious value.

Table 1
Hypothesized Factor Structure of Motor Abilities[a]

Static Muscular Strength	Manual Dexterity
grip right	ring stacking
Explosive Muscular Strength	Static Balance
broad jump	stabilometer
Muscular Strength-Endurance	Dynamic Balance
sit-ups	railwalk forward
Gross Body Coordination	Flexibility
scramble	toe touch
Cardio-Respiratory Endurance	Body Fat
physical work capacity	triceps skinfold
Limb-Eye Coordination	Body Size
pursuit motor	weight

[a]From Rarick, G.L., Dobbins, D.A., & Broadhead, G.D. *The motor domain and its correlates in educationally handicapped children,* Englewood Cliffs, NJ: Prentice-Hall, 1976.

Table 2
Psychomotor Taxonomy[a]

Reflex Movements
    segmented, intersegmental, supersegmented
Basic Fundamental Movements
    locomotor, nonlocomotor, manipulative
Perceptual Abilities
    kinesthetic, visual, auditory, tactile, coordinated
Physical Abilities
    endurance, strength, flexibility, agility
Skilled Movements
    simple, compound, complex adaptive skills
Nondiscursive Communication
    expressive, interpretive movement

[a]From Harrow, A.J. *A taxonomy of the psychomotor domain.* New York: David McKay, 1972, 96-98.

Perhaps I could add to this description of the nature and scope of APA, mention of the work of Peter (1965), who suggested a model for converting medical, psychological, and social-work diagnoses into intervention strategies. And if, to his pattern of problem, situational, and institution variables, are added an extended CA range of persons to be studied, and a variety of ecological variables, the picture becomes more complete. Thus, APA is a multidimensional area of concern, capable of multidirections for research, some directions perhaps more urgent than others. Are there priorities which could guide us in our research efforts? And does the research presented at this Symposium match up to those priorities? I hope you will agree with my view that the answer to each question is "yes."

Most of you are well aware of the recent zeit geist in this country (US Congress, 1964, 1975; US Department of Health, Education, & Welfare, 1977a, 1977b) and in the United Kingdom (Warnock, 1978) which has sought to end discrimination based on race, sex, or degree of atypical behavior. Access to facilities and to programs is the right of all. Thus, even a superficial examination of the Education for All Handicapped Children Act—PL 94-142 (US Congress, 1975) and its regulations (US Department of Health, Education, & Welfare, 1977b)—reveals distinct research priorities. Assessment concerns, the use and abuse of required documentation, parental involvement, and the necessity to find and serve those in need are but a few such examples.

Similarly, it is possible to cite other preferred research directions, such as those emanating from the 1979 Conference of the National Consortium on Physical Education and Recreation for the Handicapped (Taylor, Compton, & Johnson, 1981) held in Rochester, NY, just prior to the last International Summer Special Olympics. At that meeting a group of us, using the "Nominal Group Techniques" espoused by Delbecq and Van de Ven (1975), articulated some research priorities in physical education. It is appropriate for me to interpret these nine priorities in the wider context of all the research interests represented at this Symposium.

The Place of Physical Education in State Special Education Plans

At the Rochester conference, considerable anxiety was voiced regarding what at that time appeared to be a gross disparity in the treatment which our area of interest had received among state Special Education plans. Some states were leading at a fast pace, while others had barely begun to see the importance of providing appropriate physical education and related services to the handicapped (Kennedy Foundation, 1979). I am sure it is still important to research this issue and to press for a wider and more thorough compliance with PL 94-142 regulations (US Department of Health, Education, & Welfare, 1977b), even if problems with funding are anticipated. The sound practices involved are those of seeking, finding, evaluating, and serving all handicapped children, which transcend the existence of a law and any accompanying monies. But to have the full service requirement "on the books" provides a chance for services to be established. This is part of what we call the "trickle-down" theory. No one dealt with this research priority at the Symposium.

Home Influences on Motor Development

The discussion group acknowledged the strong association reported in the literature (Craft, 1970; Hollingshead, 1957; Stein & Susser, 1963; Wiseman, 1964) between home and family characteristics and school achievement. With forces as potent as those, it seemed important to press for greater home support as supplementing but not supplanting the work of the school or agency. Particularly critical periods for such support could be in the early childhood years, during adolescence, and during a person's postschool/agency years, though no time period lacks significance.

We believe the motor development and skills acquisition of our clients can be enhanced by such home involvement, and research in this area is strongly warranted. At this Symposium, only two studies were presented on this topic. One involved gaining parental assistance in persuading handicapped persons to use community facilities more than previously. The other study stressed the need to create parental awareness and support for whatever school or community programs existed, in order to bring about improved motivation in the child. Both studies provided insight into this issue.

Early Intervention Programming

This topic is closely related to the one previously described and provides opportunities for professionals to work in inter- and multidisciplinary settings. What is a real challenge to such professionals is also a real challenge to researchers. Because a child's early years are so important in eliciting appropriate social and intellectual development, as well as establishing control of reflexes and basic movement patterns/skills, research implications seem clear. And yet the literature on early intervention programming (Bloom, Davis, & Hess, 1965; Hunt, 1969; Smith & Bissel, 1970; Stanley, 1973; and Yinger, Ikeda, Laycock, & Cutter, 1977) is difficult to interpret, for so many design problems are reported. At this meeting, only a handful of papers was presented on this topic, and I hope that some of you were sufficiently intrigued that you become interested in researching the area yourselves. It seems rather glib to stress the importance of prevention by way of early intervention strategies, but a sizable number of our very young children are in a variety of at-risk situations; some of their problems can be diagnosed with our current methods, but they will all need our attention eventually.

Mainstreaming

None of you will be surprised by the inclusion of this topic in a list of priorities for research. It would probably have been more accurate for the discussion group to have used the phrase "least restrictive environment" as the main focus of attention was on specific educational settings (US Congress, 1975; US Department of Health, Education, & Welfare, 1977b). But bearing in mind the wide interests represented in this audience, the notion of any handicapped or disabled person fitting into the mainstream of a number of peer or community groups is useful to consider. Of particular concern to the Rochester group were the often forgotten effects or influences of a mainstreaming procedure on the nonhandicapped; their rights should be safeguarded, too.

None of the problems associated with research on this topic are easily overcome, but because such a large proportion of our clients are candidates for mainstreaming, it is a priority which cannot be overlooked. Sadly, I did not read of a single research paper which dealt in detail with mainstreaming, integration, or least restrictive environments. There were, however, oblique references to two small studies in Louisiana (Broadhead, 1981, 1982), plus the recently published work of Beuter (1981), and Rarick, McQuillan, and Beuter (1981) in California. I encourage you to research this area of concern, even if it poses many complex issues.

Physiological Parameters

An increasing awareness of the beneficial role of prescribed exercise for ameliorating a wide range of problems in humans made this research priority an obvious choice. At the research portion of this Symposium the studies on this topic focused on program effectiveness, which I shall discuss later. Measures described include percentage body fat, maximal oxygen uptake, and cardiac measures. Thus, in using such generalized descriptors the researchers made it difficult for me to determine the exact nature of their studies or the efficacy of the reported results.

Because a large number of our APA clients are likely to be included in studies of this type, I was concerned about the absence of comments indicating medical clearance for some of the subjects. But it was heartening to see an increase of research activity in this aspect of our work.

Information Processing

The members of our discussion group identified a general need for additional research activity regarding the various learning characteristics of the population we serve and study. In particular, we stressed the importance of understanding the information processing skills of handicapped and other persons. A serious drawback with some of this research has been the tasks used to help demonstrate or test the viability of theories and viewpoints. Most tasks have been somewhat contrived, laboratory-type tasks, and although I do not intend to criticize that, the willingness of some researchers to over-generalize from their data is a little perplexing. I believe that much useful knowledge has been gained from information processing studies, but the poor combination of test items with underlying theory may lack credibility among readers, most of whom are practitioners. But I applaud the recent developments seeking to use gross movement tasks to elicit responses in learning parameters. Nine presentations involved such tasks as reaction and movement time, variation of practice stimuli, and of reinforcement; this kind of work will provide useful insight into the theories and will also benefit the subject's information processing.

The Role of the Adult

The role of the professionals we place into our schools, community centers, hospitals, and institutions cannot be a passive one; the discussion group agreed that these adults can influence positive behaviors and attitudes. But whether we as professional educators build a positive enough approach into our college and university courses, and whether our former students can help to improve the attitudes among their coworkers are questions we must address.

At this Symposium researchers delivered four papers on related aspects of this topic. One paper suggested it is possible to improve the delivery of adapted physical education services by setting up a multistage training network on a regional basis. A second paper indicated ways in which teachers can upgrade their knowledge and skills at the classroom level, while alleviating anxieties that interfere with teaching effectiveness. The third study investigated ways of determining teacher effectiveness by analyzing their in-class behavior in public school special education settings. A fourth researcher de-emphasized the different behavioral characteristics of atypical persons, concentrating instead on which traits blind persons sought in their nonimpaired peers. Each of these presentations dealt with significant issues.

Test Instrumentation Issues

I think you will readily understand the Rochester group's concern with the tools of assessment, especially as they pertain to program placement and other decisions. Table 3 lists some of the assessment issues provided by PL 94-142 regulations; many research possibilities are apparent.

Table 3
Evaluation Concerns[a]

Tests and Other Evaluation Materials
- mode of communication
- conformity with directions
- validation for specific purpose/s

Parameters to Be Assessed
- all areas of educational need
- not just intelligence
- including motor abilities

Children With Known Impairments
- validity of approach

Evaluating Group
- multidisciplinary

Program Placement
- multicriterion procedures

[a]Adjusted from PL 94-142 regulations (US Department of Health, Education, & Welfare, 1977b, par. 532).

At this Symposium a quarter of the papers considered instrumentation. Most studies described and compared the performance traits of various categories of handicapped persons, emphasizing the gross motor tasks of the familiar physical fitness batteries. A smaller number dealt with basic patterns and skills, fine motor abilities, health-related traits, and water skills. Research of this type certainly can help us learn more about the populations we serve, but it is also important to acknowledge the wealth of sound, large-scale research already available (Rarick et al., 1967, 1972, 1976, 1977).

Four studies focused on test construction and validation, and could make important contributions to our literature. One paper discussed an instrument designed for use with very young children and therefore stressed fundamental motor development. Another study had included a wide range of patterns, skills, activities, and games to be used over the whole CA range. Both projects are more help to us in work with the mildly and moderately handicapped than with those more severely affected, but a third study has specifically attempted to develop an instrument for use with the severely handicapped. A fourth presentation provided a change of focus by revealing diagnostic information on a wide range of leisure functions. Perhaps the importance of these studies lies with the fact that each addresses a specific assessment concern, thus promoting the view that no test can be "all things to all people."

A small number of studies used very specific analytical and statistical techniques. Of particular interest was a paper emphasizing the value of single-subject research. This approach acknowledges the very personal nature of our work, the performance and behavior variability of the populations under examination, the importance of a one-to-one ratio for instruction, and the value of participation without comparison or competition. Three projects reported the use of multivariate analytic techniques—those which use several variables simultaneously. One study reported the use of canonical correlations for demonstrating that one group of related variables can be predicted from another set of variables. Two other studies examined the potential of discriminant analysis as a technique which can be of particular value to some of the issues concerning us: group membership, program placement, and the use of individual test items.

Although the studies on test instrumentation are of value to us in building our knowledge and expertise, another area of concern has received remarkably little attention in the APA literature and none at this Symposium: racial and cultural factors urgently need serious study in this and other aspects of our research work. Public Law 94-142 regulations provide for protection in evaluation procedures, stating:

> Testing and evaluation materials and procedures used for the purposes of

evaluation and placement of handicapped children must be selected and administered so as not to be racially or culturally discriminatory. (US Department of Health, Education, & Welfare, 1977b, par. 530b)

Program Effectiveness

Approximately one-third of our research presentations discussed the many issues involved in supplying programs to handicapped or disabled persons. Isn't it a paradox that, although as professionals we are confident that what we do is effective, we nevertheless keep asking for objective confirmation under the rigors of research? I cannot discuss the individual projects in detail, but I do want to make several general remarks which apply to research in some other areas as well as this one. And you should bear in mind that I am very sympathetic to research like this, for I have been involved in program development and evaluation for some 20 years.

In the future we should aim at designing and testing curriculum efficacy studies which are long-term—longer than the 6-12 week duration which has been well examined. The long-term behavioral and performance changes are the ones we seek, and the question of relative permanence is also worth studying. If we continue to act as though behaviors must improve and that they only improve as a result of the program, we are forgetting what our experience and literature indicate. Today is not the time to discuss the likely existence of the Hawthorne phenomenon (Roethlisberger & Dickson, 1947) or the pivotal role of teacher expectation (Rosenthal & Jacobson, 1968) in aiding behavior change, but in planning research these variables should be examined thoroughly. Likewise, for the more severely handicapped, our hopes for behavior improvement over time, in absolute or relative terms, are sometimes shattered by data which point to behavior regression; this is sad but true, as recent projects have clearly indicated (Broadhead, 1982; Rarick & McQuillan, 1979).

This group of presentations did, however, use the widest range of subjects and APA settings: the very young, the aged, the obese (no one researched the thin!) the retarded, cerebral palsied, sensory impaired, communication disordered, bedridden, and postoperation subjects. Yes, this research priority may be fraught with difficulties, but it is seldom dull.

Summary

In conclusion I want to reaffirm that the research presented here has considered many of the priorities which can be stated for APA settings and subjects. But I ask that serious consideration be given by all of us to sharpening our descriptions for characteristics of our subjects. I am sure that our knowledge far exceeds the standards we apply to our research designs. For example, in one of my recent studies and perhaps in some of yours, the phrase "moderately mentally retarded" was used to describe subjects. This term can no longer be acceptable because of the vast range of behaviors it encompasses. Using more detailed criteria will lead to a more thorough selection of subjects and more realistic data interpretations and generalizations; a larger sample size must follow.

I see these as some critical directions we must take, but speaking of directions reminds me of the person I met on a street in this cosmopolitan city. I asked, "Please can you tell me how I can get to the Mississippi River from here?" After some thought and a raising of the eyebrows, back came the reply— "If I were going to the Mississippi River, I wouldn't start from here."

What sort of an answer is that, you might ask. It is quite simply a personal answer. Where to start for the river, or on a research experience . . .? Where better than from our own interests, background, and training? Guidelines and priorities are helpful, indeed, but surely no one would want to deny that research is a very individual matter.

References

BEUTER, A.C. Effects of mainstreaming on the social interactions and motoric behaviors of normal and handicapped students in a school physical education setting. Unpublished Doctoral Dissertation. Berkeley: University of California, 1981.

BLOOM, B.S. (Ed.). *Taxonomy of educational objectives: Cognitive domain.* New York: David McKay, 1956.

BLOOM, B.S., Davis, A., & Hess, R. *Compensatory education for cultural deprivation.* New York: Holt, Rinehart, and Winston, 1965.

BROADHEAD, G.D. Physical education for previously unserved severely handicapped children. *Rehabilitation Literature,* 1981, **42**, 86-89.

BROADHEAD, G.D. A paradigm for physical education for handicapped children in the least restrictive environment. *The Physical Educator,* 1982, **39**, 3-12.

CRAFT, M. (Ed.). *Family class and education.* London, England: Longmans, 1970.

DELBECQ, A.L., & Van de Ven, A.H. *Group techniques for program planning: A guide to nominal group and Delphi processes.* Glenview, IL: Scott Foresman, 1975.

HARRIS, M.L., & Harris, C.W. A factor analytic interpretation strategy. *Educational and Psychological Measurement,* 1971, **31**, 589-606.

HARROW, A.J. *A taxonomy of the psychomotor domain.* New York: David McKay, 1972.

HOLLINGSHEAD, A.B. *Two factor index of social position.* New Haven, CT: 1965 Yale Station, 1957.

HUNT, J.M. *The challenge of incompetence and poverty.* Urbana, IL: University of Illinois Press, 1969.

JOSEPH P. Kennedy, Jr., Foundation. A telephone survey of the physical education provision of P.L. 94-142. Washington, DC: 1979.

KRATHWOHL, F.R., Bloom, B.S., & Masia, B.B. *Taxonomy of education goals: Affective domain.* New York: David McKay, 1964.

PETER, L.J. *Prescriptive teaching.* New York: McGraw-Hill, 1965.

RARICK, G.L., & Dobbins, D.A. Basic components in the motor performance of educable mentally retarded children: Implications for curriculum development. Berkeley: University of California, Department of Physical Education, Report to the USOE, 1972.

RARICK, G.L., Dobbins, D.A., & Broadhead, G.D. *The motor domain and its correlates in educationally handicapped children.* Englewood Cliffs, NJ: Prentice-Hall, 1976.

RARICK, G.L., & McQuillan, J.P. The factor structure of motor abilities of trainable mentally retarded children: Implications for curriculum development. Berkeley: University of California, Department of Physical Education, Report to the USOE, 1977.

RARICK, G.L., & McQuillan, J.P. The effects of individualized physical education instruction on selected perceptual-motor and cognitive functions of institutionalized and home-reared TMR children. Berkeley: University of California, Department of Physical Education, Report to the USOE, 1979.

RARICK, G.L., McQuillan, J.P., & Beuter, A.C. The motor, cognitive, and psychosocial effects of the implementation of Public Law 94-142 on handicapped children in school physical education programs. Berkeley: University of California, Department of Physical Education, Report to the USOSE, 1981.

RARICK, G.L., Widdop, J.H., & Broadhead, G.D. *Environmental factors associated with motor performance and physical fitness of educable mentally retarded children.* Madison, WI: University of Wisconsin, Department of Physical Education, Report to The Joseph P. Kennedy, Jr., Foundation, 1967.

ROETHLISBERGER, F.J., & Dickson, W.J. *Management and the worker.* Cambridge, MA: Harvard University Press, 1947.

ROSENTHAL, R., & Jacobson, L. *Pygmalion in the classroom.* New York: Holt, Rinehart, and Winston, 1968.

SMITH, M.S., & Bissel, J.S. Report analysis: the impact of Head Start. *Harvard Educational Review,* 1970, **40**, 51-104.

STANLEY, J.C. (Ed.). *Compensatory education for children ages two to eight.* Baltimore, MD: The Johns Hopkins University Press, 1973.

STEIN, Z., & Susser, M. The social distribution of mental retardation. *American Journal of Mental Deficiency,* 1963, **67**, 811-821.

TAYLOR, J.L., Compton, D.M., & Johnson, T.R. (Eds.). *1979-80 Proceedings: The National Consortium on Physical Education and Recreation for the Handicapped.* Lexington: University of Kentucky, Dept. HPER, 1981.

US Congress. *Civil Rights Act* (PL 88-352), 1964.

US Congress. *Education for All Handicapped Children Act* (PL 94-142), 1975.

US Department of Health, Education, and Welfare, Office of the Secretary. Non-discrimination on basis of handicap. *Federal Register,* Part IV, May 4, 1977(a).

US Department of Health, Education, and Welfare, Office of Education. Education of Handicapped Children: Implementation of part B of the education of the handicapped act. *Federal Register,* Part II, Aug. 23, 1977(b).

WARNOCK, H.M. (Chair). *Special educational needs: Report of the Committee of Enquiry into the Education of Handicapped Children and Young People. Command Paper 7212.* London, England: Her Majesty's Stationery Office, 1978.

WINNICK, J.P. *The physical fitness and performance of sensory and orthopedically impaired youth: Project Unique Training Manual.* Brockport: New York State University, 1979.

WISEMAN, S. *Education and environment.* Manchester, England: University of Manchester Press, 1964.

YINGER, J.M., Ikeda, K., Laycock, F., & Cutter, J. *Middle Start.* Cambridge, England: Cambridge University Press, 1977.

Adapted Physical Activity Quarterly

Geoffrey D. Broadhead, Editor
Claudine Sherrill, Associate Editor
Herberta M. Lundegren, Associate Editor

The *Adapted Physical Activity Quarterly (APAQ)* is a multidisciplinary journal dealing with physical activity for special populations. It includes articles originating from the disciplines of corrective therapy, gerontology, health care, occupational therapy, pediatrics, physical education, physical therapy, recreation, and rehabilitation, and deals with populations of every age. Adaptations of equipment, activity, facilities, methodology, and/or setting are all discussed within the *Quarterly*.

APAQ includes an editorial section containing commentary on current opinion, legislative and regulatory concerns, and other professional trends; a research section reporting original and replicated research using appropriate scientific methodology, as well as analytical reviews of the literature; an applications section containing applied investigations in settings often requiring unique methodologies, reports of case studies, programmatic developments involving strategies and techniques, and the design of equipment and facilities. Also included are abstracts of recently published work from around the world and a book and media review section.

Volume 1, No. 1 — January 1984

For subscription information, write to:
Human Kinetics Publishers, Box 5076, Champaign, IL 61820